NOVEL ASPECTS IN ACUTE LYMPHOBLASTIC LEUKEMIA

Edited by **Stefan Faderl**

Novel Aspects in Acute Lymphoblastic Leukemia
Edited by Stefan Faderl

Published by InTech
Janeza Trdine 9, 51000 Rijeka, Croatia

Publishing Process Manager Marina Jozipovic

Technical Editor Teodora Smiljanic

Cover Designer InTech Design Team

Additional hard copies can be obtained from orders@intechopen.com

Novel Aspects in Acute Lymphoblastic Leukemia, Edited by Stefan Faderl
p. cm.
ISBN 978-953-307-753-6

For EU product safety concerns:
IN TECH d.o.o., Prolaz Marije Krucifikse Kozulić 3, 51000 Rijeka, Croatia,
info@intechopen.com or visit our website at intechopen.com.

Meet the editor

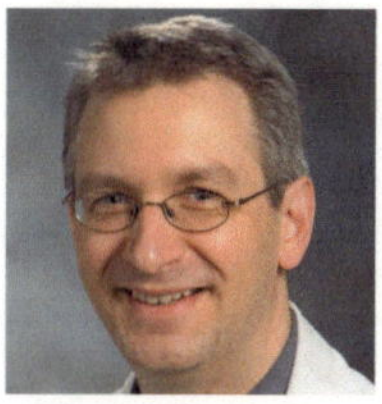

Stefan Faderl, M.D., Professor of Medicine came to M.D. Anderson in 1996. Dr. Faderl graduated from Ludwig Maximilian Medical School in Munich, Germany in 1990 and received his medical/academic degree (magna cum laude) from the same institution in 1994. Dr. Faderl is board certified in Internal Medicine and Medical Oncology. He specializes in acute and chronic leukemias. His main areas of interest include acute lymphoblastic leukemias (ALL), acute myeloid leukemias (AML), chronic lymphocytic leukemia (CLL) and its variants, as well as chronic myeloid leukemias (CML). Dr. Faderl has authored and co-authored many abstracts, articles in peer-reviewed journals and book chapters. He serves on numerous editorial boards and is a member of several professional societies such as the American Society of Hematology (ASH), the American College of Physicians (ACP), and the American Society of Clinical Oncology.

Contents

Preface

Acute lymphoblastic leukemia (ALL) is one of the great success stories in cancer medicine. Its transformation from a universally fatal disease to one which nowadays is highly curable in children extends over more than four decades. This exemplary progress is founded on a combination of factors. Starting from the vision of a few bold men who dared to make the first steps of treating patients with chemotherapy regimens that many others at the time considered to be at best ineffective and at worst un-ethical, it soon became clear that the life of patients with ALL can indeed be prolonged with this approach. Since then, clinical research in trial after trial established better and more effective therapies. At the same time, the many contributions by laboratory and translational researchers have expanded our understanding about the biology of ALL with far-reaching ramifications into the development of new drugs, the design of therapies, and an appreciation of the differences among subtypes of ALL and those between ALL in children and adults.

State-of-the-art ALL therapy can be bewildering in its complexity, yet every regimen adheres to a few basic tenets: induction therapy followed by intensified consolidation and a prolonged maintenance phase. Central nervous system (CNS) prophylaxis is a mandatory component and part of the early treatment stages of all patients. Induction therapy is based on a core group of drugs (vincristine, steroids, anthracyclines) to which various others have been added over time (asparaginase, cyclophosphamide, methorexate, cytarabine). Consolidation therapy can consist of a repetition of the induction, further intensification with added drugs, or a stem cell transplant for select patients. Maintenance extends up to three years and consists of a standard combination of vincristine, steroids, mercaptopurine, and methotrexate. CNS prophylaxis includes intrathecal chemotherapy, high-dose systemic therapy with CNS penetration (eg, cytarabine and methotrexate), and cranial radiation. With this strategy, remission rates of up to 90% and long-term disease free survival of up to 85% in children and 45% in adults are achievable.

Much progress in adult patients with ALL stems from lessons adapted from successful strategies in children. Yet, the prognosis in children remains significantly better. Explanations for this discrepancy at the expense of adults are many: decreased tolerance to intensive therapies and drugs such as asparaginase more specifically, differences in the metabolism of drugs such as methotrexate, higher expression of multi-drug resistance related proteins, and a higher likelihood to detect unfavorable cytogenetic abnormalities (eg, Ph chromosome, 11q23 translocations) whereas better prognosis karyotypes are found more rarely (eg, *ETV6-RUNX1* fusion, hyperdiploidy).

Hence, the basic structure of ALL therapy has experienced many modifications. Some important aspects of this development relate to the following:

1. Intensification of therapy in adult patients. Pediatric studies have shown better outcome among adolescents and young adults when therapy is augmented by intensifying the exposure to a group of non-myelosuppressive drugs such as vincristine, steroids, and asparaginase. This approach is now carried over in the "younger" adults to an age of up to 40 to 50 years in many ongoing clinical trials.

2. Risk-adaptation of therapy. To intensify therapy (including stem cell transplant) where necessary but avoid toxicities where possible is one of the main thrusts of clinical ALL research. Much experience has been gathered about different responses to therapy of various subtypes of ALL based on immunophenotyping and cytogenetic/molecular characteristics. An important post-treatment aspect is the measurement of minimal residual disease (MRD), the presence of which has a high positive predictive value for higher relapse likelihood in children on therapy and appears to have similar relevance in some groups of adults with ALL.

3. Incorporation of new drugs. In this respect, the most notable progress in recent years has been the success of tyrosine kinase inhibitor (TKI) therapy in *BCR-ABL*-positive ALL where early and continuous use of TKI now achieves disease-free survival rates akin to the responses of chemotherapy in patients with *BCR-ABL*-negative disease.

4. CNS prophylaxis. There has been a trend away from cranial radiation to intrathecal and systemic chemotherapy appreciating the long-term adverse events of therapeutic interventions in survivors.

The chapters in this book have been written by a diverse group of investigators throughout the world. Each of them contributes their unique knowledge and interpretation of several aspects of the biology, manifestations, and therapy of ALL. The following chapters cover aspects of the epidemiology of ALL in Hispanic patients, describe some often overlooked ophthalmologic manifestations at diagnosis and in the course of the management of ALL, and provide overviews of current therapy. Throughout several chapters investigators will elaborate on drug-resistance mechanisms, elucidate novel biological pathways and targets, and describe drugs in development. Last but not least, long-term consequences of CNS prophylaxis and therapy deal with some survivorship issues that are becoming ever more important. This book does not claim to be comprehensive but hopefully provides enough insight and information to serve as a source for knowledge and inspiration.

Stefan Faderl
Department of Leukemia, Division of Cancer Medicine,
The University of Texas, MD Anderson Cancer Center,
Houston, USA

Part 1

Epidemiology

1

Childhood Acute Leukemias in Hispanic Population: Differences by Age Peak and Immunophenotype

Juan Manuel Mejía-Aranguré et al.*
Unidad de Investigación en Epidemiología Clínica, Enfermedades Oncológicas, Enfermedades Infecciosas y Parasitarias/Hospital de Pediatria & División de Laboratorios de Vigilancia e Investigación Epidemiológica, Instituto Mexicano del Seguro Social México

1. Introduction

Childhood cancer represents 0.5–5.7% of all cancers (Birch & Blair, 1992; Smith & Gloecker, 2002). The most important kinds of cancer during childhood differ from those most frequently found in adulthood (Schellong, 1985). During infancy, the principal cancers are not epithelial, in contrast to those in the later stages of life (Miller, 1983). Therefore, it is possible that the risk factors for cancer are different during infancy than during adulthood; for children, risk factors may be present *in utero* or during the firsts months of the life (Draper, 1994).

The age peak of cancer during infancy, especially those for leukemias and lymphomas, varies among countries. Although the peak age for leukemias worldwide is principally between 2–5 years of age, a peak as late as 7–13 years of age was reported for Niger (William, 1975). In developed countries such as Germany or the United States of America (USA), the age peak for lymphomas is between 10–14 years of age, whereas in less developed countries, Mexico for example, the age peak is between 5–9 years of age (Fajardo-Gutiérrez et al., 1995; Kaatsch et al., 1995; Nully-Brown et al., 1989; Young et al., 1986).

Leukemia is the most common cancer in children under 15 years old, representing between 25–35% of all childhood cancers in most populations (Parkin et al., 1988, 1998). Leukemia is a heterogeneous group of hematopoietic malignancies, with several biologically distinct subgroups. The main subtypes of leukemia described by most cancer registries include acute lymphoblastic leukemia (ALL), representing about 80% of all leukemias; AML, with a frequency of 15%; and chronic myeloid leukemia (CML) with a frequency of 3–5% (Bathia, 2003). ALL is the most frequent leukemia in infancy (Mejía Arangure et al., 2005a). The age

---

* María Luisa Pérez-Saldivar, Rosana Pelayo-Camacho, Ezequiel Fuentes-Pananá, Carolina Bekker-Mendez, Abigail Morales-Sánchez, David Aldebarán Duarte-Rodríguez and Arturo Fajardo-Gutiérrez
Unidad de Investigación en Epidemiología Clínica, Enfermedades Oncológicas, Enfermedades Infecciosas y Parasitarias/Hospital de Pediatria & División de Laboratorios de Vigilancia e Investigación Epidemiológica, Instituto Mexicano del Seguro Social, México

peak at 2–5 years of age was reported for England after 1920, for the USA in 1940, and for Japan in 1960; during this time, this same peak was demonstrated for African-American with ALL in the USA (Greaves et al., 1993; Pratt et al., 1988; Ramot & Magrath, 1982).
We analyzed the immunophenotype of all cases of ALL registered in eight of the nine public hospitals, located in Mexico City, which attended children with ALL from January 2010 to May 2011. We showed that, for the 320 cases registered, the frequency of childhood ALL in Mexico City had two age peaks (Fig. 1), in agreement with data reported previously (Bernáldez et al., 2008; Mejía Arangure et al., 2005a). In Brazil, two peaks in ALL have also been reported (de Souza Reis et al., 2011).

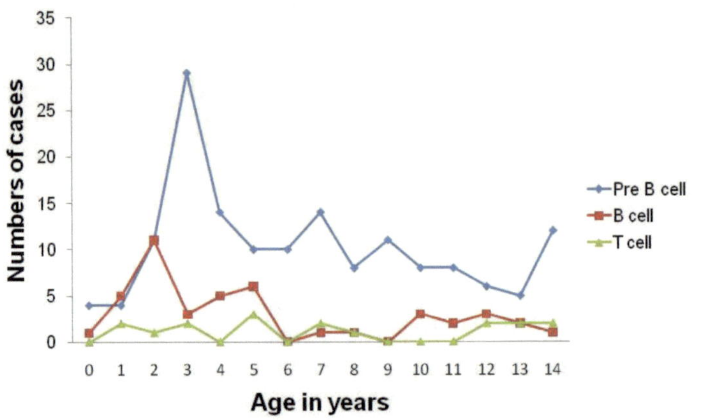

Fig. 1. Immunophenotypes in children from Mexico City during 2010-2011. The children with acute lymphoblastic leukemia have two age peaks, specially the children with Pre B cell immunophenotype.

The aim of this chapter is to present different hypotheses related to the age peak of the ALL in children. We briefly describe the ontology of B and T lymphocytes and discuss an apparent association between the genetic rearrangements involved and the age peak in leukemias. We also review data on the age peak of ALL in different countries. At the end of the chapter, we propose an hypothesis with respect to the age peak in Latin American populations and in general.

2. B- and T-cell development

After birth and throughout life, development and replenishment of lymphoid cells is a highly ordered process that starts in bone marrow (BM) with the differentiation of multipotential hematopoietic stem cells (HSC). In this multi-step process, multiple alternate lineage potentials are gradually lost and lineage commitment is coincident with gain of specialized functions. Over the last few years, remarkable advances have been made in characterizing the primitive progenitors that initiate the lymphoid program; the patterns of transcriptional activity that control decisions about the fate of early lineages and late maturation process; and the environmental signals that influence the differentiation pathway during normal hematopoiesis. Malignant early lymphoid development is currently under intense investigation, and the existence of leukemic stem cells is still a matter of debate. However, identification of cytogenetic abnormalities in cells lacking lineage markers and the unsuspected genetic diversity within individuals strongly suggests the participation of primitive cells in this disease.

2.1 From stem cells to committed B-cell progenitors

Because mature blood cells have finite life spans, they are constantly replaced from a unique cell population of HSC that resides in specialized niches in the BM (Baba et al., 2004). Within the hematopoietic system, HSC are the only cells with the ability to extensively give rise to identical daughter stem cells (self-renewal) and to differentiate into all functional blood cells (multipotency) (Seita & Weissman, 2010). The hematopoietic system is organized as a hierarchy of cell types with differing capacities for self-renewal, proliferation, and differentiation. In the pathways of this system, developing lymphoid or myeloid cells progress through critical stages of differentiation of multipotential and self-renewing HSC to multipotential early progenitors, which give rise to oligopotent progenitors. Downstream, the production of lineage-committed precursors is crucial for maturation of blood cells (Fig. 2). The lymphoid lineage consists of B, T, and natural killer (NK) cells; the myeloid lineage includes granulocytes, monocytes, macrophages, erythrocytes, megakaryocytes, and mast cells. Dendritic cells (DCs) are generated starting from the pathways of lymphoid or myeloid differentiation.

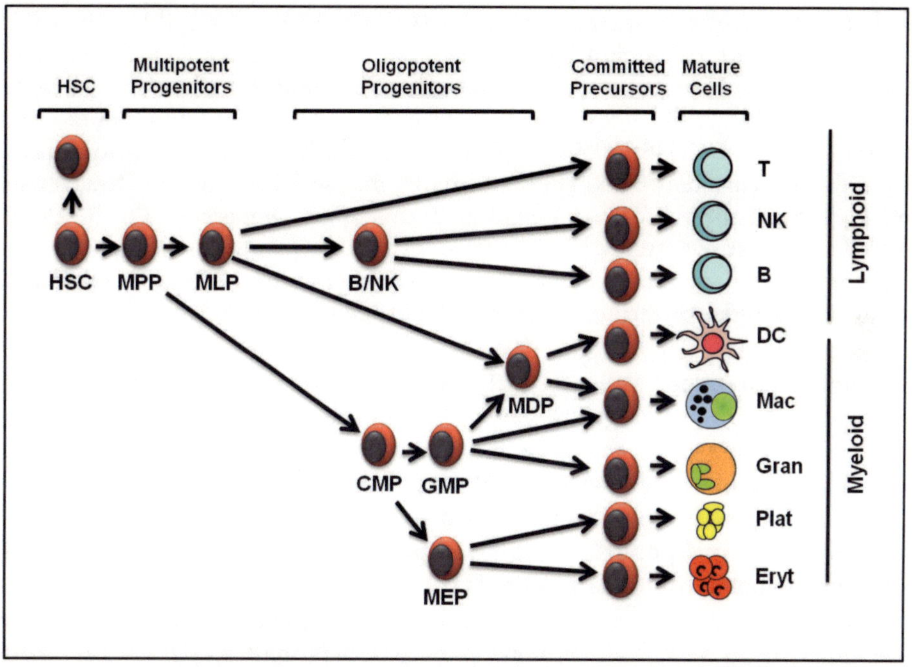

Fig. 2. Hematopoietic development in humans. The self-renewing hematopoietic stem cell (HSC) gives rise to multipotent progenitors (MPP), which have the ability to differentiate into common myeloid progenitors (CMP), and into multi-lymphoid progenitors (MLP). Mature blood cells are produced from lineage-committed precursors. The hierarchical structure of the hematopoietic system is shown. GMP, granulocyte and monocyte progenitors; MEP, megakaryocyte and erythrocyte progenitors; MDP, monocyte and dendritic cell progenitors; NK, natural killer cells; DC, dendritic cell; Mac, macrophage; Gran, granulocyte; Plat, platelets; Eryt, erythrocyte.

Current knowledge about the development of the lymphoid system is based, in great part, on the work done in mouse models, which has demonstrated that this differentiation program begins in BM in the fractions of lymphoid-primed multipotent progenitors (LMPP) and early lymphoid progenitors (ELP) capable of differentiating into T, B, NK, and conventional dendritic cells (Pelayo et al., 2005a, 2006a; Welner et al., 2008b). ELP also produce plasmacytoid dendritic cells (pDC), and interferon-producing killer dendritic cells (IKDC), both of which are key components of the innate immune response to infections (Pelayo et al., 2005b; Welner et al., 2007). The more differentiated common lymphoid progenitors (CLP) have substantially lost the possibility of differentiating into multiple lineages and efficiently generate B- and NK-cell precursors. Interestingly, HSC and early progenitors proliferate in response to systemic infection and replenish innate immune cells by using mechanisms that apparently involve interferons, tumor necrosis factor-α, and Toll-like receptors (TLR)—these last recognize viral/bacterial components. Thus, plasticity in primitive progenitor cells is sensitive to extrinsic agents that can modify differentiation fates during infection, thus supporting the idea that the stages of restriction of hematopoietic lineages are less abrupt than previously thought (Baldridge et al., 2011; Welner et al., 2008a).
In humans, the early hematopoietic progenitors are confined in the BM to a cellular compartment that expresses CD34 (Bloom & Spits, 2006). This fraction of multipotent stem cells is characterized by the phenotype $Lin^-CD34^+CD38^{-/lo}CD10^-CD45RA^-$, whereas that of the earliest lymphoid progenitors is characterized by the phenotype $Lin^-CD34^+CD38^{-/lo}CD45RA^+CD10^+$ and has been recently designated as multi-lymphoid progenitor (MLP) (Doulatov et al., 2010). While a description that fully matches the definition of mouse ELP is still missing, $Lin^-CD34^+CD38^+CD45RA^+CD10^+$ cells, which differentiate principally into B and NK cells, are considered the counterparts of mouse CLP (Fig. 2). Downstream, the sequential differentiation of lineage-restricted precursors generates Pro-B, Pre-B, and immature-B cells that eventually are exported to the peripheral lymphoid tissues. As in mice, human lymphopoiesis can undergo adjustments in cell-fate decisions under inflammatory conditions or during infections (Baldridge et al., 2011; Kim et al., 2005).

2.1.1 Biological differences between early hematopoiesis in neonatal and in adult

Some properties in hematopoietic development, including cell-cycle progression, transcription-factor networks, and growth-factor production, show substantial differences between newborns and adults (Mayani, 2010; Nguyen et al., 2010; Pelayo et al., 2006b).
During fetal and neonatal development, the hematopoietic system faces a complex set of demands, including rapid population turnover, protection against infection, and avoidance of harmful inflammatory immune responses (Levy, 2007; Pelayo et al., 2006b). After birth, there is an age-dependent maturation of the immune response; apparently, prenatal and postnatal exposure to microbial components or products may accelerate this maturation process (Levy, 2007). In response to TLR agonists, production of cytokines and chemokines is poor in early life but increases with age, though it is still limited in one-year-old infants, suggesting that the first year of life represents a critical period for the acquisition of competence by developing hematopoietic cells (Nguyen et al., 2010).
Moreover, hematopoietic stem and progenitor cells must divide extensively to generate the billions of new blood cells needed each day. Yet, little is known about the period when the expansion takes place or about the mechanisms responsible for the biological differences between fetal and adult primitive cells. However, it is widely recognized that fetal- and

neonatal-derived HSC and lymphoid progenitors possess higher proliferation and expansion potentials. Furthermore, during rebound from chemotherapy, adult progenitors acquire some, but not all, of the characteristics of fetal cells (Mayani, 2010; Pelayo et al., 2006b). Telomere dynamics, key cell-cycle mediators, and differential gene expression may account for the fetal/adult disparity. Whether the potential for high proliferation during early life makes hematopoietic precursor cells more vulnerable to gene mutations is not as yet clear, but its implication in the onset of neoplastic hematological diseases in neonates might be decisive.

2.1.2 Early steps in malignant lymphoid development

ALL is characterized by the monoclonal/oligoclonal proliferation of hematopoietic precursor cells of the lymphoid series within the BM. Although in recent years studies have reported important advances in the investigation of genetic, molecular, karyotypic, and phenotypic abnormalities that are prevalent in this disorder, the understanding of the mechanisms that damage the earliest program of lymphoid development remains poor. Results from cell cultures for early hematopoiesis, detection of specific leukemic karyotypes in primitive CD34+ cells, and data showing that cells with immature phenotypes are capable of engrafting and reconstituting leukemia in immunodeficient mice suggest that infant B cell-leukemia initiating cells have primitive characteristics (Cobaleda et al., 2000; Cox et al., 2004, 2009; Espinoza-Hernández et al., 2001) and are subject to intrinsic and extrinsic stimuli that could trigger lineage instability. On the other hand, leukemic blasts can also completely re-establish leukemic phenotypes *in vivo*, conferring them with stem-cell properties (Heidenreich & Vormoor, 2009). These conflicting results reveal that key questions regarding leukemic stem cells and lymphoid development in ALL remain unsolved. Recently, the combination of clonal studies, alterations in genetic copies, and xenotransplantation models have shown unsuspected genetic diversity, supporting the idea of multi-clonal evolution of leukemogenesis, rather than that of lineal succession (Dick, 2008). Future progress in this area will ultimately lead to an understanding of the biology of leukemia, as well as behavior and prognosis among individual groups.

2.2 Murine B-cell maturation in bone marrow

The first cells that exhibit commitment to the B-cell lineage in mice (the model in which this process is currently better understood) are B220$^+$, CD19$^+$, and CD43$^+$ pro-B cells (Allman et al., 1999). During B-cell development, the main goal is to generate functional cell populations that are capable of expressing a diverse repertoire of B-cell antigen receptors (BCR), with each clone having specificity to recognize and counteract a new or recurrent pathogen. Antigen recognition is mediated by a heterodimer of immunoglobulin (Ig) heavy chains and light chains and signaling for an antigen-induced B-cell response is mediated by the molecules Igα (CD79a) and Igβ (CD79b). Igα and Igβ exist as a disulfide-coupled heterodimer in non-covalent association with the Ig antigen-recognition element. Igα/Igβ signaling is dependent upon distinct motifs localized in the cytoplasmic tails of these proteins, the immunoreceptor tyrosine-based activation motifs (ITAM) (Cambier, 1995; Fuentes-Pananá et al., 2004b). The BCR can generate signals that lead to a variety of outcomes, depending upon the developmental stage of the B cell and the degree and persistence of receptor aggregation. Although the mature form of the BCR is present only in immature and mature B cells, genetic and biochemical studies have shown that various forms of the BCR are expressed at defined stages of B-cell development that are required for progression of B cells through several defined developmental checkpoints (Fuentes-Panańá & Monroe 2001; Fuentes-Panańá et al., 2004a).

In the pro-B stage in which the heavy chain is in the process of recombination, the signaling proteins Igα and Igβ are expressed on the cell surface and are associated with the protein calnexin, and perhaps other as yet unknown proteins, forming the so-called "pro-BCR" (Nagata et al., 1997). Pro-B cells that successfully produce an Ig heavy-chain protein transport it to the surface in association with Igα/Igβ and with the surrogate light-chain complex that is composed of λ5 and V pre-B (the pre-BCR receptor) (Karasuyama et al., 1996; Melchers et al., 1993). Surface expression of this receptor marks the transition to the pre-B stage, a step that is marked by loss of CD43 and gain of CD22 expression, by allelic exclusion of the un-recombined heavy-chain allele, and by the opening and initiation of recombination at the λ Ig light chain loci (Rolink & Melchers, 1993). A similar mechanism operates in the pre-B stage in which the successful recombination of light chain and its pairing with the Ig heavy chain and Igα and Igβ allows the assembly of the mature form of the BCR and marks the transition to the immature stage. Intimate contact between the immature-B cell and the stromal cells of the BM allows those receptors capable of recognizing self-antigens to be identified and eliminated through a variety of mechanisms collectively termed "tolerance". Non-self-reactive B cells exit to the periphery and reach the spleen where they are again tested for reactivity against self-antigens before they transition to the mature stage (von Boehmer & Melcher, 2010).

2.2.1 Heavy and light chain VDJ recombination and positive selection in BM

The main goal during the pro-B and pre-B stages is to generate a signaling-competent antigen receptor, with the progression of development conditioned by the signaling capacity of the receptor complex. The BCR Ig heavy and light chain genes are composed of constant and variable domains, the recombination of which makes BCR clonal diversity possible. The variable domain is formed by a series of segments termed variable (V), diversity (D), and joining (J) (Fig. 3A), which are brought together by a site-specific recombination process termed VDJ recombination. This is a highly ordered process during which the D and J fragments are rearranged and the V segment is then joined to the DJ fragment; these steps occur first in the heavy and then in the light chain loci (Fig. 3B) (Fuentes-Panańá et al., 2004b; Thomas et al., 2009). This process is essential for the adaptive immune function of the lymphocyte. As mentioned above, the pro-B stage is characterized by rearrangement of the Ig heavy chain and it is further divided according to the status of the rearrangement; in mice, Marshall named these sub-stages proB-A (during which the heavy chain is in the germ-line state), proB-B (during which D and J are recombined), and proB-C (during which V-DJ is recombined) (Hardy et al., 1991). In the pre-B stage, the light chain V and J fragments are recombined, first in the λ and then in the κ loci (Fig. 3A).

Unsuccessful recombination (e.g., heavy chain VDJ fragments that are not in a proper reading frame) or unsuccessful pairing of the pre-BCR components results in pro-B cells that are unable to proceed to the pre-B stage, thus leading the developing pro-B cell to apoptosis. This observation supports the concept of an active signaling role for the pre-BCR in generating the permissive signal that allows differentiation through the pre-B stage (Bannish et al., 2001; Mandal et al., 2009; Yasuda et al., 2008). A similar mechanism is thought to operate for the transition from pre-B to immature cells, which requires expression of the mature form of the BCR (Bannish et al., 2001; Mandal et al., 2009; Yasuda et al., 2008). In addition to their VDJ recombination status, all pro-B and pre-B stages can be recognized by their patterns of surface-marker expression (Hardy et al., 1991).

2.3 T-cell development

T-cell development occurs in the thymus through equivalent processes of VDJ recombination, selection against self-reactive clones, and maturation into fully functional clones (Figure 3B). Expression of the T-cell antigen receptor (TCR) on the surface of the T cell marks the transition through all developmental stages. The TCR is a complex of proteins that may be functionally divided into the antigen-binding unit formed by the β and α chains (also in a smaller fraction of T cells, the γ and δ chains) and the signaling unit formed by the CD3 chains. The β and α (and γ/δ) chains consist of constant and variable regions, with VDJ recombination taking place in the latter. There are different types of CD3 chains and each mature TCR is associated with six of them: two CD3ε, two CD3ζ, one CD3γ, and one CD3δ. The stages of T-cell development are known as the following: pro-T ($CD3^{pos}CD44^{pos}CD4^{neg}CD8^{neg}$; the TCR β chain is rearranged); pre-T ($CD3^{pos}CD44^{pos}CD25^{pos}CD4^{neg}CD8^{neg}$; the TCR α chain is rearranged); CD4 and CD8 double-positive T cells [$CD3^{pos}CD4^{pos}CD8^{pos}$; equivalent to immature/transitional B cells (the stage in which tolerance mechanisms are applied to the developing T cell)]; and CD4 or CD8 single-positive cells (mature helper or cytotoxic T cells). Pro-T and pre-T cells are further subdivided according to the status of the β and α chains rearrangements: DN1 (β chain is in germ-line configuration); DN2 (D and J rearrangement of the β chain); DN3 (V joins to DJ of the β chain); and DN4 (V and J rearrangement of the α chain). DN1, DN2, and DN3 are pro-T stage; DN4 is a pre-T stage. The progression of recombination-associated development is illustrated in Fig. 3B. Expression of pro-TCR, pre-TCR, and mature-TCR receptors mark the progression through T-cell developmental checkpoints, homologous to the positive- and negative-selection mechanisms for B cells (Love et al., 2010; Wiest, 1994, 1995).

2.4 Human B- and T-cell development

Selection processes operating on developing B and T cells of all mammals are the same; thus, B- and T-cell development in human is also mainly divided by the process of VDJ recombination and expression of antigen-recognition complexes on the cell surface and by the proliferative expansion of clones that have successfully completed the rearrangement of their receptors (Blom & Spits, 2006). However, for the human, all these processes are less well understood than are their counterparts in the murine model. Importantly in human lymphocyte development, the pro-B and pre-B sub-stages are the ones generally found to be compromised in human pediatric B-cell ALL. B-cell ALL is characterized by cells unable to progress along the differentiation pathway. The stages more often compromised are: proB-A (before heavy-chain recombination), proB-C (after heavy-chain recombination), and large pre-B stage (before light-chain rearrangement) (Fig. 3B) (Hardy et al., 1991; Rolink et al., 1991). These stages are better known in humans as early proB or pre-proB (A); proB (B); preB1 (C) (proB stage); and preB2 (large preB stage) (Fig. 3B). All these stages in human B and T cells can also be recognized by the expression of specific surface markers, a characteristic that has helped to classify the different types of pediatric ALL. In humans, B cells are recognized by the expression of CD19 and CD10; T cells by CD2, CD3, CD5, and

CD7; and, for the proliferating immature-B cells, pre-proB cells by CD34$^+$CD19$^-$CD10$^+$; preB1 by CD34$^+$CD19$^-$CD10$^+$; and preB2 by CD34$^-$CD19$^+$CD10$^+$. Immature T cells are mainly recognized by the lack of expression of CD4 and CD8 and expression of T-cell markers.

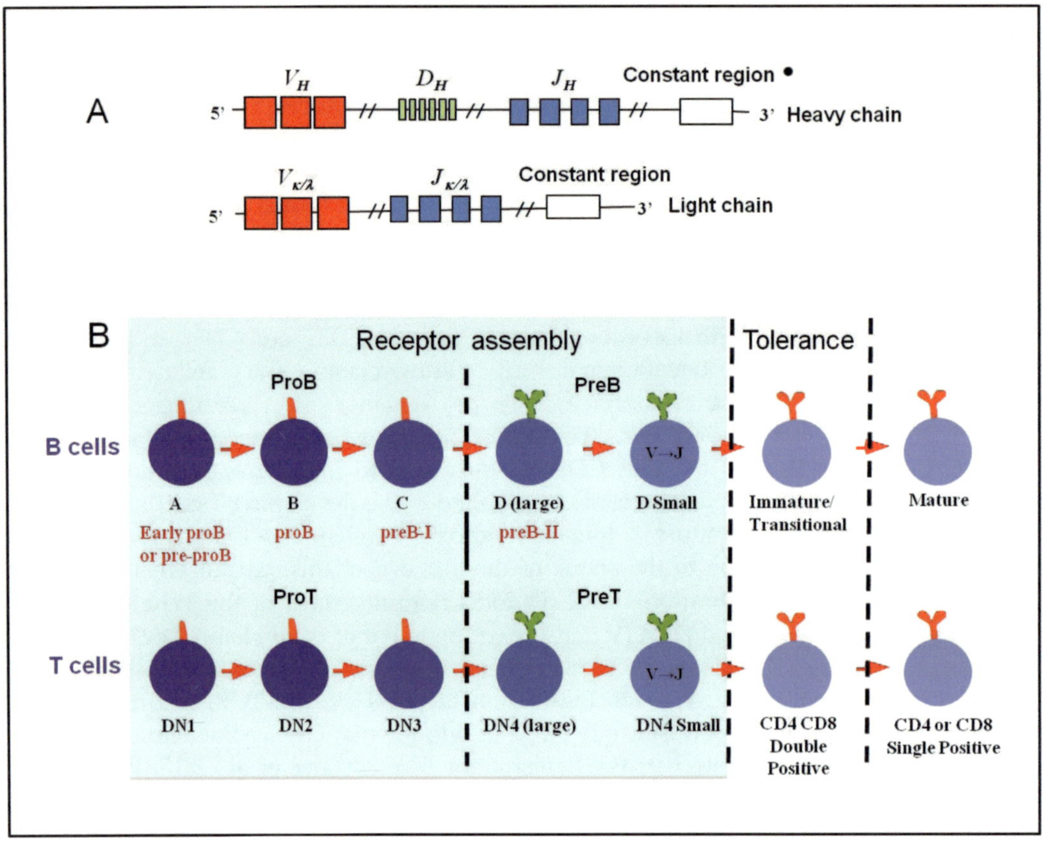

Fig. 3. B- and T-cell development. A) The Ig heavy and light chain genes are comprised of constant and variable domains; the variable domain is formed by an *n* number of segments termed variable (V), diversity (D), and joining (J) in the heavy chain and by segments V and J in the light chain. These segments are brought together by a site-specific recombination process, termed VDJ recombination, which is responsible for the extensive repertoire of BCR specificities. There are two loci for light chain, κ and λ. Here, all the loci are shown in germ-line configuration, prior to the process of VDJ recombination. B) All B- and T-cell stages can be divided according to the main processes guiding development: receptor assembly, tolerance, and activation. Receptor assembly stages (light blue box) in B and T cells are differentiated by the process of VDJ recombination in the heavy (IGH) and light (IGL) chains, which are recombined in the pro-B and pre-B stages, respectively (β and α rearrangement in pro-T and pre-T cells). The nomenclature of each sub-stage in the mouse model is shown in black letters, A-D (Marshall's) for B cells and DN1–4 for T cells; the most common human nomenclature is shown in red letters. The dashed lines separating all stages indicate checkpoints at which signaling from the preBCR and BCR is required for positive selection and progression along the B-cell maturation pathway. The proBCR, proTCR, preBCR, preTCR, and mature receptors are also illustrated in their respective stages.

3. Incidence peak of acute leukemia with specific cytogenetic aberrations in childhood

ALL is a clonal disease driven by mutations. The incidence of leukemia among children varies considerably with age. Age at diagnosis has played a relevant role in the epidemiology of these diseases and in the determination of risk groups and treatment stratification (Smith et al., 1997). The age-related incidence pattern of ALL has been established by the demonstration of the clone-specific 11q23-, t(12;21)-, as determined by blood testing (Guthrie cards), and hyperdiploidy (Gale et al., 1997; Wiemels et al., 2002).

The majority of childhood ALL cases show the emergence *in utero* of pre-leukemic cells and, postnatally, rare interactions between the immune system and childhood infections (Greaves, 2002).

The incidence rates of childhood ALL vary from country to country; in Europe and the USA, 85–90% of the cases have a B-cell-precursor phenotype (pre-B) with an incidence peak in the 2–7 years age group. For childhood T-cell ALL , lower incidence peaks have been reported (Hjalgrim et al., 2003). Most cases of pre-B ALL carry either a high hyperdiploid karyotype or the chromosomal translocation t(12;21) (p13;q22). A high hyperdiploid karyotype, which is present in 30% of pediatric patients, shows a modal chromosome number above 50, which involve trisomies of chromosomes X, 4, 6, 10, 14, 17, 18, and 21 and which, in most cases, arise by simultaneous chromosomal gain in a single abnormal mitosis (Paulsson et al., 2005). The chromosomal translocation t(12;21) (p13;q22) is found in 20–25% of cases and involves the gene *RUNX1* in chromosome region 21q22 and the gene *ETV6* in chromosome region 12p13. Both encode transcriptional factors that are essential for normal fetal hematopoiesis (Romana et al., 1995). High-hyperdiploid leukemic clones are sometimes missed by standard G-band karyotyping due to poor metaphase quality. The detection rates can be raised by extended fluorescence in situ hybridization (FISH) analyses, flow cytometry, DNA-index analyses, high-resolution comparative genomic hybridization (CGH), and comparative genomic array CHG (Kristensen et al., 2003; Nyggard et al., 2006). Translocation t(12;21) is cryptic by standard G-band karyotyping; its diagnosis is based on FISH analyses and reverse transcriptase-polymerase chain reaction (RT-PCR) (Nordgren, 2003).

Recent studies from twins with concordant leukemia suggest that a genetic event is involved in these acute leukemias: chromosomal translocations can have a prenatal origin (Ford, 1993, 1997, 1998; Gill et al., 1994; Wiemels et al., 1999a, 1999b). There is also indirect support that the prenatal origin of leukemic clones is derived from the presence of clonotypic rearrangements at the IGH and TCR loci in Guthrie spots (Fasching et al., 2000; Yagi et al., 2000). Because most of the studies have included a limited subset of leukemias, primarily those of lymphoid phenotypes, it remains an open question as to whether the prenatal origin of childhood leukemia is a possible, or a common, occurrence in other subgroups.

The most frequent translocation both in children (1–20 years of age) and in adults (older than 20 years) is t(8;21) AML1-ETO, which results in a fusion protein that disrupts the normal function of the transcription factors AML1 and ETO (Finnette et al., 1996). The incidence of leukemia with the t(8;21) AML1-ETO translocation increases slowly during childhood and is constant thereafter (Downing, 1999).

MLL/11q23 translocations are known to be involved in the leukemia of infancy, but they can also be found in older children and sometimes in the elderly (Johansson et al., 1998). MLL/11q23 translocations, of which t(11;19)(q23;p13) and t(4;11)(q21;23) are the most common, have an incident peak during first year of life; 11q23-aberrant leukemias are the second most common malignancy. When these leukemias appear in very early infancy, their prenatal origin is proven; in monozygous twins (with identical MLL-rearrangements), the concordance rate is almost 100%. This suggests that, when these mutations are present at birth, they invariably lead to overt leukemia (Greaves et al., 2003). It is not known when MLL/11q23 translocations occur in adults.

Childhood acute leukemias are clinically related, but cytogenetically different, diseases; therefore, cytogenetic subgrouping is important to understand the diversity in their etiology, natural history, and epidemiology. An understanding of the epidemiology of childhood acute leukemia is relevant in order to clarify the cytogenetic backbone of etiologic research.

4. Infectious etiology of childhood leukemia

The hypothesis concerning an infectious etiology of childhood leukemia was first raised several decades ago (Cooke, 1942). Although, to date, it has not been possible to demonstrate the involvement of one or more particular infectious agent(s), different hypotheses are still in force based on epidemiological and demographic studies that have yielded evidence about the possible participation of infectious agents in childhood leukemogenesis. Independently, Greaves (1988), Kinlen (1988), and Smith (1997) have suggested different mechanisms by which certain events of infection may explain at least some cases of childhood leukemia.

4.1 Greaves' hypothesis

More than 20 years ago, Greaves (1988) proposed the involvement of infectious agents in the etiology of childhood leukemia. In the most recent version, his hypothesis includes a model of the natural history of ALL with a minimum of two oncogenic hits (Greaves, 2002), whereby a first hit occurs *in utero* and forms a pre-leukemic clone that requires at least one secondary, postnatal carcinogenic hit to unleash the malignant transformation. According to this hypothesis of "delayed infection", the second oncogenic event could be indirectly promoted by delayed exposure to an infectious agent that causes an uncontrolled immune response and promotes the malignant, abnormal proliferation of the pre-leukemic clone.

A number of studies have shown that first-born children have a higher risk of developing leukemia. Only children and those children who do not attend daycare have been assumed to be evidence of the hypothesis, in that, by having less contact with others children and potentially less frequency of exposure to infectious agents, the probability of developing the disease increased, when compared to children outside these groups (Dockerty et al., 2001; Infante-Rivard et al., 2000; Jourdan-Da Silva et al., 2004; Perrillat, et al., 2002; Petridou et al., 1993),

Nevertheless, some research has not provided absolute support for Greaves' hypothesis: data from the Northern California study group (Ma et al., 2005) indicated that daycare attendance and ear infections during infancy are associated with a lower risk of ALL; however, this was true only for non-Hispanic children.

It should be noted that Greaves' hypothesis concerns the common form of ALL (B-cell precursor). This form comprises most of the ALL cases that peak at 2–5 years of age and that are seen in developed countries or in affluent communities that have improved their living standards and have become "more hygienic". Therefore, any relevant infection should occur in the first two years of life. Through comparison of international reports, variations in the peaks of childhood ALL have been identified. The aforementioned peak at 2–5 years of age is reduced, or even absent, for Black Africans and for other developing communities (Court & Doll, 1961; Hewitt, 1955; Ramot & Magrath, 1982, as cited in Chan et al., 2002). In Mexico, for example, two peaks have been reported; the first occurring at 2–3 years of age and the second at 6–9 (Bernaldez-Rios et al., 2008). A recent epidemiological study done in Mexico City showed that severe infections, occurring in the first year of life and requiring hospitalization, were associated with a higher risk of developing leukemia for children with Down syndrome (Flores-Lujano et al., 2009).

A possible interpretation of these results showing that infections in the first year of life represent risk factors (Cardwell et al., 2008; Roman et al., 2007) is that such infections could play a role as promoters, not as protectors, in the genesis of leukemia. In principle, this could mean that, for these groups, the infectious etiology of leukemia might be different than that proposed by Greaves.

4.2 Kinlen's hypothesis

When clusters of childhood leukemia and non-Hodgkin lymphoma were observed in the early 1980's near nuclear plants in Cumbria, England (Black, 1984), and at Dounreay, Scotland (Heasman et al., 1986), it was thought that such increase could have been a consequence of radioactive contamination by the nuclear plants, which might have caused somatic or germinal line mutations that produce cancer. However, there was no evidence of radioactive leaks (Committee on Medical Aspects of Radiation in the Environment [COMARE], 1986) or of epidemiological associations that showed greater occupational exposures of the parents (Gardner et al., 1990).

Kinlen proposed that the observed clusters of leukemia could have resulted from the unusual population mixing that occurred due to migration of workers and their families, who had travelled to work in the nuclear plants; he also hypothesized that a common, but unidentified, infectious agent could have been involved (Kinlen, 1988, 1995a). According to his proposal, cases of childhood leukemia would be a rare response from the isolated, uninfected individuals who were, therefore, susceptible to a putative infectious agent carried by these newcomers.

By extrapolating from animal leukemias caused by virus, a subtype of leukemia in adults, and by considering that childhood leukemia is not a contagious disease, Kinlen proposed that the agent involved could be a common virus causing a non-common response (Kinlen, 2011).

To date, Kinlen's working group has directed several studies, mainly in England and Scotland, and has observed a significant increase in cases of childhood leukemia where large-scale mixing between rural and urban populations occurred with unusual patterns of contact in the different communities (Kinlen et al., 1990, 1993, 1995b; Kinlen & Balkwill, 2001; Kinlen & Hudson, 1991; Kinlen & John, 1994).

Kinlen first proved his population-mixing hypothesis in the infectious etiology of childhood leukemia in Scotland, in a rural area that had received large influxes of people: the results showed a significant increase in the leukemia cases in children under five years of age (Kinlen, 1988). Another of his studies showed that excess of leukemia was higher in the 0–4 years age range; it was predominantly higher for children younger than 1 year, suggesting an infection during pregnancy (Kinlen & Hudson, 1991). From his observations, Kinlen proposed that, during population influx, adults are the main transmitters of an infectious agent and that a rare response was more likely to be made by a naive immune system; thus, in the foregoing case, population mixing could be responsible for the leukemia cases seen, even in the first year of life. Nonetheless, the author did not associate the leukemia clusters with a particular subtype of disease and interpreted that any type of childhood and infant leukemia might have a common cause.

4.3 Smith's hypothesis

A third hypothesis regarding the infectious etiology of childhood leukemia was proposed by Smith (1997). He hypothesized that some cases of ALL observed in the 2–5 years age group (B-cell precursor) could be the result of an infection that occurred during pregnancy and that was transmitted from mother to fetus.

Unlike Greaves, who postulated that infections are secondary etiological factors acting indirectly, Smith suggested that infection is one of the first hits in leukemogenesis and that a related infectious agent acts directly, i.e., the agent is able to infect the immature-B cell and to promote genomic instability, thereby leading to the transforming process. According to his model, the agent involved must be able to cross the placenta and infect the fetus without causing serious abnormalities, have limited oncogenic capacity, and produce minimal primary symptoms (Smith, 1997).

Studies that have shown that maternal infections are associated with an increased risk of ALL support this model. Lehtinen et al. (2003) showed that maternal infection with Epstein-Barr Virus (EBV) was associated with a significantly increased risk of ALL. Naumberg's work group found a similar association when the mother had lower genital tract infections (Naumberg, 2002). However, other studies have shown little or no association between infections, either by varicella or influenza during pregnancy (Little, 1999, as cited in McNally 2004), by unspecified infection in pregnancy (McKinney et al., 1999), or by recurrent maternal infections (Infante-Rivard et al., 2000), and subsequent childhood leukemia in their offspring.

Molecular screening for viruses in leukemic cells has been used as a distinct approach to explore possible mechanism(s) of direct transformation occurring *in utero* or during infancy. Smith postulated that JC polyomavirus (polyomavirus are named from the initials of the patients from whom the first isolates were made) would be a good candidate, because it met all the conditions for his model. However, to date, viral sequences from the polyomaviruses, JC or BK (a closely related virus), have not been found in leukemic cells (MacKenzie, 1999).

A number of viruses have been analyzed by different researchers. When blood or BM samples from patients diagnosed with childhood ALL were screened for members of the human herpesvirus family (HHV4, HHV6, HHV7, and HHV8), no evidence of the presence of these viruses in leukemic cells was found (MacKenzie, et al., 2001). Screenings for bovine leukemia virus (BLV) and transfusion-transmitted virus (TTV) have also been negative (Bender et al., 1988; Shiramizu et al., 2002). However, as the list of candidates has not been exhausted, massive sequencing to analyze non-human genomic components from leukemic cells, even those not previously identified, is an attractive approach.

There is evidence supporting each of the hypotheses presented here. Although the postulated mechanisms differ from each other, such hypotheses are not mutually exclusive. Because the notion of a unique carcinogenic factor is a biologically absurd assumption, the various cases of leukemia in Mexico and around the world must be triggered by a variety of agents. Given the evidence of an infectious etiology involved in childhood leukemia, the identification of this agent, or agents, remains a scientific challenge.

5. Age peak of ALL in the world: epidemiologic aspects

Industrialization, urbanization, economic growth, and technological development have brought benefits to people, making everyday tasks easier and offering accessibility to services. However, modernization and industrialization have also led to changes in the environment and in lifestyle, which have changed the pattern of diseases in adults and children over the last century. Children now face predominantly chronic and disabling diseases such as obesity, diabetes, asthma, learning disabilities, birth defects, and cancer (Suk et al., 2003).

Internationally, published studies have reported lower incidence rates of ALL in Africa, Asia, and Vietnam, with the high rates found for Hong Kong, United Kingdom (UK), USA, and Japan, thus suggesting a correlation between the reported variations in incidence of ALL and socio-economic status (Parkin, et al., 1988, 1998; Stiller, 2004). However, the highest incidence rates of ALL have been reported for Costa Rica, Mexico City, and the Hispanic populations of Los Angeles, California and of Florida in the USA. (American Cancer Society, Surveillance Research [ACSSR], 2009; Glazer et al., 1999; Mejía-Aranguré et al., 2005b; Monge et al., 2002; Surveillance Epidemiology and End Results [SEER], 2008; Wilkinson et al., 2001). Of all cases diagnosed with ALL in the 2–7 years age group in Europe and the USA, approximately 85–90% had a precursor-B (pre-B) cell immunophenotype; the remainder were classified as having either T-cell or B-cell immunophenotype (14% or 2%, respectively (Pui, 1997). Reports from the USA indicate that African-American children have half the risk of developing ALL than do White children, with a peak age of presentation of ALL between 2–6 years old (median 4 years old) and with ALL predominating in males (male:female ratio of 1.2: 1) (Eden, 2010).

Reports regarding the incidence and trend for ALL from the Surveillance Epidemiology and End Results (SEER) in the USA and the Manchester Children's Tumor Registry (MCTR) in the UK indicate that the rates have increased annually by 0.6% and 1.1%, respectively. However, recent reports indicate a modest increase of 0.4% annually for the USA (Linabery & Ross 2008) and 1–4% for Europe (McNally et al., 2001) in the group of 1–4 years old.

Of particular note in reports of cancer registries are the high incidences of ALL in Costa Rica, Mexico City, and the Hispanic populations of the USA (Table 1). For the last case, it has been suggested that, because this population tends to live in more crowded conditions and poverty that does the White population, thereby exposing this population to infectious agents that have not as yet been identified but which may promote the development of acute leukemia (Yaris et al., 2004). There are marked variations in the incidence of ALL among populations worldwide; these variations can provide valuable clues to help understand the etiology of ALL.

A review of the latest articles published about the incidence of ALL in countries around the world (Table 2), some studies reported only the incidence of acute leukemia; nevertheless we included these studies because, as 80% of leukemias are ALL, the incidence rates reported provide very important information. We considered only those works that reported incidence rate, age group, and when done, immunophenotype. In these studies, the results were generally reported by age groups: <1 year; 1–4 years; 0–4 years; 5–9 years; 10+ years; or 0–14 years. Some studies did not estimate the overall incidence rate and reported only by sex. Few studies had a graphic concerning the incidence of ALL and age, which would have better illustrated the peak incidence. Most published studies are from the Americas or Europe; few studies determined the immunophenotype of acute leukemia.

Report	Period	Age group (years)	Incidence rate per 10^6 children
United States SEER[1] (Howlader et al., 2010)	2007	0–14	35.0
CDC (NPCR)[2] (USCS[3] Working Group, 2010)	2003–2007	0–19	46.0
ACSSR[4] (American Cancer Society, 2009)	2002–2006	0–14	46.7
Florida (Wilkinson et al., 2001)	1985–1997	0–14	49.7
California (Glazer et al., 1999)	1988–1994	0–14	44.0
Mexico City IMSS[5] (Mejía-Aranguré et al., 2005b)	2006–2007	0–14	57.6
Costa Rica (Monge et al., 2002)	1981–1996	0–14	43.1

[1] Surveillance, Epidemiology and End Results Program in United States of America.
[2] Center for Disease Control, Division of Cancer Prevention and Control, National Program of Cancer Registries (NPCR).
[3] United States Cancer Statistics
[4] American Cancer Society, Surveillance Research.
[5] Instituto Mexicano del Seguro Social

Table 1. Incidence rates of lymphoid leukemias per million Mexican and Costa Rican children from cancer registries.

For the Americas, a highest incidence rate of ALL, 73.2 per 10^6 children in the 1–4 years age group, was reported for the USA for the period 1992–2004 (Linabery & Ross, 2008); the lowest incidence rate of ALL (35.5 per 10^6 children) was in Uruguay (Castillo et al., 2001), this latter report covered a different period and did not report incidence rates for different age groups. It is very important to note that, for both Brazil (de Souza Reis R et al., 2011) and Mexico City (Bernáldez-Ríos et al., 2008), the highest peak incidence of ALL was reported for the same age groups, with high (albeit distinct) incidence rates in both countries. From these data, one can speculate that these two countries share certain genetic or environmental characteristics. Although in a report from Puerto Rico (Pérez-Perdomo & Rodríguez-Figueroa, 2000), there are data only for individuals <20 years, these data were included here to provide information, not for comparative purposes. For countries in Europe, the highest incidence rate was reported for Italy (95.6 per 10^6) (Magnani et al., 2003) and Greece (82.5 per 10^6) (Petridou et al., 2008), for different periods and immunophenotypes, but for the same age group. The lowest incidence rate (35.7 per 10^6) was reported for Ireland (Stack et al., 2007).

The differences in trends across demographic subgroups provide starting points for the etiological investigation of ALL. Such research should generate testable hypotheses that include factors such as the child's birth characteristics and environmental exposures and topics such as the creation of cancer registries.

Location	Period	Type of cancer	Immuno-phenotype	Age group	Incidence rate[1]
The Americas					
North America					
USA					
SEER (Linabery & Ross, 2008)	1992–2004	ALL[2]	ND[3]	1–4	73.2
Hispanic children (Glazer et al., 1999)	1988–1994	ALL	ND	0–4	66.0
Hawaii, USA (Goodman et al., 1989)	1960–1984	ALL	ND	0–4	49.6 (M) 44.8 (F)
Mexico City (Bernáldez-Ríos et al.,	1996–2006	ALL	B-cell Precursor	3 6	65.0 50.0
Mexico City (Mejía-Aranguré et al., 2005b)	1996–2000	ALL	ND	1–4	64.6
Ontario, Canada (Agha et al., 2006)	1986 2001	AL[4]	ND	0–14	52.8 44.4
Puerto Rico (Pérez-Perdomo & Rodríguez-Figueroa et al., 2000)	1980–1991	AL	ND	<20	35.7
Central America					
Costa Rica (Monge et al., 2002)	1981–1996	ALL	ND	1–4	68.5
El Salvador (Mejía-Aranguré et al., 2005b)	1996–2000	ALL	ND	1–4	48.4
South America					
Brazil (de Souza Reis et al., 2011)	1997–2004	ALL	ND	3 6	72.8 40.0
Trinidad and Tobago (Bodkyn & Lalchandani, 2010)	2001–2006	AL	ND	0–4	49.0 (M) 27.0 (F)
Uruguay (Castillo et al., 2001)	1992–1994	ALL	ND	0–14	35.5
Asia					
Iran (Mousavi et al., 2010)	2003–2007	AL	ND	0–14	15.9 (M) 14.1 (F)

Europe					
North Europe					
Nordic Countries (Hjalgrim et al., 2003)	1998–2001	ALL	B-cell precursor	0–14	35.9
West Europe					
Ireland (Stack et al., 2007)	1994–2000	ALL	ND	0–14	35.7
Northwest England (McNally et al., 2001)	1954–1998	ALL	ND	1–4	51.2
Northwest England (McNally et al., 2000)	1995–1998	ALL	B-cell precursor	1–4	54.0
Southwest England (McKinney et al., 1993)	1984–1988	ALL	Pre-B	1–4	50.0 (M) 54.0 (F)
Yorkshire, UK (Feltbower et al., 2001)	1995–1997	ALL	B-cell precursor	1–4	46.6
Central Europe					
Eastern Germany (Spix et al., 2008)	1991–2004	ALL	ND	0–14	44.0
Germany (Kaatsch, 2010)	1988–1997	AL	ND	0–14	44.0
South Europe					
Castilla and León, Spain (González García et al., 2010)	2003–2007	AL	ND	0–4	47.6
Greece (Petridou et al., 2008)	1996–2006	ALL	B-cell precursor	1–4	82.5
Northwest Italy (Magnani et al., 2003)	1995–1998	ALL	Common Pre-B	1–4	95.6
Spain (Peris-Bonet et al., 2010)	1983–2002	AL	ND	0–14	45.9
Oceania					
Australia (Baade et al., 2010)	1997–2006	ALL	ND	0–4	84.6

[1]per 10^6 million children
[2]Acute lymphoblastic leukemia
[3]No data
[4]Acute leukemia

Table 2. The incidence of AL and ALL and the peak age in different continents expressed in cases by million.

6. Conclusions

The ontology of B and T lymphocytes demonstrates that different factors may be involved at the moment when the cell is most vulnerable to undergo an alteration that promotes the development of ALL. An important factor may be an infectious agent(s). For children with

ALL, both the presence of MLL/AF4, principally during the first year of life, and the presence of ETV6/RUNX1 in 2-6 year olds are considered causes of ALL. MLL/AF4 is sufficient to promote the development of ALL and that children born with this genetic rearrangement will always develop ALL. However, in the case of children born with the rearrangement ETV6/RUNX1, one or more additional risk factors (e.g., an exaggerated response to late common infections) would be needed to initiate leukemogenesis.

It is possible that the age peak of ALL reflects a higher degree of susceptibility with which a child is born, such as is the case with both bilateral retinoblastoma and bilateral Wilm's tumor: an earlier age peak is found in the bilateral forms of these diseases than when the retinoblastoma or Wilm's tumor is unilateral (National Wilm's Tumor Study Committee, 1999; Pastore et al., 1988; Sanders et al., 1988; Teppo et al., 1975). Thus, children with the highest susceptibility at birth should show an early age peak for ALL (say, during the firsts year of life), whereas children born with the lowest susceptibility will evidence an age peak of ALL in later years. For those children for whom it is not possible to determine their susceptibility to ALL at birth, it may be that many environmental factors are involved when the child develops ALL during the firsts year of life. That is to say, in order for a child to develop ALL, both risk factors (susceptibility at birth or degree of exposure) must be present and at least one of the two risks factors must be high.Thus, to develop ALL, a child born with a high susceptibility for developing the disease may need only a low degree of exposure to environmental factor(s), whereas a child born with low susceptibility for developing ALL will need a higher degree of exposure to environmental factor(s) (Figure 4).

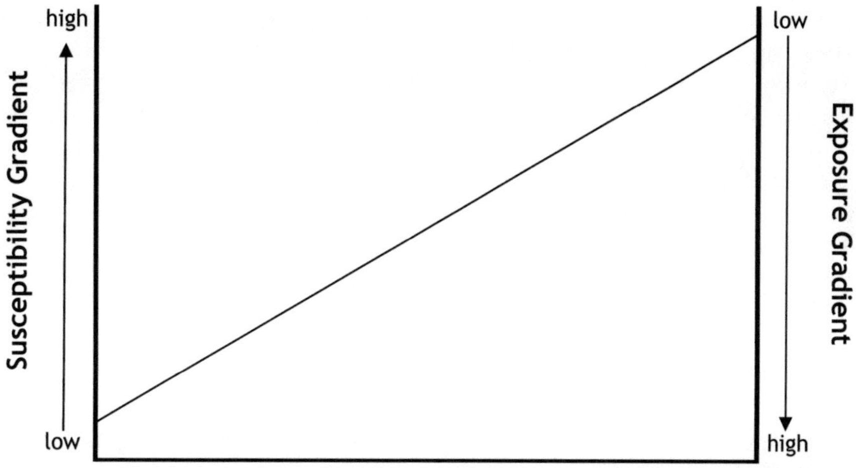

Fig. 4. Interaction between a gradient of susceptibility and a gradient of exposure to carcinogenic environmental factors. From this, to develop acute leukemia, an individual with a higher susceptibility, as determined by the interplay of genetic factors, would need a lower exposure, as determined by the interplay (unknown, possibly synergistic) of the characteristics of the exposure. Conversely, the higher the exposure, the lower the susceptibility needed to result in developing the disease.

It is possible that the two age peaks for ALL reported for children from Brazil and Mexico City reflect different etiologies, or are a result of each child's having a different etiology. It is probable that there is no one genetic rearrangement that determines susceptibility to ALL, nor one environmental factor associated with ALL. However, if the effect(s) of exposure to environmental factor(s) is(are) cumulative and if the degree of exposure to environmental factor(s) perfectly complements the degree of susceptibility with which the child was born, then the child develops ALL. The age peak of ALL permits the prediction of the degree of susceptibility with which the child was born and/or the degree of exposure to environmental factor(s) experienced by the child during the firsts years of life.

7. Acknowledgments

This work was supported by a grant (FIS/IMSS/PROT/056) from the Fondo de Investigacion en Salud, Mexico, and of projects financed by grants (2007-1-18 71223/FIS/IMSS/PROT/592 & CB-2007-1-83949/FIS/IMSS/PROT/616) from the Consejo Nacional de Ciencia y Tecnologia, Mexico, through its division for the dissemination of the results of scientific investigation. We thank Veronica Yakoleff for reviewing of the original manuscript, editorial revision, and for helpful comments. Janet Flores-Lujano did the figure 1.

8. References

Agha, M., DiMonte, B., Greenberg, M., Greenberg, C., Barr, R. & McLaughlin JR. (2006). Incidence trends and projections for childhood cancer in Ontario. *International Journal of Cancer*, Vol. 118, No. 11, (June 2006), pp. 2809-2815, ISSN 1097-0215.

Allman, D., Li, J. & Hardy, RR. (1999). Commitment to the B lymphoid lineage occurs before DH-JH recombination. *Journal of Experimental Medicine,* Vol.189, No.4, (February 1999), pp. 735-740, ISSN 0022-100.

American Cancer Society (2009). Cancer in children and adolescents, In: Cancer Facts & Figures for Hispanics/Latinos 2009-2011, Accessed on Jun 8th 2011, Available from: <http://www.cancer.org/acs/groups/content/@nho/documents/document/ffhispanicslatinos20092011.pdf.>

Baade, PD., Youlden, DR., Valery, PC., Hassall, T., Ward, L., Green, AC. & Aitken, JF. (2010). Trends in incidence of childhood cancer in Australia, 1983-2006. *British Journal of Cancer*, Vol.102, No.3, (February 2010), pp. 620-626, ISSN 1532-1827.

Baba, Y., Pelayo, R. & Kincade, PW. (2004). Relationships between hematopoietic stem cells and lymphocyte progenitors. *Trends in Immunology*, Vol.25, No.12, (December 2004), pp. 645-649, ISSN 1471-4906.

Baldridge, MT., King, KY. & Goodell, MA. (2011). Inflammatory signals regulate hematopoietic stem cells. *Trends in Immunology*, Vol.32, No.2, (February 2011), pp.57-65, ISSN 1471-4906.

Bannish, G., Fuentes-Pananá, EM., Cambier, JC., Pear, WS. & Monroe, JG. (2001). Ligand-independent signaling functions for the B lymphocyte antigen receptor and their role in positive selection during B lymphopoiesis. *Journal of Experimental Medicine*, Vol.194, No.11 (December 2001), pp. 1583-1596, ISSN 0022-100.

Bathia, S. & Robison, L. (2003). Epidemiology of leukemia in childhood, In: *Hematology of infancy and childhood*, Nathan, DG., Oski, FA. Eds., pp. (1081-1100), Saunders, ISBN 978-1-4160-9977-2, Philadelphia.

Bender, AP., Robison, LL., Kashmiri, SV., McClain, KL., Woods, WG., Smithson, WA., Heyn, R., Finlay, J., Schuman, LM., Renier, C. & Gibson, R. (1988). No involvement of bovine leukemia virus in childhood acute lymphoblastic leukemia and non-

Hodgkin's lymphoma. *Cancer Research*. No.48, Vol.10, (May 1988), pp. 2919-2922, ISSN 0008-5472.

Bernaldez-Rios, R., Ortega-Alvarez, MC., Perez-Saldivar, ML., Alatoma-Medina, NE., Del Campo-Martinez, Mde L., Rodriguez-Zepeda, Mdel C., Montero-Ponce, I., Franco-Ornelas, S., Fernandez-Castillo, G., Nuñez-Villegas, NN., Taboada-Flores, MA., Flores-Lujano, J., Argüelles-Sanchez, ME., Juarez-Ocaña, S., Fajardo-Gutierrez, A. & Mejia-Arangure, JM. (2008). The age incidence of childhood B-cell precursor acute lymphoblastic leukemia in Mexico City. *Journal of Pediatric Hematology/ Oncology*, Vol. 30, No. 3, (March 2008), pp. 199-203, ISSN 1536-3678.

Birch, J. & Blair, V. (1992). The epidemiology of infant cancers. *British Journal of Cancer*; Vol. 66, No. Suppl. 18, (August 1992), pp. 2-4, ISSN 0007-0920.

Black, D. (1984). Investigation of the Possible Increased Incidence of Cancer in West Cumbria, London. *Proceedeings of Report of the Independent Advisory Group*. HMSO. London.

Blom, B. & Spits, H. (2006). Development of human lymphoid cells. *Annual Review of Immunology*, Vol.24 (April 2006), pp. 287-320, ISSN 0732-0582.

Bodkyn, C. & Lalchandani, S. (2010). Incidence of childhood cancer in Trinidad and Tobago. *West Indian Medical Journal*, Vol.59, No.5, (October 2010), pp. 465-468, ISSN 0043-3144.

Cambier, J. C. (1995). Antigen and Fc receptor signaling. The awesome power of the immunoreceptor tyrosine-based activation motif (ITAM). *Journal of Immunology*, Vol.155, No.7, (October 1995) pp. 3281–3285, ISSN 0022-1767.

Cardwell, CR., McKinney, PA., Patterson, CC., & Murray, LJ., (2008). Infections in early life and childhood leukaemia risk: a UK case-control study of general practitioner records. *British Journal of Cancer*, Vol.99, No.9, (November 2008), pp. 1529-1533, ISSN 0007-0920.

Castillo, L., Fluchel, M., Dabezies, A., Pieri, D., Brockhorst, N. & Barr, R. (2001). Childhood cancer in Uruguay: 1992-1994. Incidence and mortality. *Medical and Pediatric Oncology*, Vol.37, No.4, (October 2001), pp. 400-404, ISSN 0098-1532.

Chan, LC., Lam, TH., Li, CK., Lau, YL., Li, CK., Yuen, HL., Lee, CW., Ha, SY., Yuen, PM., Leung, NK., Patheal, SL., Greaves, MF. & Alexander, FE. (2002). Is the timing of exposure to infection a major determinant of acute lymphoblastic leukaemia in Hong Kong? *Paediatric Perinatal Epidemiology*, Vol.16, No.2, (April 2002), pp. 154-165, ISSN 0269-5022.

Cobaleda, C., Gutiérrez-Cianca, N., Pérez-Losada, J., Flores, T., García-Sanz, R., González, M. & Sánchez-García, I. (2000). A primitive hematopoietic cell is the target for the leukemic transformation in human philadelphia-positive acute lymphoblastic leukemia. *Blood*, Vol.95, No.3, (February 2000) pp. 1007-1013, ISSN 0006-4971.

Committee on Medical Aspects of Radiation in the Environment (COMARE). First Report Proceedings of The Implications of the New Data on the Releases From Sellafield in the 1950s for the Conclusions of the Report on the Investigation of the Possible Increased Incidence of Cancer in West Cumbria (Department of Health, 1986)

Cooke, V. (1942). The incidence of acute leukemia in children. *The journal of the American Medical Association*, Vol.119, No.7, (June 1942), pp. 547–550, ISSN 00987484.

Court, WM. & Doll, R. (1961). Leukaemia in childhood and young adult life. Trends in mortality in relation to aetiology. *British Medical Journal,* Vol.1, No.5231, (April 1961), pp. 981–988, ISSN 09598138.

Cox, CV., Diamanti, P., Evely, RS., Kearns, PR. & Blair, A. (2009). Expression of CD133 on leukemia-initiating cells in childhood ALL. *Blood,* Vol.113, No.14, (April 2009), pp.3287-3295, ISSN 0006-4971.

Cox, CV., Evely, RS., Oakhill, A., Pamphilon, DH., Goulden, NJ. & Blair, A. (2004). Characterization of acute lymphoblastic leukemia progenitor cells. *Blood,* Vol.104, No.9, (November 2004), pp. 2919-2925, ISSN 0006-4971 de Souza Reis R, Sr., de Camargo, B., de Oliveira Santos, M., de Oliveira, JM., Azevedo Silva, F. & Pombo-de-Oliveira, MS. (2011). Childhood leukemia incidence in Brazil according to different geographical regions. *Pediatric blood & Cancer,* Vol.56, No.1, (January 2011), pp. 58-64, ISSN 1545-5017.

Dick, J.E. (2008). Stem cell concepts renew cancer research. *Blood,* Vol.112, No.13, (December 2008), pp. 4793-4807, ISSN 0006-4971.

Dockerty, JD., Draper, G., Vincent, T., Rowan, SD. & Bunch, KJ. (2001). Case-control study of parental age, parity and socioeconomic level in relation to childhood cancers. *International Journal of Epidemiology,* Vol.6, No.30, (December 2001), pp. 1428-1437, ISSN 0300-5771.

Doulatov, S., Notta, F., Eppert, K., Nguyen, LT., Ohashi, PS. & Dick, JE. (2010). Revised map of the human progenitor hierarchy shows the origin of macrophages and dendritic cells in early lymphoid development. *Nature Immunology,* Vol.11, No.7, (July 2010), pp. 585-593, ISSN 1529-2908.

Downing, JR. (1999). The AML1-ETO chimeric transcription factor in acute myeloid leukaemia. Biology and clinical significance. *British Journal of Haematology,* Vol.106, No.2, (August 1999), pp. 296-308, ISSN 1365-2141.

Draper, G., Kroll, M. & Stiller, C. (1994). Childhood cancer. *Cancer Surveys;* Vol.19-20, (April 1994), pp. 493-517, ISSN 0261-2429.

Eden, T. (2010). Aetiology of childhood leukaemia. *Cancer Treatment Reviews,* Vol.36, No.4, (June 2010), pp. 286-297, ISSN 0305-7372.

Espinoza-Hernández, L., Cruz-Rico, J., Benítez-Aranda, H., Martínez-Jaramillo, G., Rodríguez-Zepeda, MC., Vélez-Ruelas, MA. & Mayani, H. (2001). In vitro characterization of the hematopoietic system in pediatric patients with acute lymphoblastic leukemia. *Leukemia Research,* Vol.25, No.4, (April 2001), pp. 295-303, ISSN 0145-2126.

Fajardo-Gutiérrez, A., Mejía-Aranguré, M., Gómez-Delgado, A., Mendoza-Sánchez. H., Garduño-Espinosa, J. & Martínez-García, MC. (1995). Epidemiología de las neoplasias malignas en niños residentes del Distrito Federal (1982-1991). *Boletín Médico del Hospital Infantil de México,* Vol.52, No.9, (September 2005), pp. 513-522, ISSN 1665-1146.

Fasching, K., Panzer, S., Haas, OA., Marschalek, R., Gadner, H. & Panzer-Grumayer, ER. (2000). Presence of clone-specific antigen receptor gene rearrngement at birth indicates an in utero origin of diverse types of early childhood acute lymphoblastic leukemia. *Blood,* Vol.95, No.8, (April 2000), pp. 2722-2724, ISSN 1528-0020.

Feltbower, RG., Moorman, AV., Dovey, G., Kinsey, SE. & McKinney, PA. (2001). Incidence of childhood acute lymphoblastic leukaemia in Yorkshire, UK. *The Lancet*, Vol.358, No.9279, (August 2001), pp. 385-387, ISSN 0140-6736.

Finnette, BA., Posseno, T. & Albertini, RJ. (1996). V(D)J recombinase-mediated HPRT mutations in peripheral blood lymphocytes of normal childrens. *Cancer Research*, Vol.56, No.6, (March 1996), pp. 1405-1412, ISSN 1538-7445.

Flores-Lujano, J., Perez-Saldivar, ML., Fuentes-Pananá, EM., Gorodezky, C., Bernaldez-Rios, R., Del Campo-Martinez, MA., Martinez-Avalos, A., Medina-Sanson, A., Paredes-Aguilera, R., De Diego-Flores Chapa, J., Bolea-Murga, V., Rodriguez-Zepeda, MC., Rivera-Luna, R., Palomo-Colli, MA., Romero-Guzman, L., Perez-Vera, P., Alvarado-Ibarra, M., Salamanca-Gómez, F., Fajardo-Gutierrez, A. & Mejía-Aranguré, JM. (2009). Breastfeeding and early infection in the aetiology of childhood leukaemia in Down syndrome. *British Journal of Cancer*, Vol.101, No.5, (September 2009), pp. 860-864, ISSN 0007-0920.

Ford, AM., Bennett, CA., Price, CM., Bruin, MC., Van Wering, ER. & Greaves, M. (1998). Fetal origins of the TEL-AML1 fusion gene in identical twins with leukemia. *Proceedings of the National Academy of Scinces of United States of America*, Vol.95, No.8, (April 1998), pp. 4584-4588, ISSN 1091-6490.

Ford, AM., Pombo-de-Oliveira, MS., McCarthy, KP., MacLean, JM., Carrico, KC., Vincent, RF. & Greaves, M. (1997). Monoclonal origin of concordant T-cell malignancy in identical twins. *Blood*, Vol.89, No.1, (January 1997), pp. 281-285, ISSN 1528-0020.

Ford, AM., Ridge, SA., Cabrera, ME., Mahmoud, H., Steel, CM., Chan, LC. & Greaves, M. (1993). In utero rearrangements in the trithorax-related oncogene in infant leukemias. *Nature*, Vol.363, No.6427, (May 1993), pp. 358-360, ISSN 1476-5551.

Fuentes-Pananá, EM., & Monroe, J. G. (2001). Ligand-dependent and -independent processes in B-cell-receptor-mediated signaling. *Springer Seminars in immunopathology*, Vol.23, No.4, (December 2001), pp. 333-350, ISSN 1863-2297.

Fuentes-Pananá, EM., Bannish, G. & Monroe, J. G. (2004a). Basal B-cell receptor signaling in B lymphocytes: mechanisms of regulation and role in positive selection, differentiation, and peripheral survival. *Immunological Reviews*, Vol.197, No.1, (January 2004), pp. 26-40, ISSN 0105-2896.

Fuentes-Pananá, EM., Bannish, G. & Monroe, J. G. (2004b). Basal Igα/Igβ signals trigger the coordinated initiation of preBCR-dependent processes. *Journal of Immunology*, Vol.173, No.2, (July 2004), pp. 1000-1011, ISSN 0022-1767.

Gale, KB., Ford, AM., Repp, R., Borkhardt, A., Keller, C., Eden, OB. & Greaves, MF. (1997). Backtracking leukemia to birth: identification of clonotypic gene fusion sequences in neonatal blood spots. *Proceedings of the National Academy of Scinces of United States of America*, Vol.94, No.25, (December 1997), pp. 13950-13954, ISSN 1091-6490.

Gardner, MJ., Snee, MP., Hall, AJ., Powell, CA., Downes, S. & Terrell, JD. (1990). Results of case–control study of leukaemia and lymphoma among young people near Sellafield nuclear plant in West Cumbria. *British Medical Journal*, Vol.300, No.6722, (February 1990), pp. 423–429, ISSN 0959-8138.

Gill Super, HJ., Rothberg, PG., Kobayashi, H., Freeman, AL., Diaz, MO. & Rowly, JD. (1994). Clonal Nonconstitutional rearrangements of the MLL gene in infant twins with acute lymphoblastic leukemia: in utero chromosome rearrangement of 11q23. *Blood*, Vol.83, No.3, (May 1994), pp. 641-644, ISSN 1528-0020.

Glazer, ER., Perkins, CI., Young, JL. Jr., Schlag, RD., Campleman, SL. & Wright, WE. (1999). Cancer among Hispanic children in California, 1988-1994: comparison with non-Hispanic white children. *Cancer,* Vol.86, No.6, (September 1999), pp. 1070-1079, ISSN 1097-0142.

González García, H., Quirós, AB., Crespo, CV., Meléndez, PG., Gómez, ST. & Sanz, JC. (2010). Incidence of childhood cancer in the autonomous region of Castilla y León in Spain (2003-2007). *Anales de Pediatría (Barcelona, Spain),* Vol.73, No.4, (October 2010), pp. 169-179, ISSN 1695-9531.

Goodman, MT., Yoshizawa, CN. & Kolonel, LN. (1989) Incidence trends and ethnic patterns for childhood leukaemia in Hawaii: 1960-1984. *British Journal of Cancer,* Vol.60, No.1, (July 1989), pp. 93-97, ISSN 1532-1827.

Greaves, M. (2002). Childhood leukemia. *British Medical Journal,* Vol.324, No.7332, (February 2002), pp. 283-287, ISSN 1468-5833.

Greaves, M., Maia, AT., Wiemels, JL. & Ford, AM. (2003). Leukemia in twins; lessons in natural history. *Blood,* Vol.102, No.7, (October 2003), pp. 2321-2333, ISSN 1528-0020.

Greaves, MF. (1988). Speculations on the cause of childhood acute lymphoblastic leukemia. *Leukemia,* Vol.2, No.2, (February 1988), pp. 120-125, ISSN 1476-5551.

Greaves, MF., Colman, SM., Beard, MEJ., Bradstock, K., Cabrera, ME., Chen, PM., Jacobs, P., Lam-Po-Tang, PR., MacDougall, LG. & Williams, CK. (1993). Geographical distribution of acute lymphoblastic leukemia subtypes: Second report of the collaborative group study. *Leukemia,* Vol.7, No.1, (January 1993), pp. 27-34, ISSN 1476-5551.

Hardy, RR., Carmack, CE., Shinton, SA., Kemp, JD. & Hayakawa, K. (1991). Resolution and characterization of pro-B and pre-pro-B cell stages in normal mouse bone marrow. *Journal of Experimental Medicine,* Vol.173, No.5, (May 1991), pp. 1213-1225, ISSN 0022-1007.

Heasman, MA., Kemp, IW., Urquhart, JD. & Black, R. (1986). Childhood leukaemia in northern Scotland. *Lancet,* Vol.327, No.8475, (February 1986), pp. 266, ISSN 0140-6736.

Heidenreich, O. & Vormoor, J. (2009). Malignant stem cells in childhood ALL: the debate continues! *Blood,* Vol.113, No.18, (April 2009), pp. 4476-4477, ISSN 0006-4971.

Hewitt, D. (1955). Some features of leukaemia mortality. *British Journal of Preventive and Social Medicine,* Vol.9, No.2, (April 1955), pp. 81–88, ISSN 0007-1242.

Hjalgrim, LL., Rostgaard, K., Schmiegelow, K., Söderhäll, S., Kolmannskog, S., Vettenranta, K., Kristinsson, J., Clausen, N., Melbye, M., Hjalgrim, H. & Gustafsson, G. (2003). Age-and sex-specific incidence of childhood leukemia by immunophenotype in the Nordic countries. *Journal of the National Cancer Institute,* Vol.95, No.20, (October 2003), pp. 1539-1544, ISSN 1460-2105.

Howlader, N., Noone, AM., Krapcho, M., Neyman, N., Aminou, R., Waldron, W., Altekruse, SF., Kosary, CL., Ruhl, J., Tatalovich, Z., Cho, H., Mariotto, A., Eisner, MP., Lewis, DR., Chen, HS., Feuer, EJ., Cronin, KA. & Edwards, BK. (2010). *SEER Cancer Statistics Review, 1975-2008,* National Cancer Institute. Bethesda, MD. Retrieved from <http://seer.cancer.gov/csr/1975_2008/>

Infante-Rivard, C., Fortier, I. & Olsen, E. (2000). Markers of infection, breast-feeding and childhood acute lymphoblastic leukaemia. *British Journal of Cancer,* Vol.83, No.11, (December 2000), pp. 559–1564, ISSN 0007-0920.

Johansson, B., Moorman, AV., Haas, OA., Watmore, AE., Cheung, KL., Swanton, S. & Secker-Walker, LM. (1998). Hematologic malignancies with t(4;11)(q21;q23)-a cytogenetic, morphologic, immunophenotypic and clinical study of 183 cases. European 11q23 Workshop participants. *Leukemia*, Vol.12, No.5, (May 1998), pp. 779-787, ISSN 1476-5551.

Jourdan-Da Silva, N., Perel, Y., Méchinaud, F., Plouvier, E., Gandemer, V., Lutz, P., Vannier, JP., Lamagnére, JL., Marguerítte, G., Boutard, P., Robert, A., Armari, C., Munzer, M., Millot, F., De Lumley, L., Berthou, C., Rialland, X., Pautard, B., Hémon, D. & Clavel, J. (2004). Infectious diseases in the first year of life, perinatal characteristics and childhood acute leukaemia. *British Journal of Cancer*, Vol.90, No.1, (January 2004), pp. 139–145, ISSN 0007-0920.

Kaatsch, P. (2010). Epidemiology of childhood cancer. *Cancer Treatment Reviews*, Vol.36, No.4, (June 2010), pp. 277-285, ISSN 0305-7372.

Kaatsch, P., Haaf, G. & Michaelis, J. (1995). Childhood malignancies in Germany. Methods and results of a nationwide registry. *European Journal of Cancer*, Vol.31A, No.6, (June 1995), pp. 993-999, ISSN 0959-8049.

Karasuyama, H., Rolink, A. & Melchers, F. (1996). Surrogate light chain in B cell development. *Advances in Immunology*, Vol.63, No.2, (1996), pp. 1-41, ISSN 0065-2776.

Kim, JM., Kim, NI., Oh, YK., Kim, YJ., Youn, J. & Ahn, MJ. (2005). CpG oligodeoxynucleotides induce IL-8 expression in CD34+ cells via mitogen-activated protein kinase-dependent and NF-kB-independent pathways. *International Immunology*, Vol.17, No.12, (December 2005), pp. 1525-1531, ISSN 0953-8178.

Kinlen, L. (2011). Childhood leukaemia, nuclear sites, and population mixing. British Journal of Cancer, Vol.104, No.1, (January 2011), pp. 12-18, ISSN 0007-0920.

Kinlen, LJ., O'Brien, F., Clarke, K., Balkwill, A. & Matthews, F. (1993). Rural population mixing and childhood leukaemia: effects of the North Sea oil industry in Scotland, including the area near Dounreay nuclear site. *British Journal of Cancer*, Vol.306, No.6880, (March 1993), pp. 743–748, ISSN 0007-0920.

Kinlen, L. (1988). Evidence for an infective cause of childhood leukaemia: comparison of a Scottish New Town with nuclear reprocessing sites in Britain. *The Lancet*, Vol.2, No.8624, (December 1988), pp. 1323–1327, ISSN 0140-6736.

Kinlen, L. (1995a). Epidemiological evidence for an infective basis in childhood leukaemia. *British Journal of Cancer*, Vol.71, No.1, (January 1995), pp. 1–5, ISSN 0007-0920.

Kinlen, LJ. & Balkwill, A. (2001). Infective cause of childhood leukaemia and wartime population mixing in Orkney and Shetland, UK. *Lancet*, Vol.357, No.9259, (March 2001), pp. 357-858, ISSN 0140-6736.

Kinlen, LJ. & Hudson, C. (1991). Childhood leukaemia and poliomyelitis in relation to military encampments in England and Wales in the period of national military service, 1950 –63. *British Medical Journal*, Vol.303, No.6814, (November 1991), pp. 1357–1362, ISSN 0959-8138.

Kinlen, LJ. & John, SM. (1994). Wartime evacuation and mortality from childhood leukaemia in England and Wales in 1945–9. *British Medical Journal*, Vol.309, No.6963, (November 1994), pp. 1197–1202, ISSN 0959-8138.

Kinlen, LJ., Clarke, K. & Hudson, C. (1990). Evidence from population mixing in British New Towns of an infective basis for childhood leukaemia. *Lancet*, Vol.3368, No.715, (September 1990), pp. 577–582, ISSN 0140-6736.

Kinlen, LJ., Dickson, M. & Stiller, CA. (1995b). Childhood leukaemia and non-Hodgkin's lymphoma near large rural construction sites, with a comparison with Sellafield nuclear site. *British Medical Journal*, Vol.310, No.6982, (March 1995), pp. 763–768, ISSN 0959-8138.

Kristensen, T., Wesenberg, F., Jonsoon, OG., Carlsen, NT., Forestier, E., Kirchhoff, M., Lundsteen, C. & Schmiegelow, K. (2003). High resolution comparative genomic hybridisation yields at high detection rate of chromosomal aberrations in childhood acute lymphoblastic leukemia. *European Journal of Haematology*, Vol.70, No.6, (June 2003), pp. 363-372, ISSN 1600-0609.

Lehtinen, M., Koskela, P., Ogmundsdottir, H., Bloigu, A., Dillner, J., Gudnadottir, M., Hakulinen, T., Kjartansdottir, A., Kvarnung, M., Pukkala, E., Tulinius, H & Lehtinen, T. (2003). Maternal herpesvirus infections and risk of acute lymphoblastic leukemia in the offspring. *American Journal Epidemiology*, Vol.58, No.3, (August 2003), pp. 207-213, ISSN 0002-9262.

Levy, O. (2007). Innate immunity of the newborn: basic mechanisms and clinical correlates. *Nature Reviews Immunology*, Vol.7, No.5, (May 2007), pp. 379-390, ISSN 1474-1733.

Linabery, AM. & Ross, JA. (2008). Trends in childhood cancer incidence in the U.S. (1992-2004). *Cancer*, Vol. 112, No.2, (January 2008), pp. 416-432, ISSN 1097-0142.

Little, J. (August 15, 1999). Epidemiology of Childhood Cancer. (1st edition), International Agency for Research on Cancer Scientific Publications, ISBN-10 9283221494, ISBN-13 978-9283221494, Lyon, France

Love, P. E., & Hayes, S. M. (2010). ITAM-mediated signaling by the T-cell antigen receptor. *Cold Spring Harbor Perspectives in Biology*, Vol.2, No.6, (June 2010), pp. 1-11, ISSN 1943-0264.

Ma, X., Buffler, PA., Wiemels, JL., Selvin, S., Metayer, C., Loh, M., Does, MB. & Wiencke, JK. (2005). Ethnic difference in daycare attendance, early infections, and risk of childhood acute lymphoblastic leukemia. *Cancer Epidemiology, Biomarkers & Prevention*, Vol.14, No.8. (August 2005), pp. 1928-1934, ISSN 1055-9965.

MacKenzie, J., Gallagher, A., Clayton, RA., Perry, J., Eden, OB., Ford, AM., Greaves, MF. & Jarrett, RF. (2001). Screening for herpesvirus genomes in common acute lymphoblastic leukemia. *Leukemia*, Vol.15, No.3, (March 2001), pp. 415-421, ISSN 0887-6924.

MacKenzie, J., Perry, J., Ford, AM., Jarrett, RF. & Greaves, M. (1999). JC and BK virus sequences are not detectable in leukaemic samples from children with common acute lymphoblastic leukaemia. *British Journal of Cancer*, Vol.81, No.5, (November 1999), pp. 898-899, ISSN 0007-0920.

Magnani, C., Dalmasso, P., Pastore, G., Terracini, B., Martuzzi, M., Mosso, ML. & Merletti, F. (2003). Increasing incidence of childhood leukemia in Northwest Italy, 1975-98. *International Journal of Cancer*, Vol. 105, No. 4, (July 2003), pp. 552-557, ISSN 1097-0215.

Mandal, M., Powers, S. E., Ochiai, K., Georgopoulos, K., Kee, B. L., Singh, H. & Clark, M. R. (2009). Ras orchestrates exit from the cell cycle and light-chain recombination during early B cell development. *Nature Immunology*, Vol.10, No.10, (October 2009), pp. 1110-1117, ISSN 1529-2908.

Mayani, H. (2010). Biological differences between neonatal and adult human hematopoietic stem/progenitor cells. *Stem Cells and Development*, Vol.19, No.3, (March 2010), pp. 285-298, ISSN 1547-3287.

McKinney, PA., Alexander, FE., Cartwright, RA., Scott, CS. & Staines, A. (1993). Acute lymphoblastic leukaemia incidence in the UK by immunophenotype. *Leukemia*, Vol. 7, No. 10, (October 1993), pp. 1630-1634, ISSN 1476-5551.

McKinney, PA., Juszczak, E., Findlay, E., Smith, K. & Thomson, CS. (1999). Pre- and perinatal risk factors for childhood leukaemia and other malignancies: a Scottish case control study. *British Journal of Cancer*, Vol.80, No.11, (August 1999), pp. 1844-1851, ISSN 0007-0920.

McNally, RJ. & Eden, TO. (2004). An infectious aetiology for childhood acute leukaemia: a review of the evidence. *British Journal of Haematology*, Vol.127, No.3, (November 2004), pp. 243-263, ISSN 0007-1048.

McNally, RJ., Birch, JM., Taylor, GM. & Eden, OB. (2000). Incidence of childhood precursor B-cell acute lymphoblastic leukaemia in north-west England. *The Lancet*, Vol.356, No.9228, (August 2000), pp. 485-486, ISSN 0140-6736.

McNally, RJ., Cairns, DP., Eden, OB., Kelsey, AM., Taylor, GM. & Birch, JM. (2001). Examination of temporal trends in the incidence of childhood leukaemias and lymphomas provides aetiological clues. *Leukemia*, Vol.15, No.10, (October 2001), pp. 1612-1618, ISSN 1476-5551.

Mejía-Aranguré, JM., Flores Aguilar, H., Juárez Muñoz, I., Vázquez Langle, J., Games Eternod, J., Pérez Saldívar, ML., Ortega Alvarez, MC., Rendón Macías, ME. & Gutiérrez, AF. (2005a). Age of onset of different malignant tumors in childhood. *Revista Médica del Instituto Mexicano del Seguro Social*, Vol.43, No.1, (January-February 2005), pp. 25-37, ISSN 0443-5117.

Mejía-Aranguré, JM., Bonilla, M., Lorenzana, R., Juárez-Ocaña, S., de Reyes, G., Pérez-Saldivar, ML., González-Miranda, G., Bernáldez-Ríos, R., Ortiz-Fernández, A., Ortega-Alvarez, M., Martínez-García, Mdel C. & Fajardo-Gutiérrez, A. (2005b). Incidence of leukemias in children from El Salvador and Mexico City between 1996 and 2000: population-based data. *Bio Medical Central Cancer*, Vol.4, No.5, (April 2005), pp. 33, ISSN 1471-2407.

Melchers, F., Karasuyama, H., Haasner, D., Bauer, S., Kudo, A., Sakaguchi N., Jameson B. & Rolink A. (1993). The surrogate light chain in B-cell development. *Immunology Today*, Vol.14, No.2, (February 1993), pp. 60-68, ISSN 0167-5699.

Miller, RW. & Myers, MH. (1983). Age distribution of epithelial and non-epithelial cancers. *Lancet*, Vol.2, No.8361, (November 1983), pp. 1250, ISSN 0140-6736.

Monge, P., Wesseling, C., Rodríguez, AC., Cantor, KP., Weiderpass, E., Reutfors, J., Ahlbom, A. & Partanen, T. (2002). Childhood leukaemia in Costa Rica, 1981-96. *Paediatric and Perinatal Epidemiology*, Vol.16, No.3, (July 2002), pp. 210-218, ISSN 1365-3016.

Mousavi, SM., Pourfeizi, A. & Dastgiri, S. (2010). Childhood cancer in Iran. *Journal of Pediatric Hematology/Oncology*, Vol.32, No.5, (July 2010), pp. 376-382, ISSN 1536-3678.

Nagata, K., Nakamura, T., Kitamura, F., Kuramochi, S., Taki, S., Campbell, K. S. & Karasuyama, H. (1997). The Ig alpha/Igbeta heterodimer on mu-negative proB cells is competent for transducing signals to induce early B cell differentiation. *Immunity*, Vol.7, No.4, (October 1997), pp. 559-570, ISSN 1074-7613.

National Wilm's Tumor Study Committee (1991). Wilm's tumor: status report, 1990. *Journal of Clinical Oncology*, Vol.9, No.5, (May 1991), pp. 877-887, ISSN 1527-7755.

Naumberg, E., Bellocco, R., Cnattingius, S., Jonzon, A. & Ekbom, A. (2002). Perinatal exposure to infection and risk of childhood leukemia. *Medical and Pediatric Oncology*, Vol.38, No.6, (June 2002), pp. 391-397, ISSN 0098-1532.

Nguyen, M., Leuridan, E., Zhang, T., De Wit, D., Willems, F., Van Damme, P., Goldman, M. & Goriely, S. (2010). Acquisition of adult-like TLR4 and TLR9 responses during the first year of life. *Plos One*, Vol.5, No.4, (April 2010), pp. e10407, ISSN 1932-6203.

Nordgren, A. (2003). Hidden aberrations diagnosed by interphase fluorescence in situ hybridization and spectral karyotping in childhood acute lymphoblastic leukemia. *Leukemia and Lymphoma*, Vol.44, No.12, (March 2003), pp. 2039-2053, ISSN 1029-2403.

Nully-Brown, P., Hertz, H., Olsen, JH., Yssing, M., Scheibel, E. & Jensen, OM. (1989). Incidence of childhood cancer in Denmark 1943-1984. *International Journal of Epidemiology*, Vol.18, No.3, (September 1989), pp. 546-555, ISSN 1464-3685.

Nyggard, U., Larsen, J., Kristensen, TD., Wesenberg, F., Jonsson, OG., Carlsen, NT., Forestier, E., Kirchhoff, M., Larsen, JK., Schmiegelow, K. & Christensen, IJ. (2006). The sensitivity of G-band karyotyping, flow cytometric DNA index and comparative genomic hybridization in detection of high hiperdiploidy in childhood acute lymphoblastic leukemia. *Journal of Pediatric Hematology/Oncology*, Vol.28, No.3, (March 2006), pp. 134-140, ISSN 1536-3678.

Parkin, D.M., Kramárová, E., Draper, G.J., Masuyer, E., Michaelis, J., Neglia J., Qureshi, S. & Stiller, CA (Eds.). (1998) *International Incidence of Childhood Cancer: Volume 2*, IARC Scientific Publications No. 144). International Agency for Research on Cancer, ISBN 9789283221449 , Lyon France.

Parkin, DM., Stiller, CA., Draper, GJ. & Bieber, CA. (1988). The international incidence of childhood cancer. *International Journal of Cancer*, Vol.42, No.4, (October 1988), pp. 511-520, ISSN 1097-0215.

Pastore, G., Carli, M., Lemerle, J., Tournade, MF., Voute, PA. Rey, A., Burgers, JMV., Zucker, JM., Burger, D., Kraker, JD. & Delemarre, JFM. (1988). Epidemiological features of Wilms' tumor: Results of studies by the International Society of Pediatric Oncology (SIOP). *Medical and Pediatric Oncology*, Vol.16, No.1, (1988), pp. 7-11, ISSN 1096-911X.

Paulsson, K., Mörse, H., Fioretos, T., Behrendtz, M., Strömbeck, B. & Johansson, B. (2005). Evidence for a single-step mechanism in the origin of hyperdiploid childhood acute lymphoblastic leukemia. *Genes Chromosomes and Cancer*, Vol.44, No.2, (October 2005), pp. 113-122, ISSN 1098-2264.

Pelayo, R., Hirose, J., Huang, J., Garrett, KP., Delogu, A., Busslinger, M. & Kincade, PW. (2005b). Derivation of 2 categories of plasmacytoid dendritic cells in murine bone marrow. *Blood*, Vol.105, No.11, (June 2005), pp. 4407-4415, ISSN 0006-4971.

Pelayo, R., Miyazaki, K., Huang, J., Garrett, KP., Osmond, DG. & Kincade, PW. (2006b). Cell cycle quiescence of early lymphoid progenitors in adult bone marrow. *Stem Cells*, Vol.24, No.12, (December 2006), pp. 2703-2713, ISSN 1549-4918.

Pelayo, R., Welner, R., Perry, SS., Huang, J., Baba. Y., Yokota, T. & Kincade, PW. (2005a). Lymphoid progenitors and primary routes to becoming cells of the immune system. *Current Opinion in Immunology*, Vol.17, No.2, (April 2005), pp. 100-107, ISSN 0952-7915.

Pelayo, R., Welner, RS., Nagai, Y. & Kincade, PW. (2006a). Life before the pre-B cell receptor checkpoint: specification and commitment of primitive lymphoid progenitors in adult bone marrow. *Seminars in Immunology*, Vol.18, No.1, (February 2006), pp. 2-11, ISSN 1044-5323.

Pérez-Perdomo, RV. & Rodríguez-Figueroa, L. (2000). Characteristics of cancer patients under age 20 at a population-based registry, Puerto Rico, 1980-1991. *Puerto Rico Health Sciences Journal*, Vol.19, No.2, (June 2000), pp. 123-129, ISSN 0738-0658.

Peris-Bonet, R., Salmerón, D., Martínez-Beneito, MA., Galceran, J., Marcos-Gragera, R., Felipe, S., González, V. & Sánchez de Toledo Codina, J. (2010). Spanish Childhood Cancer Epidemiology Working Group. Childhood cancer incidence and survival in Spain. *Annals of Oncology*, Vol.21, No.Suppl 3, (May 2010), pp. 103-110, ISSN 1569-8041.

Perrillat, F., Clavel, J., Auclerc, MF., Baruchel, A., Leverger, G., Nelken, B., Philippe, N., Schaison, G., Sommelet, D., Vilmer, E. & Hémon, D. (2002). Day-care, early common infections and childhood acute leukaemia: a multicentre French case-control study. *British Journal of Cancer*, Vol.86, No.7, (April 2002), pp. 1064–1069, ISSN 0007-0920.

Petridou, E., Kassimos, D., Kalmanti, M., Kosmidis, H., Haidas, S., Flytzani, V., Tong, D. & Trichopoulos, D. (1993). Age of exposure to infections and risk of childhood leukaemia. *British Medical Journal*, Vol.307, No.6907, (September 1993), pp. 774, ISSN 09598138.

Petridou, ET., Pourtsidis, A., Dessypris, N., Katsiardanis, K., Baka, M., Moschovi, M., Polychronopoulou, S., Koliouskas, D., Sidi, V., Athanasiadou-Piperopoulou, F., Kalmanti, M., Belechri, M., La Vecchia, C., Curado, MP. & Skalkidis, I. (2008). Childhood leukaemias and lymphomas in Greece (1996-2006): a nationwide registration study. *Archives of disease in childhood*, Vol.93, No.12, (December 2008), pp. 1027-1032, ISSN 1468-2044.

Pratt, JA., Velez, R., Brender, JD. & Manton, KG. (1988). Racial differences in acute lymphoblastic leukemia mortality and incidence trends. *Journal of Clinical Epidemiology*, Vol.41, No.4, (August 1988), pp. 367-371, ISSN 0895-4356.

Pui, CH. (1997). Acute lymphoblastic leukemia. *Pediatric Clinics of North America*, Vol.44, No.4, (August 1997), pp. 831-846, ISSN 0031-3955.

Ramot, B. & Magrath, I. (1982). Hypothesis: the environment is a major determinant of the immunological sub-type of lymphoma and acute lymphoblastic leukaemia in children. *British Journal of Haematology*, Vol.50 No.2, (February 1982), pp. 183–189, ISSN 0007-1048.

Rolink, A., Kudo, A., Karasuyama, H., Kikuchi, Y. & Melchers, F. (1991). Long-term proliferating early pre B cell lines and clones with the potential to develop to surface Ig-positive, mitogen reactive B cells in vitro and in vivo. *The EMBO Journal*, Vol.10, No.2, (February 1991), pp. 327-336, ISSN 0261-4189.

Rolink, A. & Melchers, F. (1993). B lymphopoiesis in the mouse. *Advances in Immunology*, Vol.53, (1993), pp. 123-156, ISSN 0065-2776.

Roman, E., Simpson, J., Ansell, P., Kinsey, S., Mitchell, CD., McKinney, PA., Birch, JM., Greaves, M. & Eden, T. (2007). Childhood acute lymphoblastic leukemia and infections in the first year of life: a report from the United Kingdom Childhood Cancer Study. *American Journal of Epidemiology*, Vol.165, No.5, (March 2007), pp. 496–504, ISSN 0002-9262.

Romana, SP., Poiret, H., Leconiat, M., Flexor, MA., Mauchauffé, M., Jonveaux, P., Macintyre, EA., Berger, R. & Bernard OA. (1995). High frequency of t(12:21) in childhood B-lineage acute lymphoblastic leukemia. *Blood*, Vol.86, No.11, (December 1995), pp. 4263-4269, ISSN 1528-0020.

Sanders, BM., Draper, GJ. & Kingston, JE (1988). Retinoblastoma in Great Britain 1969-80: incidence, treatment, and survival. *The British Journal of Ophthalmology*, Vol.72, No.8, (August, 1988), pp. 282-286, ISSN 1468-2079.

Schellong, G. (1985). What's new in pediatric oncology? Epidemiology, treatment principles and prognosis in childhood malignancies. *Pathology, Research and Practice*, Vol.179, No.3, (January 1985), pp. 425-428, ISSN 0344-0338.

Seita, J. & Weissman, I.L. (2010). Hematopoietic stem cell: self-renewal versus differentiation. *Wires Systems Biology and Medicine*, Vol.2, No.6, (November/December 2010), pp. 640-653, ISSN 1939-005X.

Shiramizu, B., Yu, Q., Hu, N., Yanagihara, R. & Nerurkar, VR. (2002). Investigation of TT virus in the etiology of pediatric acute lymphoblastic leukemia. *Pediatric Hematology and Oncology*, Vol.19, No.8, (December 2002), pp. 543-551, ISSN 1077-4114.

Smith, MA., Chen, T. & Simon, R. (1997). Age-specific incidence of acute lymphoblastic leukemia in U.S. children: in utero initiation model. *Journal of the National Cancer Institute*, Vol.89, No.20, (October 1997), pp. 1542-1544, ISSN 1460-2105.

Smith, MA. & Gloecker RL. (2002). Childhood cancer: incidence, survival, and mortality. In: *Principles and practice of pediatric oncology*, Pizzo PA, Poplack DG., pp. 1-12, Lippincott Williams & Wilkins Publishers, ISBN 0-7817-2658-1, Philadelphia.

Smith, M. (1997). Considerations on a possible viral etiology for B-precursor acute lymphoblastic leukemia of childhood. *Journal of Immunotherapy*, Vol.20, No.2, (March 1997), pp. 89-100, ISSN 1053-8550.

Spix, C., Eletr, D., Blettner, M. & Kaatsch, P. (2008). Temporal trends in the incidence rate of childhood cancer in Germany 1987-2004. *International Journal of Cancer*, Vol.122, No.8, (April 2008), pp. 1859-1867, ISSN 1097-0215.

Stack, M., Walsh, PM., Comber, H., Ryan, CA. & O'Lorcain, P. (2007). Childhood cancer in Ireland: a population-based study. *Archives of disease in childhood*, Vol.92, No.10, (October 2010), pp. 890-897, ISSN 1468-2044.

Stiller, CA. (2004). Epidemiology and genetics of childhood cancer. *Oncogene*, Vol.23, No.38, (August 2004), pp. 6429-6444, ISSN 1476-5594.

Suk, WA., Murray, K. & Avakian, MD. (2003). Environmental hazards to children's health in the modern world. *Mutation Research*, Vol.544, No.2-3, (November 2003), pp. 235-242, ISSN 0027-5107.

Teppo, L., Salonen, T. & Hakulinen, T. (1975). Incidence of childhood cancer in Finland. *Journal of the National Cancer Institute*, Vol.55, No.5, (November 1975), pp. 1065-1067, ISSN 1460-2105.

Thomas, L. R., Cobb, R. M. & Oltz, E. M. (2009). Dynamic regulation of antigen receptor gene assembly. *Advances in Experimental Medicine and Biology*. Vol.650, (June 2009),

pp. 103-115, ISSN 0065-2598. U.S. Cancer Statistics Working Group. (2010). *United States Cancer Statistics: 1999–2007 Incidence and Mortality Web-based Report*. Atlanta: U.S. Department of Health and Human Services, Centers for Disease Control and Prevention and National Cancer Institute. Retrieved from < www.cdc.gov/uscs>
von Boehmer, H. & Melcher, F. (2010). Checkpoints in lymphocyte development and autoimmune disease. *Nature Immunology*, Vol.11, No.1, (January 2010), pp. 14-20, ISSN: 1529-2908.

Welner, RS., Pelayo, R. & Kincade, PW. (2008a). Evolving views on the genealogy of B cells. *Nature Reviews Immunology*, Vol.8, No.2, (February 2008), pp. 95-106, ISSN 1474-1733.

Welner, RS., Pelayo, R., Garrett, KP., Chen, X., Perry, SS., Sun, XH., Kee, BL. & Kincade, PW. (2007). Interferon-producing dendritic cells (IKDC) arise via a unique differentiation pathway from primitive c-kit^{hi}CD62L^{+} lymphoid progenitors. *Blood*, Vol.109, No.11, (June 2007), pp. 4825-4831, ISSN 0006-4971.

Welner, RS., Pelayo, R., Nagai, Y., Garrett, KP., Wuest, TR., Carr, DJ., Borghesi, LA., Farrar, MA. & Kincade, PW. (2008b). Lymphoid precursors are directed to produce dendritic cells as a result of TLR9 ligation during Herpes infection. *Blood*, Vol.112, No.9, (November 2008), pp. 3753-3761, ISSN 0006-4971.

Wiemels, JL., Ford, AM., Van Weiring, ER., Postma, A. & Greaves, M. (1999b). Protracted and variable latency of acute lymphoblastic leukemia after TEL-AML1 gene fusion in utero. *Blood*, Vol.94, No. 3, (August 1999), pp. 1057-1062, ISSN 1528-0020.

Wiemels, J., Cazzaniga, G., Daniotti, M., Eden, OB., Addison, GM., Masera, G., Saha, V., Biondi, A. & Greaves, M. (1999a). Prenatal origin of acute lymphoblastic leukaemia in children. *Lancet*, Vol.354, No.9189, (October 1999), pp. 1499-1503, ISSN 0140-6736.

Wiest, D. L., Kearse, K. P., Shores, E. W. & Singer, A. (1994). Developmentally regulated expression of CD3 components independent of clonotypic T cell antigen receptor complexes on immature thymocytes. *Journal of Experimental Medicine*, Vol.180, No.4, (October 1994) pp. 1375-1382, ISSN 0022-100.

Wiest, D. L., Burgess, W. H., McKean, D., Kearse, K. P. & Singer, A. (1995). The molecular chaperone calnexin is expressed on the surface of immature thymocytes in association with clonotype-independent CD3 complexes. *The EMBO Journal*, Vol.14, No.14, (July 1995), pp. 3425-3433, ISSN 0261-4189.

Wilkinson, JD., Fleming, LE., MacKinnon, J., Voti, L., Wohler-Torres, B., Peace, S. & Trapido, E. (2001). Lymphoma and lymphoid leukemia incidence in Florida children: ethnic and racial distribution. *Cancer*, Vol.91, No.7, (April 2001), pp. 1402-1408, ISSN 1097-0142.

William, AO. (1975). Tumors of childhood in Ibadan, Nigeria. *Cancer*, Vol.36, No.2, (August 1975), pp. 370-378, ISSN 1097-0142.

Yagi, T., Hibi, S., Tabata, Y., Kuriyama, K., Teramura, T., Hashida, T., Shimizu, Y., Takimoto, T., Todo, S., Sawada, T. & Imashuku, S. (2000). Detection of clonootypic IGH and TCR rearrangements in the neonatal blood spots of infants and children with the B-cell precursors acute lymphoblastic leukemia. *Blood*, Vol.96, No.1, (July 2000), pp. 264-268, ISSN 1528-0020.

Yaris, N., Mandiracioglu, A. & Büyükpamukcu, M. (2004). Childhood cancer in developing countries. *Journal of Pediatric Hematology/ Oncology*, Vol.21, No.3, (April-May 2004), pp. 237-253, ISSN 1536-3678.

Yasuda, T., Sanjo, H., Pagès, G., Kawano, Y., Karasuyama, H., Pouysségur, J., Ogata, M. & Kurosaki, T. (2008). Erk kinases link pre-B cell receptor signaling to transcriptional events required for early B cell expansion. *Immunity*, Vol.28, No.4, (April 2008), pp. 499-508, ISSN 1074-7613.

Young, Jl., Gloeckler, RL., Silverberg, E., Horm, JW. & Miller R. (1986). Cancer incidence, survival, and mortality for children younger than age 15 years. *Cancer*, Vol.58, No.2Suppl, (July 1986), pp. 598-602, ISSN 1097-0142.

Part 2

NK Cell Leukemia

2

Natural Killer Cell Leukemia: Diagnosis, Pathogenesis and Treatment

Shoko Kobayashi
Kohseichuo Hospital
Japan

1. Introduction

Natural Killer(NK) cell nenoplasm is heterogeneous disease group. In the latest World Health Organization(WHO) classification of tumors of hematopoietic and lymphoid tissue(2008), disease entities considered as NK cell deviation are 1) Aggressive NK cell leukemia (ANKL), 2) NK cell lymphoblastic leukemia/lymphoma, 3) Extranodal NK/T-cell lymphoma, nasal. While several NK related diseases are proposed and investigated actively, optical treatment of NK cell neoplasms remains uncertain. However, several new chemoagents and transplantation are now in progress.

2. Natural killer cell

2.1 Definition

Natural killer(NK) cells are the first lymphoid cells deployed in the defense against tumors and viral infection(Sun, 2010). Their activity is regulated by the interplay between inhibitory receptors, most of which recognize MHC class I molecules on target cells, and activating receptors which bind various ligands. Because NK cells originate from progenitor cells that can give rise to either NK or T cells; NK cells are phenotypically and immunologically similar to T cells. NK cells express T cell-associated markers, including CD2, cytoplasmic CD3(cCD3), CD7 and CD8, subsets of cytotoxic T cells and also express the NK-associated markers, CD16, CD56 and CD57. NK cells do not rearrange the T-cell receptor (TCR) genes. Early in development, NK-cell progenitors express no specific markers. Some markers that might be considered relatively more specific with NK progenitors, such as CD94 or CD161 are no commonly tested.

Important inhibitory receptors are members of the immunoglobulin-like receptor (KIR) family as well as CD94/NKG2 heterodimers. Examples for activating receptors are NKG2D (CD314), DNAM-1 (CD226) and the well-characterized natural cytotoxicity receptors (NCRs), NKp30(CD337), NKp44 (CD336) and NKp46 (CD335). Activating receptors such as NKG2D, recognize ligands that are not usually expressed by healthy cells but rather expressed by infected cells. The inhibitory receptors of NK cells interact with specific MHC class I molecules; for example, CD94/NKG2 binds to HLA-E, and KIR binds to HLA-B. The major constituents of cytotoxic granules are perforin and granzyme B.

2.2 Development

Because NK cells exhibit considerable immunophenotypic similarity to T cells, they are thought to originate from a bipotent NK/T-progenitor cell. Moreover, human CD34(+) hematopoietic progenitors develop into NK cells in vitro in the presence of cytokines, hydrocortisone and stromal cells through the recruitment of myeloid precursors(Grzywacz, 2011). Cells at more advanced stages of myeloid differentiation (those with higher levels of CD13 and macrophage colony-stimulating factor receptor [M-CSFR]) could also differentiate into NK cells in the presence of cytokines (interleukin-7, interleukin-15, stem cell factor, and fms-like tyrosine kinase-3 ligand), stromal cells, and hydrocortisone. NK cells derived from myeloid precursors (CD56(-)CD117(+)M-CSFR(+)) showed more expression of KIR.

3. Natural killer cell neoplasm

3.1 Diagnosis

Accurate diagnosis of NK-cell neoplasm requires analysis of clinical presentation and of cell/tumor morphology, immunophenotype, and genotype(Oshimi, 2007). Expression of at lease one NK cell marker(CD56, CD16, or CD57), lack of expression of surface CD3, B-cell antigen(CD19, ad CD20) and MPO and other lineage markers and/or TCR Ig genes in germline configuraion in tumors are diagnostic factors. During the early stages of NK cell neoplasm, tumor cells do not express any tumor-specific markers or they express markers also found in T cell acute lymphoblastic leukemia (ALL), including CD7, CD2, CD5, and cCD3. Therefore it is difficult to distinguish between T- cell ALL and NK-cell tumors may be difficult. Later-stage but more specific markers, such as CD16, are rarely expressed in NK cell leukemia while some markers, such as CD94 and CD161, that might be considered relatively more specific expressed on NK progenitors. However, even now, it is difficult for us to distinguish NK cell neoplasm from myeloid neoplasms and T-cell neoplasms. It is hoped that wider availability of more specific NK markers including panels of antibodies against KIRs.

3.2 Classification

In the latest World Health Organization(WHO) classification of tumors of hematopoietic and lymphoid tissues(2008), acute leukemia with phenotype of NK cells includes(Swerdlow, 2008); 1) Aggressive NK cell leukemia (ANKL) and 2) NK cell lymphoblastic leukemia/lymphoma. Other NK cell neoplasm and related disease are reported in literature; 1) extranodal NK/T-cell lymphoma, nasal, 2) Myeloid/NK leukemia, and 3) Other CD56-positive neoplasm(Oshimi, 2007).

3.2.1 Aggressive NK cell leukemia (ANKL)

ANKL is a catastrophic disease(Suzuki, 2010; Ham, 2010). ANKL has no gender preference, with the median age of presentation being in the third decade. ANKL is more prevalent among Asians than other ethnic populations. Circulation neoplastic cells varying morphologically form large granular lymphocytes to frank blast, may be present despite treatment. The neoplastic cells are CD2+, surface CD3-, CD3e+, CD56+, and positive for cytotoxic molecules. Immunophenoytpe is identical to that of extranodal type is identical to that of extranodal NK/T-cell lymphoma, except that CD16 is frequently positive. Patients have generally only been unwell for a few weeks, presenting with significant weight loss, jaundice and a high fever. Skin infiltration, lymphoadenopaty and hepatosplenomegaly are common. Severe anemia and throm Survival measured in some weeks. It is unclear whether aggressive NK-cell leukemia represents the leukemic counterpart of extranodal NK/T-cell lymphoma. Strong association with Epstein-Barr virus(EBV) suggests a mechanism of pathogenesis.

3.2.2 NK cell lymphoblastic leukemia/lymphoma

This neoplasm has been very difficult to define, because of considerable confusion in the literature(Swerdlow, 2008). WHO proposed that the diagnosis of precursor NK lymphoblastic leukemia/lymphoma may be considered in a case that expresses CD56 along with immature T cell-associated markers such as CD7, CD2 or even including cCD3, provided the tumor lacks B-cell and myeloid markers, and that theT cell and Ig receptor genes are in the germline configuration. Clinical features associated with these NK neoplasms are not well known. Previously we reported a 69-year-old man with NK cell lymphoblastic leukemia/lymphoma(Kobayashi, 2010). He presented with skin and bone marrow involvement upon initial diagnosis. Neoplastic cells were blastic in appearance with a CD3-, CD4-, CD8-, CD7-, CD16-, CD56+ and HLA-DR+ phenotype. Molecular studies showed germline configuration of both immunoglobulin H and T cell receptor genes, and negative results for Epstein-Barr virus-encoded small RNA (EBER).
Optimal treatment of this disease has not been determined. The presence or absence of P-glycoprotein(P-gp) on tumor cells is one factor that influences the choice of anti-cancer drugs(Egashira, 1999).

3.2.3 Extranodal NK/T-cell lymphoma, nasal

Extranodal NK cell lymphomas(ENKL) are more prevalent in Asia, Mexico, and Central and South America and are characterized by extranodal presentation and an aggressive clinical course(Schmitt, 2011; Yok-Lam, 2011; Suzuki, 2009; Ng, 2011). Two types of ENKL (nasal and extranasal ENKL) were reported. Because they share the same histology, the WHO classification groups both nasal and extranasal ENKL in the same category. However, nasal and extranasal ENKL have different clinical manifestations, treatment approaches and prognosis.
International Peripheral T-cell lymphoma Project showed the clinical characteristics of both NK cell lymphoma among 1153 new adult cases of peripheral/T-cell lymphoma at 22 centers in 13 countries(Au, 2009). 136 cases (11.8%) of extranodal NK/T-cell lymphoma were identified (nasal 68%, extranasal 26%, aggressive/unclassifiable 6%). There were no differences in age, sex, ethnicity, or immunophenotypic profile between the nasal and extranasal cases, but the latter had more adverse clinical features. The median overall survival (OS) was better in nasal compared with the extranasal cases in early- (2.96 vs 0.36 years) and late-stage disease (0.8 vs 0.28 years). Among nasal cases, both the International Prognostic Index and Korean NK/T-cell Prognostic Index were prognostic. In addition, Ki67 proliferation greater than 50%, transformed tumor cells greater than 40%, elevated C-reactive protein level (CRP), anemia (< 11 g/dL) and thrombocytopenia (< 150 x 10(9)/L) predicts poorer OS for nasal disease. No histologic or clinical feature was predictive in extranasal disease.
The strong association of EBV was observed, with type II latency pattern(EBNA-1+, EBNA-2+, LMP1+), and commonly showed a 30-base pair deletion in the latent membrane protein-

1(LMP-1) gene(Swerdlow, 2008). Genome-wide gene expression profiling of extranodal NK/T lymphoma(NKTL) showed genes differentially expressed between NKTL and normal NK cells revealed significant enrichment for cell cycle-related genes and pathways, such as PLK1, CDK1, Aurora-A, activation of Myc and nuclear factor kappa B (NF-κB), and deregulation of p53. A significant percentage of NKTLs (n = 33) overexpressed c-Myc (45.4%), p53 (87.9%), NF-κB p50 (67.7%) and survivin(97%)(Huang, 2010). It is possible to propose a model of NKTL pathogenesis where deregulation of p53 together with activation of Myc and NF-κB, possibly driven by EBV LMP-1, results in the cumulative up-regulation of survivin. Down-regulation of survivin with Terameprocol (EM-1421, a survivin inhibitor) results in reduced cell viability and increased apoptosis in tumour cells, suggesting that survivin may be a potential oncoregulative gene in NKTL. Overexpressed PDGFRA, deregulation of the AKT, JAK-STAT, and nuclear factor-kappaB , RelA and recurrent copy number aberrations (AKT3 [1q44], IL6R [1q21.3], CCL2 [17q12], TNFRSF21 [6p12.3]) was reported (Ng, 2011).
The common cytogenetic abnormality of ENKL is del(6)(q21q25)or i(6)(p10). Integrative analysis also evidenced deregulation of the tumor suppressor HACE1 in the frequently deleted 6q21 region(Zhang, 2007). HACE1 is novel E3 ubiquitin ligase, frequently downregulated in human tumors. Genetic inactivation of HACE1 in mice results in the development of spontaneous, late-onset cancer. A second hit from either environmental triggers or genetic heterozygosity of another tumor suppressor, p53, markedly increased tumor incidence in a Hace1-deficient background. Re-expression of HACE1 in human tumor cells directly abrogates in vitro and in vivo tumor growth, whereas downregulation of HACE1 via siRNA allows non-tumorigenic human cells to form tumors in vivo. Mechanistically, the tumor-suppressor function of HACE1 is dependent on its E3 ligase activity and HACE1 controls adhesion-dependent growth and cell cycle progression during cell stress through degradation of cyclin D1.

3.2.4 Myeloid/NK leukemia

The entity of myeloid/NK-cell acute leukemia may be of precursor NK origin, however myeloid/NK-cell acute leukemia cannot be distinguished form acute myeloid leukemia with minimal differentiation(Tang, 2008). Reportedly, myeloid/NK cell precursor acute leukemia (MNKPL) give rise to blasts that are cytochemically myeloperoxidase negative (MPO(-)) and phenotypically CD56(+)CD3(-)CD7(+)CD34(+) and have myeloid antigens(Guan, 2011). In contrast, myeloid/NK cell acute leukemia (MNKL) give rise to blasts that are cytochemically MPO(dim) and phenotypically CD56(+), CD16(-), CD3(-), CD)33(+)HLA-DR(-). Several cases of childhood NK leukemia, four MNKPL and one MNKL, were reported in China. The extramedullary involvement that usually occurs in cases of adult MNKPL was not observed in these cases of childhood MNKPL. Those with MNKPL were treated using a protocol designed for childhood high-risk ALL containing cytarabine, mitoxantrone, etoposide, l-asparaginase, and methotrexate depending on the myeloid and lymphoid characteristics of the MNKPL. They responded slowly to chemotherapy and were in complete remission (CR), except one who died from pneumonia while in CR. Therefore, protocols that combine agents used against acute myeloid leukemia with agents used against ALL are apparently effective against childhood MNKPL.
A 6-year-old Japanese child was reported to be myeloid/NK cell precursor acute leukemia (MNKL)(Shiba 2010). The patient was treated by cord blood transplantation from an HLA 1-

locus mismatched unrelated donor after chemotherapy comprising cytosine arabinoside, idarubicin, etoposide, and L-asparaginase. The nonsense mutation, C7412A, resulting in S2471X, where X is a terminal codon, in the PEST domain of NOTCH1 were observed, suggesting a possible role in the leukemogenesis of MNKL.

In addition, CD7+ and CD56+ myeloid/natural killer cell precursor acute leukemia was proposed(Suzuki, 1997; Suzuki, 2005, Piichowska, 2007). Striking extramedullary involvement was evident at initial presentation, with peripheral lymphadenopathy and/or mediastinal masses. Expression of CD7, CD33, CD34, CD56, and frequently HLA-DR, but not NK, T-cell, and B-cell markers was observed. Myeloperoxidase was negative. Almost all presented germline configurations of the TCR β and γ chain genes and Ig heavy chain gene. Despite intensive chemotherapy, including allogeneic bone marrow transplantation, most persued fatal courses within 41 months. Forty-nine patients with CD7(+) CD56(+) acute myeloid leukemia were analyzed(Suzuki, 1997). There were 17 patients with a classification of M0, which corresponded to MNKPL, and 32 patients with an AML classification other than M0 (i.e., M1-M7; 9 each for M1 and M2, 1 for M3, 3 for M4, 4 for M5, and 6 for M7). The age distribution was similar in both groups, but the MNKPL group, i.e., CD7(+) CD56(+) M0, had significantly more males than the CD7(+) CD56(+) M1-M7 group. The disease localization and the hematological manifestations were different between the groups; specifically, the patients with MNKPL presented with lower white blood cell counts and fewer circulating leukemic blasts, less anemia, less thrombocytopenia, and more frequent extramedullary involvement. The prognosis was poor in both groups. These findings suggest that extramedullary involvement of myeloid/NK cell precursor acute leukemia is not directly derived from the presence of CD7 and CD56 antigens on leukemic cells. The poor prognosis of CD7(+) CD56(+) M1-M7 suggests that this phenotype may act as a prognostic factor for AML, but this assertion should be confirmed in further clarification.

3.2.5 Other CD56 positive neoplasm

CD56 has been recognized as a sensitive marker for NK cells and has become popular for identifying NK cell neoplasms. Approximately 200 CD56+ hematopoietic neoplasms with immature features have been reported in the literature under different names. It is difficult to determine whether these tumors are of a truly derived from NK cells. For example, tumors that were previously defined as "blastic NK lymphoma" are now classified into two entities: 1) blastic plasmacytoid dendritic cell neoplasm; and 2) NK cell lymphoblastic leukemia/lymphoma(Pilichowska, 2007). The identification of the cell type, blastic plasmacytoid dendritic cell led to the definition of a new disease entity of blastic plasmacytoid dendritic cell neoplasm.

Recently a new disease category, NK-cell enteropathy, was proposed based eight patients with atypical NK-cell lymphoproliferative lesions that mimicked NK- or T-cell lymphoma(Mansoor, 2011). These patients presented with vague gastrointestinal symptoms and with lesions involving stomach, duodenum, small intestine, and colon. Biopsies revealed a mucosal infiltrate of atypical cells with an NK-cell phenotype (CD56(+)/TIA-1(+)/Granzyme B(+)/cCD3(+)).EBER was negative, and TCR-γ gene rearrangement showed no evidence of a clonal process. Some patients received aggressive chemotherapy followed by auto HSCT. Five patients were followed without treatment. However, no patient developed progressive disease or died of lymphoma.

While a distinct disease entity, "lymphomatoid gastropahty (LyGa)", was proposed based on the analysis of 10 other patients with unrecognized self-limited NK-cell proliferation in the stomach(Takeuchi, 2010). Endoscopy showed elevated lesion(s). The cells were $CD2^{+/-}$, $sCD3^-$, $cCD3^+$, $CD4^-$, $CD5^-$, $CD7^+$, $CD8^-$, $CD16^-$, $CD20^-$, $CD45^+$, $CD56^+$, $CD117^-$, $CD158a^-$, $CD161^-$, T cell-restricted intracellular antigen-1^+, granzyme B^+, $perforin^+$, Epstein-Barr early RNA^-, T-CR $\alpha\beta^-$, and TCR $\gamma\delta^-$. Most lesions underwent self-regression. Three cases relapsed, but none of the patients died. LyGa is proposed as a pseudomalignant process because of its clinical characteristics.

4. Pathogenesis

4.1 EBV

NK cell neoplasms are strongly related with latent EBV infection.

EBV is a ubiquitous human gamma-herpesvirus that preferentially establishes latent infection in viral infected B-lymphocytes(Pizzigallo, 2010). The structure of EBV shows a linear double-stranded DNA, an capside, 162 capsomers and an envelope. The EBV genome encodes nearly 100 viral proteins. During viral replication, these proteins play a fundamental role in regulating the expression of viral genes, replicating viral DNA, forming structural components of the virion, modulating the host immune response, and forcing these cells immortal. The receptor for the virus on epithelial cells and B lymphocytes is the CD21 molecule, which is also the receptor for the C3d component of complement. The major histocompatibility complex (MHC) class II molecule serves as cofactor for the infection of B cells.

Cellular infection from EBV could have two possible outcomes. A lytic infection occurs wherein virions are produced and the host cell is lysed. Lytic infection typically occurs in epithelial cells and partly in plasma cells. EBV may induce a latent infection by generating an episome, the circular EBV genome, that is located in the nucleus of host lymphocytes.

The response of CD8-positive (CD8+) cytotoxic T-cells is crucial to control the primary infection, and these cells show a predominant role in infectious mononucleosis(IM), being present in the circulation and tissues in very high numbers. These cells probably give rise to most of the symptoms and signs of IM as a result of massive production of cytokines, including lymphotoxin, tumor necrosis factor-α, interleukin (IL)-1β and IL-6. That CD8+ T cells are essential for recovery from IM is exemplified by the consequence of primary EBV infection.

The latent viral infections in which the virus persists in a form unable to be identified through standard methods. The mechanisms of EBV latency have been carefully examined both because they represent the virus strategy to elude the response of the immune system of the host, and because they are correlated with those oncologic conditions associated to the viral persistence, particularly lymphoma and lymphoproliferative disorders. During latency, resting memory B cells represent the site of persistence of EBV within the body. In normal adults, from 1 to 50 B cells per million in the circulation are infected with EBV, and the number of latently infected cells remains stable over years.

There are different programs of EBV latency that are probably associated with different viral strategies aimed at surviving host immunological responses, and some of these programs have been correlated with malignancies typically associated with viral persistence. Four latency programs was proposed(Table I, II). In the first form, only EBNA-1 and EBER are expressed, whereas in the second form EBNA-1, LMP-1, LMP-2, and EBER are expressed. In the third pattern, all the latency genes are expressed. A fourth pattern of latency is seen in B cells obtained from the peripheral blood of healthy persons infected with EBV in the past, in which only EBER and LMP-2, and in some studies, EBNA-1 RNA have been detected. Burkitt's lymphoma is characterized by the type 1 of the latency program, the nasopharyngeal carcinoma, Hodgkin's lymphoma and peripheral T cell lymphoma by the type 2. The type 3 of the latency program should characterize other lymphoproliferative diseases induced by EBV in immunocompromised hosts as well as the IM. These mechanisms are involved virological factors associated with EBV antigenic characteristics, host factors with particular regard to the genetic and immune systems and environmental co-factors. Of the nearly 100 viral genes that are expressed during replication, only 10 are expressed in latently infected B cells in vitro: two types of nontranslated RNA, six nuclear protein and two membrane proteins. Among several viral proteins, EBNA1 and LMP1 are important in tumorigenesis.

4.1.1 EBV nuclear antigen 1 (EBNA-1)

EBV latent infection, and its associated oncogenic potential, is dependent on genome maintenance functions of EBV nuclear antigen 1 (EBNA-1), one of six EBNAs expressed from a common promoter(Wp and then Cp) upon infection of naive B cells. EBNA1 initiates latent viral replication in B cells maintains the viral genome copy number, and regulates transcription of to the EBV-encoded latent genes. These activity are mediated through the ability of EBNA1 to bind viral-DNA.

Resistance to apoptosis is an important in tumorigenic process. EBNA1 forms a complex with Sp1 or Sp1-like proteins bound to their cis-element at the survivin promoter. This interaction enhances the activity of the complex and up-regulates survivin. Knockdown of survivin and EBNA1 showed enhanced apoptosis in EBV -infected cells and thus supports a role for EBNA1 in suppressing apoptosis in EBV-infected cells(Ian, 2008).

Cell proliferation was inhibited in an EBV-positive ENKL cell line by RNA interference (RNAi)-mediated silencing of EBNA1. Silencing of EBNA1 expression by RNAi inhibited cell growth, increased the expression of the p27 protein, and caused cell cycle arrest in G(1).

Gene	Protein	Function
BKRF1	EBNA-1	viral genome maintenance transcription of EBV latent genes B cell immortalization
BKRF1	EBNA-2	B cell immortalization
BLF-BERF	EBNA-3	B cell immortalization
BNLF1	LMP-1	oncoprotein
BNLF2	LMP-2	prevents cell lytic-cycle entry
BCRF1	EBER1,2	regulates PKC activity
BARF0	Bam HIA transcripts	not known

Table 1. EBV latent viral genes

4.1.2 Latent membrane protein-1(LMP-1)

EBV encodes a viral oncogene, LMP1 (latent membrane protein-1). LMP1 is expressed in EBV-associated lymphoma and is essential for B-cell transformation and for disruption of cellular signal transduction(Dellis, 2009). LMP1 acts by constitutive activating multiple signaling pathway, including the NK-kB pathway. In extranodal NK/T-cell lymphoma, nasal type, deletion of 30 bp in the LMP-1 gene are reported, but the molecular and pathogenic significance of these deletions is not clear.

	EBNA-1	EBNA-2	EBNA-3	LMP-1	LMP-2	EBER	Disease
Type 1	+	-	-	-	-	+	Burkitt's lymphoma
Type 2	+	-	-	+	+	+	Nasopharyngea carcinoma Hodgkin's disease
Type 3	+	+	+	+	+	+	Lymphoproliferative disease Infectious mononucleosis
others	+	-	-	-	+	+	Healthy carieer

Table 2. Expression of EBV latent genes in disease

4.2 Cytogenetics

Several cytogenetic abnormalities have been reported in ENKL cases(Schmitt, 2011).
Reported abnormal chromosomal gains are 1q21–q44, 2q13-q14, 2q31.1–q32.2, 6p25–p11.1, 7q11.2–q34, 7q35-q36, 17q21.1, 20pter-qter、 while abnormal chromosomal losses are 6q16–q25, 11q23.1, 11q24-q25, 13q14.11, 17p13.3
The genes for responsible for above abnormalities have been investigated and are speculated to be EBV LMP2-TR; survival/apoptosis related: CCND3, SERPINB9, FASL, or TNFAIP3; angiogenesis related: HGFR (MET), VEGFR2, VEGFA, or HIF1α; cell signaling pathway related: JAK-STAT, AKT, NOTCH, WNT, or PDGF; tumor-suppressor gene related: del6q21(PRDM1, ATG5, AIM1, or HACE1); and other pathways/genes: TP53, TP73, or AURKA.

5. Staging

A standard staging system for NK-T-cell lymphomas is lacking. Moreover, the Ann-Arbor staging system is probably unsatisfactory for NK/T-cell lymphomas.
Involvement of bone marrow(BM) is an important staging and prognostic factor(Huang, 2005). A study was done to evaluate the use of EBER -1 in situ hybridization (EBER-1 ISH) to detect occult micrometastasis in the bone marrow (BM) of patients with nasal NK/T-cell lymphoma. Conventional morphologic examinations failed to identify any lymphoma involvement in the BM specimens obtained at initial staging. However, some BM specimens were positive for EBER-1. A lower survival rate was seen in patients with BM positive for EBER-1-positive BM specimens, and only the BM EBER-1 ISH result was shown to be an independent variable predicting overall survival in stage I / II patients, suggesting that EBER-1 positivity in BM is the major determinant of a poor prognosis. These findings indicate that EBER-1-positive BM specimens are an important indicator of a poor prognosis, and based on this study, BM EBER-1 ISH evaluation is recommended for accurate staging.

6. Prognosis; Prognostic factors

To improve the stratification of patients for treatment, some prognostic models have been applied to NK-cell neoplasms.

The International Prognostic Index(IPI), taking into account the stage, age, performance status, number of extranodal sites and the LDH level, is evidently useful for assess the prognosis of patients with NK-cell lymphoma(Lee, 2006).

Clinical features and prognosis of 22 with ANKL and 150 with ENKL patients was reviewed(Suzuki, 2010). The ENKLs consisted of 123 nasal and 27 extranasal (16 cutaneous, 9 hepatosplenic, 1 intestinal and 1 nodal) lymphomas. Multivariate analysis showed that four factors (non-nasal type, stage, performance status and numbers of extranodal involvement) were significant prognostic factors. Using these four variables, an NK prognostic index was successfully constructed. Four-year overall survival of patients with zero, one, two and three or four adverse factors were 55%, 33%, 15% and 6%, respectively.

Korean prognostic index (K-IPI) was analyzed as a prognostic model specifically for ENKL(Lee, 2006). Prognostic factors for survival were "B" symptoms, stage, LDH level, and regional lymph nodes. K-IPI identified four different risk groups: group 1, no adverse factor; group 2, one factor; group 3, two factors; and group 4, three or four factors. The K-IPI showed a superior prognostic discrimination when compared with the IPI. Notably, when the K-IPI system was used, 7% of patients were in group 1; 31% were in group 2; 20% were in group 3, and 22% were in group 4; in contrast, 81% of patients were categorized as low or low-intermediate risks using IPI.

In nasal NK/T-cell lymphoma, measurement of circulating plasma EBV DNA is reportedly useful for evaluating the prognosis of patients(Hsieh, 2007).

7. Treatment

1 Chemotherapy
   a) L-asparaginase
   b) Methotrexate
   c) combination regimen SMILE
2 Hematopoietic stem cell transplantation(HSCT)
3 New therapeutic strategies
   a) Bortezomib
   b) Pegasparaginase
   c) Kinase inhibitor
   d) Antibody treatment
4 Radiation

Table 3. Treatment of NK neoplasm

7.1 Chemotherapy

7.1.1 L-asparaginase containing regimen

The poor treatment results of conventional chemotherapy reatments for NK cell neoplasm are often attributed to the high expression level of the drug-exporting protein P-glycoprotein, which results in the multidrug-resistance(MDR) phenotype(Jaccard, 2009). L-asparaginase(L-asp), an enzyme that hydrolyzes serum L-asp, induces asparagine starvation of tumors with low expression of asparagine synthetase. This results in rapid inhibition of protein synthesis and delayed inhibition of DNA and RNA synthesis in lymphocytes.

Thirty-three Chinese patients with midline NK/T-cell lymphoma nasal-type were received L-asp based salvage regimen for 2 approximately 6 cycles (median 3 cycles) plus locoregional radiation. Seventeen of the 33 CHOP failures (51.5 %) (L-asp group) reached CR(Yong, 2006). The 5-year overall survival (OS) rates were 55.9% for L-asp group. On univariate analysis, disease stage, fever symptom and performance status were significant factors influencing overall survival. On multivariate analysis, only disease stage and fever symptom remained as independently significant factors influencing OS.

The multicentric French retrospective study of 15 patients with relapsed, refractory, or disseminated disease, treated with L-asp - containing regimens(Jaccard, 2009). All but two of the patients had an objective response to L-asp-based treatment. Seven patients reached complete remission and only two relapsed. These data confirm the excellent activity of L-asp-containing regimens in refractory extranodal NK/T-cell lymphoma and also aggressive NK-cell leukemia. The results indicated that L-asp based regimen might be a promising new salvage or even first-line chemotherapeutic regimen for NK-cell neoplasms..

7.1.2 Methotrexate (MTX)

To overcome the drug resistance of P-glycoprotein, multiple clinical trials were conducted. We report a case of a 69-year-old man with NK cell lymphoblastic leukemia /lymphoma who was treated mainly with methotrexate (MTX) (Kobayashi, 2010). He presented with skin and bone marrow involvement at onset. Neoplastic cells were blastic in appearance with a CD3-, CD4-, CD8-, CD7-, CD16-, CD56+ and HLA-DR+ phenotype. Molecular studies showed germline configuration of both immunoglobulin JH and T cell receptor genes and negative results for EBER. He was treated with standard ALL-targeting induction therapy, followed by one cycle of high-dose MTX(HD-MTX) as consolidation therapy. However, the disease recurred during the standard ALL maintenance therapy. Three cycles of HD-MTX were effective in achieving a second complete remission and he then received low dose MTX as maintenance therapy. The disease remained well-controlled for 4 years. MTX is one component of SMILE (methotrexate, ifosfamide, dexamethasone, etoposide, L-asparaginase) therapy. This encouraging result warrants further investigation of MTX either as a single agent or in a combination regimen as a first-line treatment for patients with NK cell malignancies.

7.1.3 Combination chemotherapy: SMILE

Japanese investigators treated advanced extranodal NK lymphoma with SMILE (Methotrexate, Ifosfamide, Dexamethasone, Etoposide, L-asparaginase) therapy(Yamaguchi, 2008). For newly diagnosed stage IV or relapsed/refractory ENKL, the overall response rate was 74% and the CR rate was 40%.

Another study with patients had newly diagnosed stage IV, relapsed or refractory diseases after first-line chemotherapy, were 15-69 years of age, and had satisfactory performance scores (0-2) (Jaccard, 2011). For the six enrolled patients, the overall response rate was 67% and the complete response rate was 50%. Its safety and efficacy require further evaluation.

To explore an effective salvage regimen, phase I pilot study of combination chemotherapy with methotrexate, ifosfamide, l-asparaginase and dexamethasone (MILD), which are unaffected by MDR1-encoded P-glycoprotein, was tested in 18 patients(Tsukune, 2010). Among them, eleven had T/NK-cell malignancies, six had B-cell malignancies, and one had a blastic plasmacytoid dendritic cell neoplasm. Of the 14 patients evaluated, three achieved CR, and four showed a partial response(PR). The overall response rate was 57%. All seven responders had T/NK-cell malignancies. MILD therapy was feasible and presented acceptable toxicity in patients with refractory or lethal lymphoid malignancies.

7.2 Hematopoietic Stem Cell Transplantation (HSCT)

Because of the poor prognosis, many groups have favored the use of early transplantation of NK-cel neoplasms (Murashige. 2005:Suzuki, 2006; Ennishi, 2011; Ichikawa, 2010).

Autologous HSCT has been evaluated in stage I/II disease in first or second CR, or chemosensitive relapse, and primary or secondary refractory disease without marrow involvement. The disease status pre-HSCT significantly affected overall survival. For most patients with stage I/II disease, the definite advantage of auto HSCT in first CR is questionable. However, based on a retrospective analysis, auto HSCT may be beneficial in a subgroup of patients in CR1 who have a high risk of relapse. HSCT is generally indicated in lymphoma patients achieving second CR, however further controlled trials are required to examine whether this also applies to NK/T-cell lymphoma. There is no survival advantage of auto HSCT in patients with advanced or refractory disease. Allogeneic HSCT, with the potential benefit of graft-versus-lymphoma (GVL) effect, is an option for patients with advanced disease. The GVL effect is further enhanced by the expression of EBV antigen on tumor cells. Small series have shown that it is a potentially curative option.

The retrospective analysis studied the potential survival benefits of HSCT for ENKL compared with a historical control group. Forty-seven patients from 3 previously published series of HSCT were matched according to NK/T cell lymphoma International Prognostic Index (NK-IPI) risk groups and disease status at transplantation. After a median follow-up of 116.5 months, the median survival time was not determined for the HSCT group, but it was 43.5 months for the control group. In patients who were in CR at the time of HSCT or at surveillance after remission, disease-specific survival rates were significantly higher in the HSCT group compared with the control group (disease-specific 5-year survival rate, 87.3% for HSCT vs 67.8% for non-HSCT). In contrast, in subgroup analysis on non-CR patients at the time of HSCT or non-HSCT treatment, disease-specific survival rates were not significantly prolonged in the HSCT group compared with the control group (1-year survival rate, 66.7% for HSCT vs 28.6% for non-HSCT). The impact of HSCT on the survival of all patients was significantly retained at the multivariate level with a 2.1-fold reduced risk of death. HSCT seems to confer a survival benefit in patients who attained CR on postremission consolidation therapy. These findings suggest that patients in CR with high NKIPI risk scores at diagnosis should receive full consideration for HSCT.

Among NK neoplasm, ANKL is a highly aggressive lymphoproliferative disease. a few case reports have suggested that allo-HSCT can be curative. For example, a report of a young

woman with ANKL showing central nervous system invasion, who has been in complete remission for more than a year after allo-HSCT following two courses of intravenous chemotherapy and several rounds of intrathecal chemotherapy(Ichikawa, 2010).
However, most of the reported cases have been performed from HLA-identical sibling donors, and data on alternative HSCT sources including matched unrelated donor and umbilical cord blood are very limited.

7.3 Radiation

For localized diseases, radiation therapy is reportedly effective. For example, the addition of radiotherapy for early-stage nasal NK cell lymphoma cases yielded survival benefit (P = .045)(Suzuki. 2010).

7.4 New therapeutic strategies

7.4.1 Bortezomib

Basic studies showed that LMP1 activates nuclear factor-κB (NF-κB) and that NF-κB is activated in extranodal natural killer (NK)/T-cell lymphoma, nasal type(Shen, 2008). Bortezomib is known to be effective for diseases involving NF-κB activation, such as multiple myeloma. Recently, bortezomib was reported to induce apoptosis of EBV-transformed B cells.
Twenty three patients with previously untreated NK/T-cell lymphoma initially treated with cyclophosphamide, vincristine, doxorubicin and prednisone (CHOP) or CHOP-based chemotherapy were examined by immunohistochemistry for three NF-κB subunits(p65, p50 and p52), which are involved in either the canonical or alternative pathway. NF-κB activation through the alternative pathway is frequently observed in NK/T-cell lymphoma and associated with chemoresistance and poor survival. In vitro, bortezomib treatment decreased the viability of NK cell lines. The decreased viability in response to bortezomib treatment was abrogated by a pan-caspase inhibitor. Additionally, cleavage of caspases and polyadenosine diphosphate -ribose polymerase, increased expression of phosphorylated IκB, and decreased expression of inhibitor of apoptotic proteins were detected by immunoblotting in bortezomib-treated cell lines. Administration of bortezomib to peripheral blood mononuclear cells from two patients with EBV-associated lymphoproliferative diseases show a greater killing effect on EBV-infected cells. These results indicate that bortezomib killed T or NK lymphoma cells by inducing apoptosis.
A Phase I study of Bortezomib + CHOP treatment were conducted with 13 patients with advanced, aggressive T-cell or NK/T-cell lymphoma(Lee, 2008). The overall CR rate in all patients was 61.5% and showed no severe side effects. Bortezomib can be safely combined with CHOP chemotherapy and constitutes an active regimen.

7.4.2 Pegaspargase

Pegaspargase selected the pegylated form to achieve more prolonged continuous asparagine depletion as well as for ease of administration as it requires only a single treatment every 2–3 weeks(Reyes, 2008). Pegaspargase were reported an effective treatment for two patients with aggressive, extended, and refractory to CHOP chemotherapy. Pegaspargase is worth considering development of combination regimens and possibly front-line regimens.

7.4.3 Kinase inhibitor

The EBV oncoprotein LMP1 reportedly activates the phosphatidylinositol-3 kinase (PI3K)/Akt pathway to induce cell survival(Jeon, 2007). The intrinsic level of pAkt was higher in EBV-positive NK cells than in EBV-negative NK cells. Geldanamycin (GA) and its derivative, 17-allylamino-17- demethoxygeldanamycin (17-AAG), are PI3K and Akt inhibitors that exhibit anti-tumor activity by degrading HSP90 client proteins, including Akt. The administration of GA and 17-AAG resulted in apoptosis of NK cells, accompanied by Akt and pAkt down-regulation, caspase 3 activation, and mitochondrial membrane potential disruption. Apoptosis of NK cells was also induced by LY294002 (a PI3K inhibitor) or Akt inhibitor II. More results both in vitro and in vivo are necessary to determine the efficacy of kinase inhibitors for treating NK neoplasms.

7.4.4 Antibody treatment

The immunoconjugate I MGN901 (huN901-DM1; ImmunoGen, Cambridge, MA,USA) is composed of the composed of the humanized monoclonal IgG1 antibody, huN901, and the maytansinoid drug, DM1, which binds CD56 with high affinity(Ishitsuka, 2009). IMGN901 is a tumour-activated prodrug because the conjugation of DM1 to huN901 renders the cytotoxic drug inactive until it reaches the target site. The conjugate is then internalized and releases DM1, which inhibits tubulin polymerization and causes cell death. IMGN901 has been demonstrated to be safe and show promising efficacy in small cell lung cancer, CD56-positive small cell carcinoma and multiple myeloma in phase I/II clinical studies. An in vitro study demonstrated that IMGN901 was cytotoxic for a CD56-positive NK cell line and fresh tumour cells derived from a patient with an NK-cell malignancy in vitro. These results indicate that IMGN901 represents a promising novel and targeted approach to improve patient outcomes for patients with NK cell malignancies. The activity of IMGN901 should be further validated in clinical trials.

8. Conclusion

The classification of NK cell neoplasms with overlapping features will remain controversial, particularly when EBV is absent. In order to establish more definitive and widely accepted diagnostic criteria for NK-cell neoplasms, more accurate diagnostic tools are needed. For proper treatment stratification of NK cell neoplasms, randomized clinical trials are waited, although conducting meaningful clinical trials is difficult because NK-cell neoplasms are rare.

9. References

Au WY, Weisenburger DD, Intragumtornchai T, et al.; International Peripheral T-Cell Lymphoma Project.(2009) Clinical differences between nasal and extranasal natural killer/T-cell lymphoma: a study of 136 cases from the International Peripheral T-Cell Lymphoma Project. *Blood.* Vol 113. No 17. pp.3931-7.

Dellis O, Arbabian A, Brouland JP, et al.(2009) Modulation of B-cell endoplasmic reticulum calcium homeostasis by Epstein-Barr virus latent membrane protein-1. *Mol Cancer.* Vol.8, pp.59-73.

Egashira M, Kawamata N, Sugimoto K, et al.(1993) P-glycoprotein expression on normal and abnormally expanded natural killer cells and inhibition of P-glycoprotein function by cyclosporin A and its analogue, PSC833. *Blood.* Vol. 93. No. 5. pp.599-606

Ennishi D, Maeda Y, Fujii N, et a;.(2011) Allogeneic hematopoietic stem cell transplantation for advanced extranodal natural killer/T-cell lymphoma, nasal type. *Leuk Lymphoma.* 2011 May 23. [Epub ahead of print]

Guan XQ, Xu L, Ke ZY, et.al(2011) Five Chinese pediatric patients with leukemias possibly arising from immature natural killer cells: clinical features and courses. *Pediatr Hematol Oncol. Vol* 28. No.3. pp187-93.

Grzywacz B, (2011) Natural killer-cell differentiation by myeloid progenitors. *Blood.* Vol.117, No.13, pp. 3548-58.

Ham MF,& Ko YH.(2010) Natural killer cell neoplasm: biology and pathology. *Int J Hematol.* Vol.92, No.5. pp.681-9.

Hsieh PP, Tung CL, Chan AB, et al.(2007) EBV viral load in tumor tissue is an important prognostic indicator for nasal NK/T-cell lymphoma. *Am J Clin Pathol. Vol* 128. No.4. pp.579-84.

Huang WT, Chang KC, Huang GC, et al.(2005) Bone marrow that is positive for Epstein-Barr virus encoded RNA-1 by in situ hybridization is related with a poor prognosis in patients with extranodal natural killer/T-cell lymphoma, nasal type. *Haematologica.* Vol. 90.No. 8. pp.1063-9.

Huang Y, de Reyniès A, de Leval L, et al.(2010) Gene expression profiling identifies emerging oncogenic pathways operating in extranodal NK/T-cell lymphoma, nasal type. *Blood.* Vol 115. No.6. pp1226-37.

Ian MX, Lan SZ, Cheng ZF, et.al(2008) Suppression of EBNA1 expression inhibits growth of EBV-positive NK/T cell lymphoma cells. *Cancer Biol Ther. Vol* 7. No.10. pp1602-6.

Ichikawa S, Fukuhara N, Yamamoto J, , et al.(2010) Successful allogeneic hematopoietic stem cell transplantation for aggressive NK cell leukemia. *Intern Med.* Vol 49, No.17. pp.1907-10.

Ishitsuka K, Jimi S, Goldmacher VS, et al.(2009) Targeting CD56 by the maytansinoid immunoconjugate IMGN901 (huN901-DM1): a potential therapeutic modality implication against natural killer/T cell malignancy. *Blood.* Vol 114. No.15. pp.3265-75.

Jaccard A, Petit B, Girault S, et al.(2009) L-asparaginase-based treatment of 15 western patients with extranodal NK/T-cell lymphoma and leukemia and a review of the literature. *Ann Oncol. Vol* 20. No.1, pp.110-6.

Jaccard A, Gachard N, Marin B, et al; GELA and GOELAMS Intergroup.(2011) Efficacy of L-asparaginase with methotrexate and dexamethasone (AspaMetDex regimen) in patients with refractory or relapsing extranodal NK/T-cell lymphoma, a phase 2 study.*Blood. Vol* 117. No.6. pp.1834-9.

Jeon YK, Park CH, Kim KY, et al.(2007) The heat-shock protein 90 inhibitor, geldanamycin, induces apoptotic cell death in Epstein-Barr virus-positive NK/T-cell lymphoma by Akt down-regulation.*J Pathol.* Vol 213, No.2, pp.170-9.

Kobayashi S, Teramura M, Arai M, et al.(2010) Successful salvage treatment of blastic natural killer cell lymphoma with methotrexate. *Int J Hematol.* Vol.92, No.4, pp.634-7.

Lee J, Suh C, Park YH, , et al.(2006) Extranodal natural killer T-cell lymphoma, nasal-type: a prognostic model from a retrospective multicenter study. *J Clin Oncol.* Vol. 24, No.4. pp.612-8.

Lee J, Suh C, Kang HJ, et al.(2008) Phase I study of proteasome inhibitor bortezomib plus CHOP in patients with advanced, aggressive T-cell or NK/T-cell lymphoma. *Ann Oncol. Vol* 19. No.12, pp.2079-83.

Mansoor A, Pittaluga S, Beck PL, et.al(2011) NK-cell enteropathy: a benign NK-cell lymphoproliferative disease mimicking intestinal lymphoma: clinicopathologic features and follow-up in a unique case series. *Blood.* Vol.117. No.5. pp1447-52.

Murashige N, Kami M, Kishi Y, et al.(2005) Allogeneic haematopoietic stem cell transplantation as a promising treatment for natural killer-cell neoplasms. *Br J Haematol.* Vol.130, No.4. pp.561-7.

Ng SB, Selvarajan V, Huang G, Zhou J, Feldman AL, Law M, et al.(2011) Activated oncogenic pathways and therapeutic targets in extranodal nasal-type NK/T cell lymphoma revealed by gene expression profiling.*J Pathol. Vol* 223. No.4. pp.496-510.

Oshimi K, Kawa K, Nakamura S, et al; NK-cell Tumor Study Group.(2005) NK-cell neoplasms in Japan.*Hematology.* Vol.10, No.3, pp.237-45.

Oshimi K.(2007) Progress in understanding and managing natural killer-cell malignancies. *Br J Haematol.* Vol.139, No.4, pp.532-44.

Pilichowska ME, Fleming MD, Pinkus JL, et.al.(2007) CD4+/CD56+ hematodermic neoplasm ("blastic natural killer cell lymphoma"): neoplastic cells express the immature dendritic cell marker BDCA-2 and produce interferon. *Am J Clin Pathol.* Vol 128, No.3. pp445-53.

Pizzigallo E, Racciatti D, and Gorgoretti V(2010) EBV Chronic Infections *Mediterr J Hematol Infect Dis.* Vol.2. No.1:e2010022.

Reyes VE Jr, Al-Saleem T, Robu VG, et al.(2008) Extranodal NK/T-cell lymphoma nasal type: efficacy of pegaspargase. Report of two patients from the United Sates and review of literature. *Br J Haematol.* Vol.141, No.1. pp.129-31.

Schmitt C, Sako N, Bagot M et.al.(2011) Extranodal NK/T-Cell Lymphoma: Toward the Identification of Clinical Molecular Targets. *J Biomed Biotechnol.* :790871.

Shen L, Au WY, Wong KY, et al.(2008) Cell death by bortezomib-induced mitotic catastrophe in natural killer lymphoma cells. *Mol Cancer Ther.* Vol 7. No.12. pp.3807-15.

Shiba N, Kanazawa T, Park MJ, et al.(2010) NOTCH1 mutation in a female with myeloid/NK cell precursor acute leukemia. *Pediatr Blood Cancer.* Vol 55. No.7. pp1406-9.

Sun, JC.(2010) Re-educating natural killer cells. *J Exp Med.* Vol.207, No.10, pp.2049-52.

Suzuki R, Yamamoto K, Seto M, et al.(1997) CD7+ and CD56+ myeloid/natural killer cell precursor acute leukemia: a distinct hematolymphoid disease entity. *Blood. Vol* 90. No.6. pp.2417-28.

Suzuki R, Suzumiya J, Oshimi K.(2009) Differences between nasal and extranasal NK/T-cell lymphoma. *Blood.* 113(17):3931-7.

Suzuki R, Ohtake S, Takeuchi J, et al.(2010) The clinical characteristics of CD7+ CD56+ acute myeloid leukemias other than M0. *Int J Hematol.* Vol.91, No.2.pp.303-9.

Suzuki R, Nakamura S, Suzumiya J, et al.(2005) Blastic natural killer cell lymphoma/leukemia (CD56-positive blastic tumor). *Cancer Vol.*104, No.5,pp.1022-31

Suzuki R, Suzumiya J, Nakamura S, et al. NK-cell Tumor Study Group.(2006) Hematopoietic stem cell transplantation for natural killer-cell lineage neoplasms. *Bone Marrow Transplant.* Vol.37. No.4, pp.425-31.

Suzuki R, Suzumiya J, Yamaguchi M, et al.(2010); NK-cell Tumor Study Group. Prognostic factors for mature natural killer (NK) cell neoplasms: aggressive NK cell leukemia and extranodal NK cell lymphoma, nasal type.

Suzuki R.(2010) Treatment of advanced extranodal NK/T cell lymphoma, nasal-type and aggressive NK-cell leukemia.*Int J Hematol.* Vol.92.No.5. pp.697-701.

Swerdlow SH, et al. (2008) WHO classification of tumours of haematopoietic and lymphoid tissues. Fourth edition, Lyon, IARC Press. *Ann Oncol.* Vol.21. No.5. pp.1032-40.

Takeuchi K, Yokoyama M, Ishizawa S, et al. Lymphomatoid gastropathy: a distinct clinicopathologic entity of self-limited pseudomalignant NK-cell proliferation. *Blood.* Vol.116, No.25. pp.5631-7.

Tang G, Truong F, Fadare O. et.al (2008) Diagnostic challenges related to myeloid/natural killer cells, a variant of myeloblasts. *Int J Clin Exp Pathol. Vol* 1. No.6. pp544-9.

Tsukune Y, Isobe Y, Yasuda H, et al.(2010) Activity and safety of combination chemotherapy with methotrexate, ifosfamide, l-asparaginase and dexamethasone (MILD) for refractory lymphoid malignancies: a pilot study.*Eur J Haematol.* Vol.84. No.4. pp.310-5.

Yamaguchi M, Suzuki R, Kwong YL, et al.(2008) Phase I study of dexamethasone, methotrexate, ifosfamide, L-asparaginase, and etoposide (SMILE) chemotherapy for advanced-stage, relapsed or refractory extranodal natural killer (NK)/T-cell lymphoma and leukemia.*Cancer Sci. Vol* 99. No.5. pp.1016-20.

Yok-Lam K.(2011) The Diagnosis and Management of Extranodal NK/T-Cell Lymphoma, Nasal-Type and Aggressive NK-Cell Leukemia.*J Clin Exp Hematop.* Vol.51, No.1, pp.21-8.

Yong W, Zheng W, Zhu J, Zhang Y, Wei Y, Wang X, et al.(2006) Midline NK/T-cell lymphoma nasal-type: treatment outcome, the effect of L-asparaginase based regimen, and prognostic factors.*Hematol Oncol.* Vol 24, No.1. pp.28-32.

Zhang L, Anglesio MS, O'Sullivan M, Zhang F, Yang G, Sarao R, et al.(2007) The E3 ligase HACE1 is a critical chromosome 6q21 tumor suppressor involved in multiple cancers.*Nat Med.* Vol.13. No.9. pp1060-9.

Part 3

Clinical Manifestations of Acute Lymphoblastic Leukemia

3

Ophthalmological Manifestations in Acute Lymphoblastic Leukemia

Javier Mateo[1], Francisco J. Ascaso[1], Esther Núñez[1], Carlos Peiro[1], Gonzalo González[2] and José A. Cristóbal[1]
[1]Department of Ophthalmology,
[2]Department of Pediatrics, "Lozano Blesa" University Clinic Hospital, Zaragoza
Spain

1. Introduction

The aim of the present chapter is to review the different ophthalmological signs and symptoms that can be observed in acute lymphoblastic leukemia and the importance of the examination of these patients by an ophthalmologist whenever an ocular affectation is suspected.

Acute lymphoblastic leukemia is a malignant neoplasm caused by the proliferation of poorly differenciated precursors of the lymphoid cells, which are known as blast cells. Blast cells replace the normal elements of the bone marrow, decreasing the production of normal blood cells and, therefore, causing anemia, thrombocytopenia and neutropenia. They can also infiltrate other organs, such as liver, spleen, lymph nodes or, less frequently, central nervous system. (Florensa et al, 2006; Ribera & Ortega, 2003; Sharma et al, 2004)

Acute lymphoblastic leukemia is the most common type of leukemia in children, although it is also seen in adult patients. If blood test results are abnormal or the doctor suspects leukemia despite normal cell counts, a bone marrow aspiration and biopsy are the next steps. Treatment is based on chemotherapy, radiotherapy and bone marrow transplantation. (Ribera & Ortega, 2003; Ortega, 2006; Ribera, 2006)

The dominant clinical feature of these diseases is usually bone marrow failure caused by accumulation of blast cells although any organ can be infiltrated. Furthermore, signs and symptoms of acute lymphoblastic leukemia can be secondary to the toxicity of chemotherapy and/or radiotherapy, graft versus host reaction following bone marrow transplantation, or infections due to immunosuppression. They can include fever, weakness, fatigue, breathlessness, opportunistic infections, weight loss, anorexia, easy bruising and bleeding, thrombosis, edema of the lower limbs and the abdomen, swollen liver or spleen, lymphadenopathy, or bone pain. (Florensa et al, 2006; Ribera & Ortega, 2003; Ortega, 2006)

Ophthalmological signs in patients suffering from leukemia were first described as "leukemic retinopathy" by Liebreich in 1863. (Campos-Campos et al, 2004; Guyer et al, 1989)

Reports of patients with acute lymphoblastic leukemia presenting with visual symptoms as the initial sign of the disease are rare (Kim et al, 2010). However, ocular changes in acute lymphoblastic leukemia are common. They have been reported to occur in up to 90% of patients with this disease (Kincaid & Green, 1983; Mesa, 2003).

The improvement of the survival of patients suffering from acute lymphoblastic leukemia has increased the incidence of ocular manifestations they develop. Ocular involvement is associated with a higher frequency of bone marrow relapses and central nervous system compromise weeks or months later, which means a poor prognosis and a low survival rate. (Ohkoshi & Tsiaras, 1992) Leukemic relapses are often diagnosed after ocular presentation. A lot of lesions are asymptomatic and the patient is diagnosed in a routine examination by an ophthalmologist. (Ribera & Ortega, 2003; Sharma et al, 2004; Ribera 2006) Therefore, it is important to consider an ophthalmic evaluation at the time of diagnosis of acute leukemia in adults and children.

The treatment of the ocular manifestations is complicated, as the penetration of the chemotherapic drugs to the eye is quite difficult, even when they are injected intrathecally. Radiotherapy is also used for the treatment. (Ribera & Ortega, 2003; Ortega, 2006; Ribera, 2006).

All the structures of the eye and its adnexal structures can be affected by acute lymphoblastic leukemia. Ophthalmic involvement in acute lymphoblastic leukemia can be classified into two major categories: primary or direct leukemic infiltration of the ocular structures; and secondary or indirect involvement. These secondary changes may be the result of hematologic abnormalities such as anemia, thrombocytopenia, leucopenia, and hyperviscosity. Likewise, opportunistic infections due to immunosuppression -particularly viral, protozoal and fungal infections- and the leukemia treatment itself may secondarily involve the ocular system (Rosenthal, 1983; Wu et al, 2006), as well as graft-versus-host reaction or toxicity of the chemotherapy or radiotherapy. (Sharma et al, 2004; Rosenthal, 1983).

2. Primary manifestations

2.1 Orbit and eyelids

All the structures of the orbit, including lacrimal glands, eyelids, soft tissues and extraocullar muscles, may become affected in the course of acute lymphoblastic leukemia.

Orbital infiltration or a mass formation may cause exophtalmos and/or diplopia. Leukemic cells may infiltrate the soft tissues, extraocuar muscles or lacrimal glands. All kinds of leukemia can affect the orbit, but it is more common in acute lymphoblastic leukemias. (Cardone et al, 2006; Sharma et al, 2004) The symptoms are not different from those caused by other orbital masses, so the diagnosis is usually made after a biopsy of the mass and anatomopathological study. (Abdelouahed et al, 2005).

When the eyelids are involved, they can suffer edema, inflammation, chemosis and pain.

2.2 Conjunctiva

Primary manifestations of conjunctiva involvement in acute lymphoblastic leukemia are caused by direct infiltration by blast cells. Hyperemia and edematization of the lower subpalpebral conjunctiva can be an unusual initial sign of acute lymphoblastic leukemia (Rosenthal, 1983). Infiltrates can also be seen, preferably around vessels (Fernández et al, 1999) or in the form of a conjunctival mass. (Cook & Bartley, 1997)

2.3 Sclera

Scleral infiltration is common during Acute lymphoblastic leukemia, around the episcleral vessels. It is usually asymptomatic and can be an autopsy finding (Sharma et al, 2004;

Burton et al, 2005). Sometimes, a slceral infiltration can simulate a scleritis. Recurrent episcleritis has been associated to adult T-cell leukemia. (Goto et al, 1993)

2.4 Cornea

Because cornea is an avascular structure, it is hardly ever affected by a direct leukemic infiltration. Occasionally there can be ring-shaped corneal ulcers, subepithelial limbal infiltrates and peripheral ulcers. (Taylor, 1997; Rosenthal, 1983; Eiferman et al, 1988).

2.5 Anterior chamber and iridocorneal angle

The space between cornea and lens may be affected in the form of anterior uveitis, pseudohypopyon or spontaneous hyphema.

Most types of leukemias may show protean ocular manifestations ranging from leukemic retinopathy to involvement of the iris and anterior chamber (Decker & Burnstine, 1993). Clinically evident infiltration of the iris by leukemic cells is not common. It occurs associated with the involvement of choroid and ciliary body. It is characterized by a change in iris color, and a pseudohypopyon, which is grey/yellow in color (Perry & Mallen, 1979). In acute lymphoblastic leukemia, hypopyon has been estimated at 2.5 to 18% of relapsed cases, depending on the stage of the disease (Decker & Burnstine, 1993; Yi et al, 2005; Wetzler & Lincoff, 2000; Ramsay & Lightman, 2001).

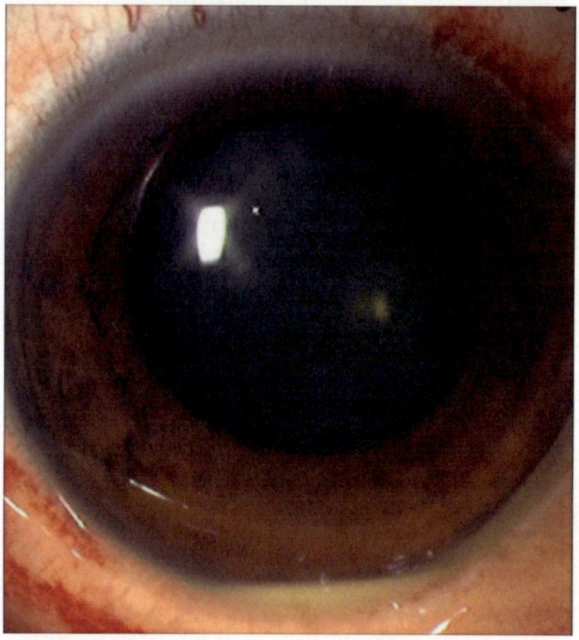

Fig. 1. Sterile hypopion/pseudohypopion in a patient with acute lymphoblastic leukemia.

Although leukemias have been identified as the cause of uveitis in only 5% of paediatric uveitis cases (Soylu et al, 1997), a hypopyon in a child would make us suspicious of a masquerade syndrome. Anterior chamber involvement in cases of acute lymphoblastic leukemia relapse is typically bilateral (Yi et al, 2005). The mechanisms by which the cells migrate into the anterior chamber are not clear.

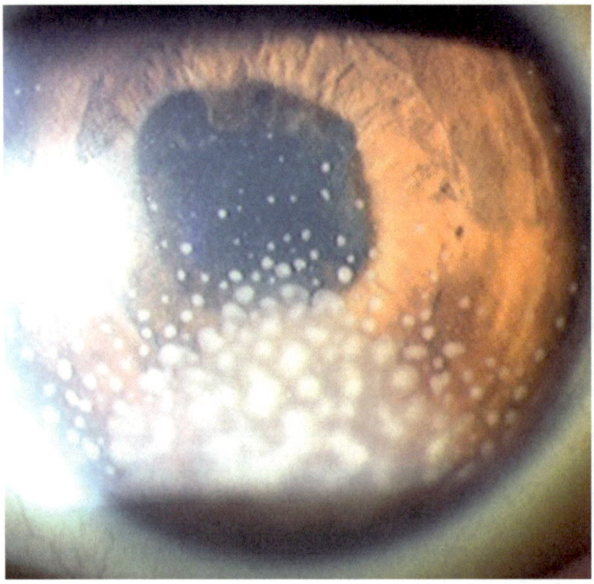

Fig. 2. Corneal precipitates in a case of uveitis secondary to acute lymphoblastic leukemia.

On histopathological examination, the iris may show diffuse involvement, especially at the root and sphincter. An iris biopsy can give us the diagnosis of leukemia (Campos-Campos et al, 2004). The intraocular pressure can be high enough to cause signs and symptoms of acute glaucoma with normal depth of anterior chamber (Wolintz et al, 1971). The raised intraocular pressure is probably due to infiltration of the trabecular meshwork (Rowan & Sloan, 1976).

Prompt anterior chamber paracentesis, and pathological studies should be done in such cases where history of leukemia is present even though other systemic investigations might indicate remission. Complete ocular examination including slit-lamp examination should be performed in all leukemic patients periodically. Early diagnosis is the aim to detect such extramedullary relapses so that timely referral and effective treatment can be initiated. (Campos-Campos et al, 2004)

In children, spontaneous hyphema is also a presentation of leukemia (Perry & Mallen, 1979). Usually clinically apparent involvement of the iris and anterior segment occurs with acute lymphoblastic leukemia (Rowan & Sloan, 1976; Fonken & Ellis, 1966). It may also occur less commonly with chronic lymphocytic leukemias (Martin, 1968) and myeloid leukemias (Perry & Mallen, 1979).

Any ophthalmic manifestation in children with leukemia should be detected and treated early. Radiotherapy is warranted in infiltration of the anterior chamber. The presence of ocular or central nervous system involvement indicates poor prognosis in acute childhood leukemia.

2.6 Retina

The retina is involved in leukemia very commonly. It is estimated that up to 70% of all patients with leukemia show fundus changes during the course of their disease (Alemayehu et al, 1996). Early manifestations are venous dilatation and tortuosity (Ballantyne & Michaelson, 1970).

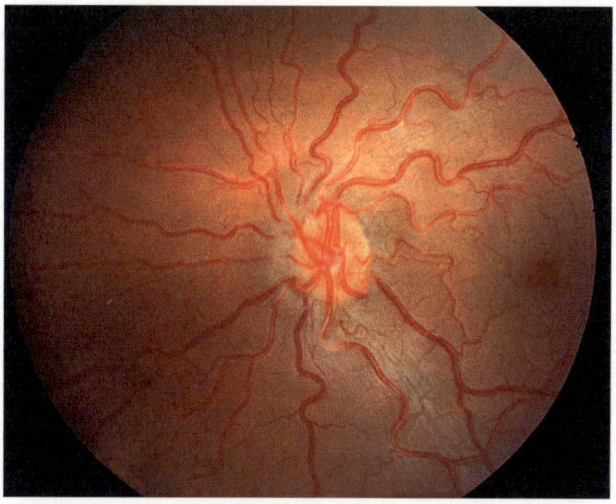

Fig. 3. Vascular congestion and tortuosity in a leukemic retinopathy

Other common retinal manifestations of acute lymphoblastic leukemia include retinal vascular sheathing, superficial retinal or intraretinal hemorrhages, and cotton wool spots, comprising what is called leukemic retinopathy (Rosenthal, 1983; Kincaid & Green, 1983; Park et al, 2000). Vascular occlusions have also been reported.

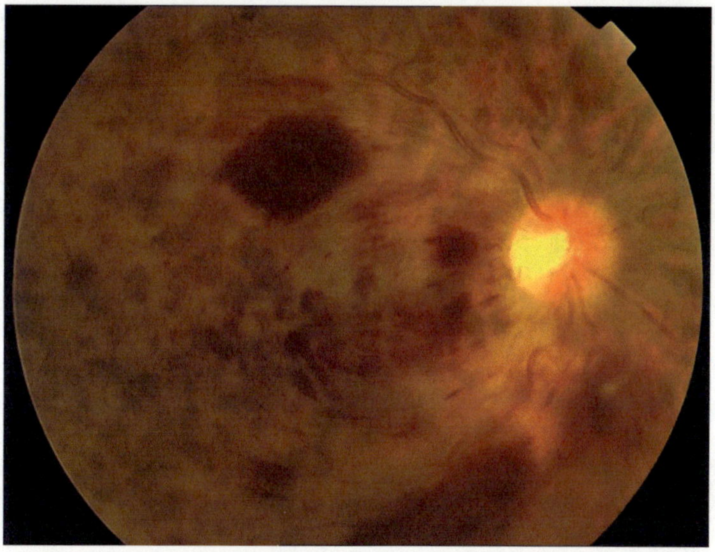

Fig. 4. Central retinal vein occlusion in a patient with hyperviscosity.

Retinal hemorrhages, usually in the posterior pole, may occur in all levels of the retina, but especially in the inner layers with focal destruction. They may be round or flame-shaped hemorrhages and often has a white component in the center. This white area consists of leukemic cells and debris, platelet-fibrin aggregates, or septic emboli (Abdallah et al, 2005). We may also see vitreous haemorrhages coming from retinal bleedings.

Infiltrates and aggregates of leukemic cells are usually seen with surrounding hemorrhage (Kuwabara & Aiello, 1964). Large leukemic infiltrates can cause total retinal detachment presenting as an isolated relapse (Primack et al, 1995). Smaller infiltrates tend to be perivascular. Subretinal infiltration in leukemia has been referred as subretinal hypopyon (Schworm et al, 1995). Cotton wool spots can be seen and are probably due to ischemia from anemia, hyperviscosity, or leukemic infiltration.

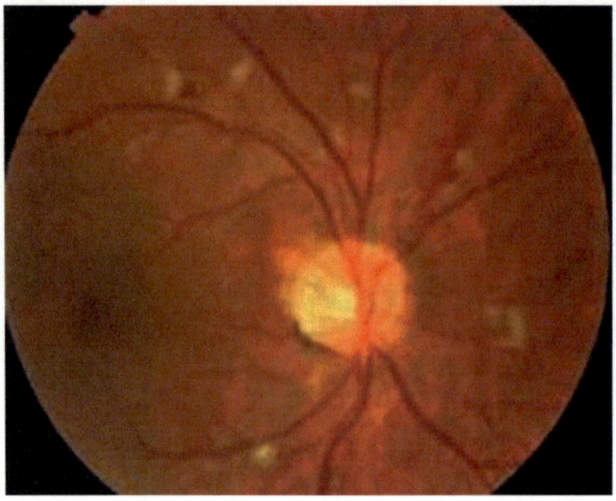

Fig. 5. Cotton-wool spots in a case of acute lymphoblastic leukemia.

Less frequent manifestations include microaneurysms which tend to be peripheral. The presence of microaneurysms is probably related to increased viscosity from elevated white blood cell count, and does not correlate with the hemoglobin level or platelet count (Jampol et al, 1975).

The internal limiting membrane generally acts as an effective barrier to leukemic cell infiltration (Kuwabara & Aiello, 1964). However, leukemic cells occasionally invade the vitreous body, possibly emerging from the optic nerve head. So, a bilateral dense cellular infiltration has been reported (Reese & Guy, 1993; Swartz & Schumann, 1980; Zhioua et al, 2001), resulting in a significant bilateral visual loss, and a vitrectomy may be necessary.

Although less commonly, serous retinal detachment, has been reported in only a few cases of acute lymphoblastic leukemia world-wide (Kincaid & Green, 1983; Tang et al, 1988; Stewart et al, 1989; Dahreddine et al, 2004), especially as a presenting sign of the disease or the first sign of relapse (Yang & Yu, 2009; Kim et al 2010).

Most of the reported cases of acute lymphoblastic leukemia with serous retinal detachment have involved younger patients (Reddy & Menon, 1998; Miyamoto et al, 2000; Malik et al, 2005) and are reported to be shallow in the posterior pole (Stewart et al, 1989; Miyamoto et al, 2000). Serous retinal detachment may develop as a result of choroidal involvement by leukemic cells or due to incompetence of the outer blood-retinal barrier inducing retinal pigment epithelial changes (Stewart et al, 1989; Hine & Kingham, 1979). The differential diagnosis of serous retinal detachment includes Vogt-Koyanagi-Harada disease, central serous chorioretinopathy, uveal effusion syndrome, age-related macular degeneration, choroidal hemangioma and metastatic neoplasm. The choroid is the most frequently involved ocular tissue in leukemia. Leukemic cell infiltration or hematologic disturbances may cause partial occlusion of the choriocapillaries and delay of choroidal circulation. The fact that systemic chemotherapy induced a rapid remission of exudative retinal detachment, consistent with previous reports, suggests leukemic cell infiltration as the underlying pathology (Yang & Yu, 2009). With an appropriate and early treatment, that can include systemic chemotherapy and radiotherapy, serous retinal detachment may resolve completely with good recovery of visual acuity (Kim et al, 2010).

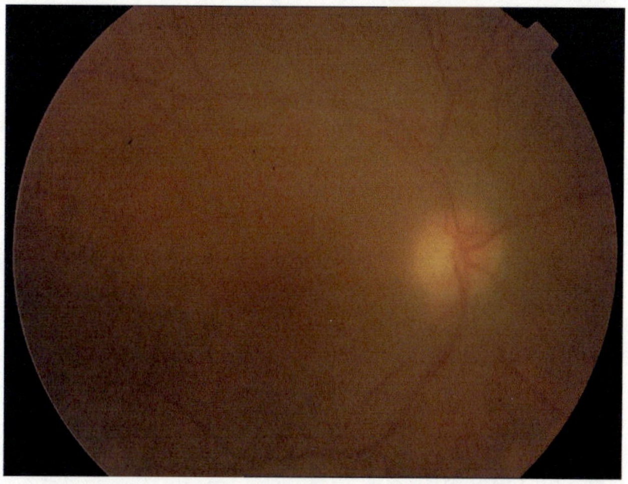

Fig. 6. Leukemic cells' infiltration of the vitreous body.

2.7 Choroid

The choroid is the most commonly affected ocular tissue, but choroidal involvement is often not clinically apparent. Sometimes choroidal and orbital leukemic infiltrate mimic advanced retinoblastoma. There can be a diffuse or perivascular involvement. When it is affected, the overlying retina can show alterations such as photoreceptor damage, retinal pigment epithelium atrophy or serous retinal detachment, usually affecting the posterior pole. (McManaway & Neely, 1994; Campos-Campos et al, 2004)

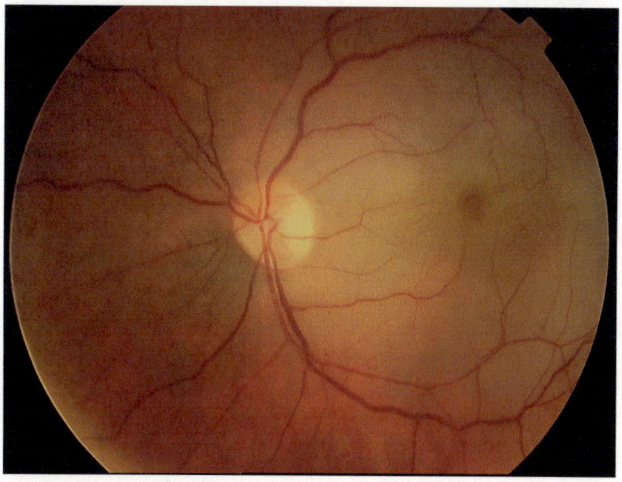

Fig. 7. Posterior pole serous detachment.

Uveal effusion syndrome is caused mainly by disruption of the transscleral outflow of intraocular fluid. Cytological examination of the choroidal fluid may detect atypical lymphoid cells (Kase et al, 2010; Campbell et al, 1990; Schmiegelow et al, 1988). Leukemic infiltration of the choroid may cause a serous detachment of the retina, which is often bilateral. The fluoroangiographic aspect is similar to what is observed in acute choriocapillaris occlusion. (De Laey & De Gersem, 1989)

2.8 Optic nerve

The optic nerve is usually involved in central nervous system leukemia. It can happen in up to 13 to 18% of leukemias. Central nervous system involvement is becoming more frequent as new, more effective treatments have allowed an improvement of the survival of patients suffering from acute lymphoblastic leukemia (Arruga, 2000; Nikaido et al, 1988). The symptoms of central nervous system leukemia depend on the rise of the intracranial pressure and the affectation of the cranial nerves. They can include lethargy, nausea, vomiting, seizures and ocular symptoms such as blurred vision, loss of visual acuity or diplopia, when the cranial nerves III, IV or VI are affected. Sometimes the affectation of the optic nerve is asymptomatic and only papilloedema can be found. (Ribera & Ortega, 2003; Lin et al, 2004; Sharma et al, 2004; Mayo et al, 2002)

Papilloedema is the most frequent sign of optic nerve involvement. It can be due to direct infiltration of the nerve by leukemic cells, increased intraocular person, or swelling because of retrolaminar leukemic invasion. However, optic nerve can also be affected without the presence of papilloedema. (Joshi et al, 2009; Mateo et al, 2007; Bhatt et al 2008; Cleveland & Gelfand, 2009)

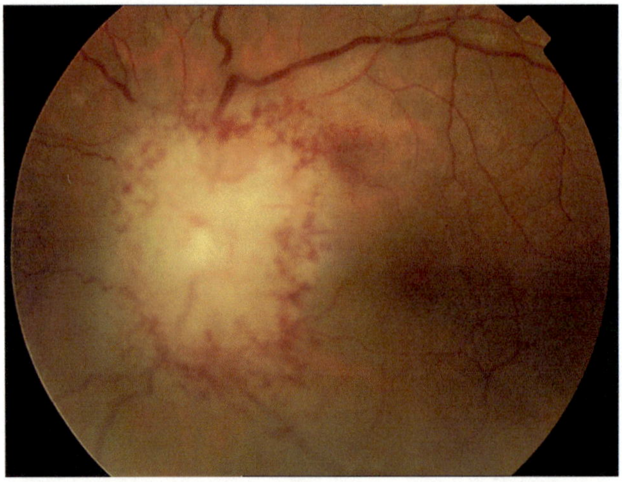

Fig. 8. Massive papilloedema in a patient with acute lymphoblastic leukemia.

The affectation of the optic nerve usually happens during the evolution of acute lymphoblastic leukemia, but it can also be the first sign of acute lymphoblastic leukemia or of extramedullary relapse after remission. (Mesa et all 2003) It always means a poor prognosis for the patient, especially if it happens when the patient is still receiving treatment, rather than after it. (Lo Curto et al, 1996; Bhatt et al, 2008; Schocket et al, 2003)

The treatment of optic nerve involvement is quite difficult, as the optic nerve is relatively unaffected by systemic chemotherapy and serves as a sanctuary of acute lymphoblastic leukemia. It usually includes intratecal chemotherapy and radiotherapy. (Bandyopadhyay et al, 2010; Lo Curto et al, 1996)

3. Secondary manifestations

3.1 Orbit and eyelids

The structures of the orbit can show affectation after remission or secondary to chemotherapy, radiotherapy or graft versus host reaction. In immunocompromised patients, also opportunistic infections can happen.

Lacrimal glands are affected frequently, either by direct infiltration by leukemic cells, graft versus host reaction or radiation, causing a tear dysfunction and dry eye. If severe, it can cause conjunctival and corneal problems such as queratoconjunctivitis sicca, corneal ulcers which can even lead to a corneal perforation and endophtalmitis. (Sharma et al, 2004; Im & Yoon, 2010).

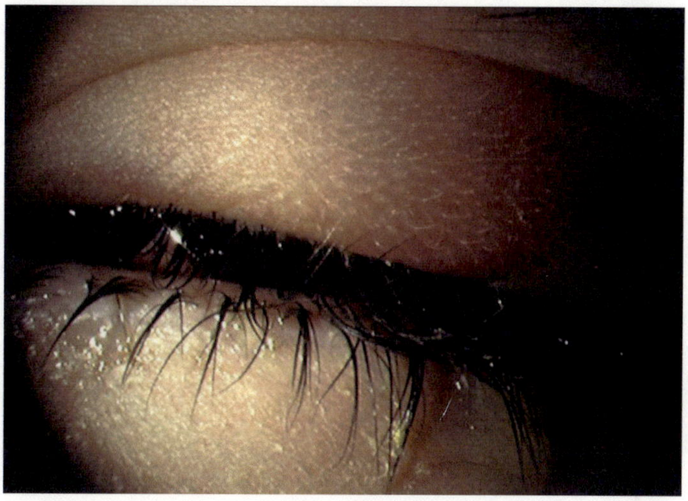

Fig. 9. Preseptal cellulitis in an immunocompromised patient.

Infectious diseases such as preseptal cellulitis or acute dacryocystitis can be seen in immunocompromised patients. They should be treated with both antibiotics and chemotherapy, as soon as possible, to avoid further complications. (Im & Yoon, 2010; Wirostko et al, 1999)

3.2 Conjunctiva

Secondary manifestations to blood disorders are not common. Hyperviscosity can produce vascular anomalies in the conjunctiva, wich are more frequent in chronic leukemias. (Swartz & Jampol, 1975)

The most common involvement of the conjunctiva comes from conjunctivitis secondary to dry eye after a graft versus host reaction. The bone marrow transplantation, in which allogeneic bone marrow obtained from a HLA-matched donor is used, can be a part of the treatment of acute lymphoblastic leukemia. The patients treated are predisposed to suffer a graft against host disease. The incidence of ocular affectation is variable according to the series, reaching to achieve 81.8% of cases, and it is considered a marker of poor prognosis.

Keratoconjunctivitis sicca secondary to graft versus host reaction is difficult to manage. In the acute phase, there are four stages of severity: hyperemia, chemosis, pseudomembranous conjunctivitis with complete loss of conjunctival epithelium and finally, compromise of the corneal epithelium. (Jabs et al, 1989; Sanders, 2002; Uchino et al, 2006) Its presence is related to vital prognosis with a mortality rate of 90% for stages 2 through 4 (Coskuncan 1994, Ohkoshi 1992).

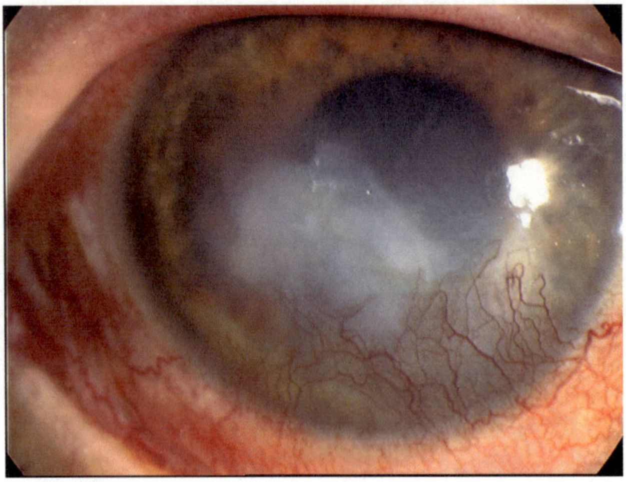

Fig. 10. Conjunctivitis sicca and corneal opacification in a patient with severe dry eye.

Dysfunction of the meibomian glands is another common manifestation of chronic graft against host disease. It is estimated that up to half of patients receiving allogeneic bone marrow transplantation are going to develop a dry eye 6 months later. (Ogawa & Kuwana, 1999)

An almost pathognomonic sign of passage to chronicity is the appearance of fibrous lines in the tarsal conjunctiva (Mondéjar et al, 2001). The severe dryness and the progressive superficial keratinization evolve towards the formation of ectropion, cicatricial lagophthalmos and a palpebral lichenification. A major impact of this is the emergence of severe and recurrent corneal erosions and ulcerations, which can even evolve to the drilling of trophic or infectious origin. (Mittelviefhaus & Auw-Hadrich, 2003)

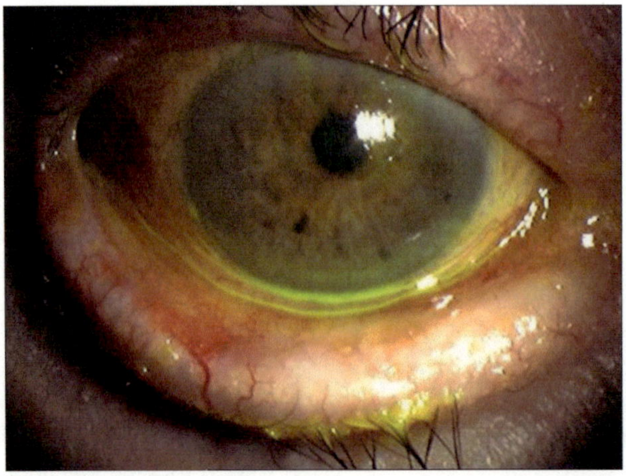

Fig. 11. Ectropion in a severe dry eye patient.

Other secondary manifestations are those due to complications of the antileukemic treatment and opportunistic ocular infections. Direct toxicity of methotrexate is associated with the appearance of keratoconjunctivitis. The immunosuppression attached to marrow failure typical of the leukemia and the secondary to chemotherapy, favours infections by different microorganisms. (Fernández et al 1999; Cogan, 1977)

3.3 Sclera

Occasionally, immunocompromised patients suffer opportunistic infectious scleritis.

3.4 Cornea

Some drugs used for chemotherapy can produce corneal toxicity: citarabine produces corneal toxicity by interfering with epithelium´s synthesis of DNA. (Fernandez et al, 1999; Mondéjar et al, 2001)

Keratoconjunctivitis sicca is the most common manifestation of graft versus host reaction. In the more severe cases, keratitis, corneal ulcers or corneal opacification are not uncommon. (Jabs et al, 1989; Uchino et al, 2006) The appearance of calcareous corneal degeneration in patients with severe dry eye in graft against host disease has also been described. In these cases the deposit of calcium salts occurs in all the layers of the cornea. (Lavid et al, 1995) However, sometimes there is a rapid development of extracellular deposits of calcium at subepithelial level, causing the appearance of acute calcium keratopathy that is located in the interpalpebral zone (Carreras & Muiños, 1996). Given the frequency and severity of these alterations of the ocular surface, it is important a close monitoring of all patients who received bone marrow transplant and especially those who develop a graft against host disease aimed at early detection.

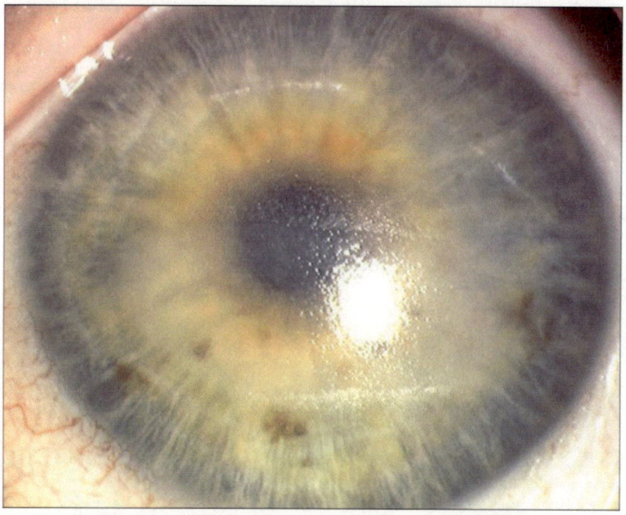

Fig. 12. Corneal opacification secondary to severe keratocojunctivitis sicca.

In patients suffering from secondary immunosupression, infections by microorganisms such as herpes and fungi are favoured. Some secondary manifestations are keratitis, corneal thinning, ulcers and even corneal melting and perforation. (Fernández et al, 1999; Cogan, 1977).

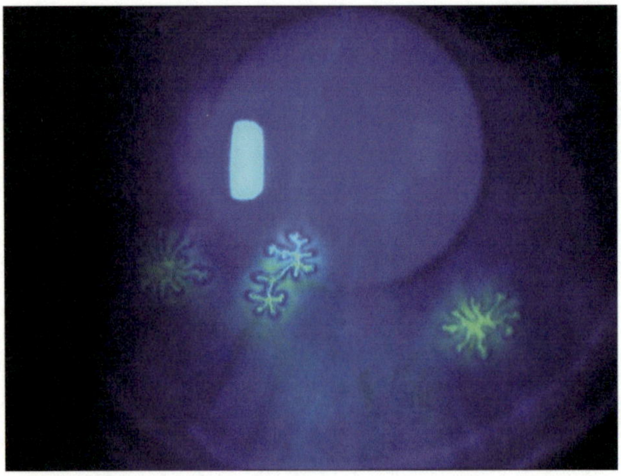

Fig. 13. Herpetic corneal ulcers.

3.5 Anterior chamber and iridocorneal angle

Extramedullary relapse of acute leukemias may masquerade as hypopyon uveitis (Ayliffe, 1995). Primary relapse of acute leukemia in the anterior segment is not uncommon (Ayliffe, 1995; Jancovic et al, 1995; MacLean et al, 1995; Soylu et al, 1997).

It is possible an ischemia of the anterior segment secondary to anaemia or hyperviscosity. It might cause corneal edema, conjunctival chemosis, visual loss, anterior uveitis, increased intraocular pressure, cataracts and eye pain. (Sharma et al, 2004)

Cataracts may also develop as a consequence of the use of stereoids, chemotherapy drugs or radiotherapy, or after ischemia caused by hyperviscosity or anaemia. (Elliott et al, 1985; Sharma et al 2004)

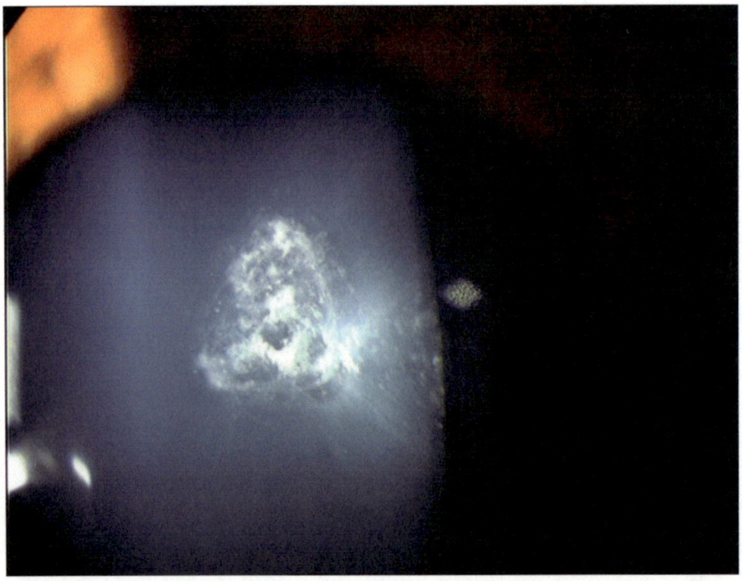

Fig. 14. Subcapsular cataract caused by the use of corticosteroids.

3.6 Retina

Patients with acute leukemia are susceptible to unusual and potentially life-threatening opportunistic infections that may involve the retina, especially during periods of neutropenia, which result both from the underlying disease as well as chemotherapy. These patients are susceptible to a wide variety of infections by viral (Cytomegalovirus, herpes virus), fungal (Candida, Aspergillus), protozoal, and bacterial organisms (Cogan, 1977). Cytomegalovirus infection is among the common viral infections in the immunocompromised hosts (Shibata et al, 1997). However, the prevalence of cytomegalovirus antigenemia and disease in patients with hematological malignancies who are not transplant recipients or HIV infected is largely unknown and is thought to be low (Taha et al, 2010). The virus invades the retina, causing necrosis, vascular sheathing, hemorrhage, and combined exudative and rhegmatogenous retinal detachment (Meredith et al, 1979).

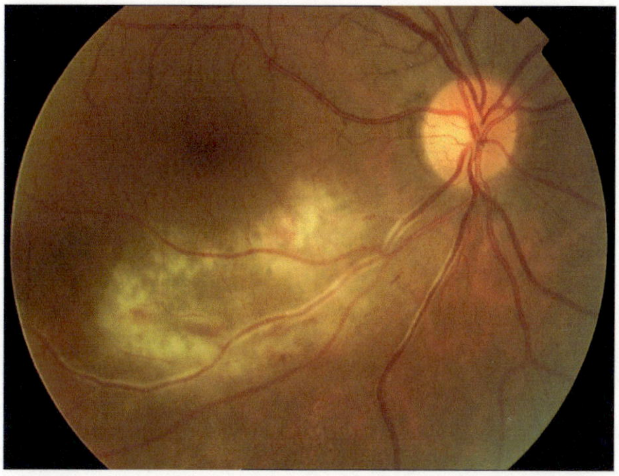

Fig. 15. Opportunistic infection by cytomegalovirus in a patient with neutropenia.

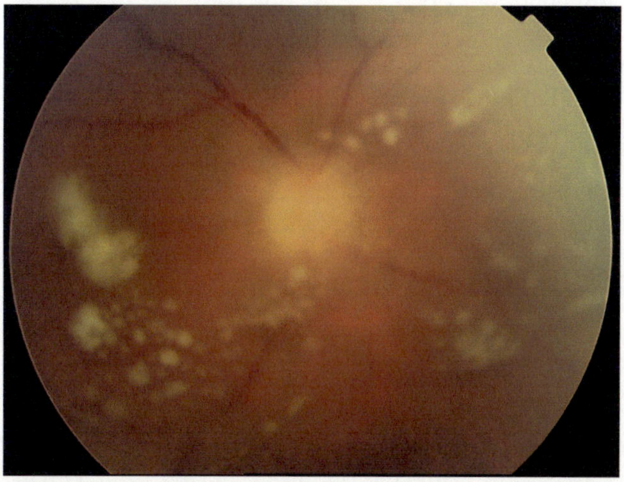

Fig. 16. Vitritis caused by Candida infection.

Other viruses (herpes simplex, varicella zoster, and mumps) may also cause necrotizing retinitis in immunocompromised hosts (Cogan, 1977). Herpes zoster can also cause peripheral corneal ulcer, keratitis, and scleritis (Walton & Reed, 1999). Mumps virus has been reported to be a cause of granulomatous uveitis (Al-Rashid & Cress, 1977). Fungi are common causes of ocular infection in leukemias. Candida, especially Candida albicans, is among the common infections in this subset of patients; when it involves the retina, it typically appears as focal, deep white lesions that can be singular or multiple. It may extend into the vitreous and cause uveitis and retinitis with characteristic cotton balls in the vitreous (Cogan, 1977). The rate of developing chorioretinitis in patients with candidemia has reduced markedly since the 1990's due to the early identification of candidemia in blood cultures coupled with a trend of early empiric antifungal therapy (Ninane et al, 1979). Aspergillus is also a common fungal infection in leukemic patients (Ellis & Little, 1973).

3.7 Choroid

Choroid secondary affectation is much less common than primary. Retinochoroidal infarction has been detected during the treatment of acute lymphoblastic leukemia. (Kato et al, 2006).

3.8 Optic nerve

Secondary optic nerve affectation include toxicity of chemotherapy, antibiotics or radiotherapy, ischemia after anaemia or hyperviscosity, and opportunistic infections in immunocompromised patients. (Joshi et al, 2009; Bhatt et al 2008; Cleveland & Gelfand, 2009).

4. Conclusion

Ophthalmological manifestations in patients suffering acute lymphoblastic leukemia are very common, partly thanks to the improvement of the survival because of the new and more efficient treatments, appearing in as much as 90% of the patients. They usually occur during the evolution of the illness, but they can be its first manifestation or the first sign of relapse after remission. (Kincaid & Green, 1983; Mesa, 2003)

Ocular involvement can be caused by direct infiltration by leukemic cells or be secondary to anemia, thrombocytopenia, leucopenia, hyperviscosity and opportunistic infections in immunosuppressed patients. All the structures of the eye can be affected, as well as the orbit, the eyelids and the lacrimal glands. (Sharma et al, 2004)

The treatment of the ocular manifestations is difficult, because the effect of chemotherapy in the eye is very limited. Radiotherapy is frequently used for the treatment. (Ribera & Ortega, 2003; Ortega, 2006; Ribera, 2006)

Every patient suffering acute lymphoblastic leukemia should get a complete ophthalmological exam regularly, to detect and treat eye problems in order to preserve vision and, even more important, in patients who are in remission, to diagnose relapses as soon as possible, because an early treatment can improve the patient's vital prognosis. (Mateo et al, 2007)

5. References

Abdallah E, Hajji Z, Mellal Z, Belmekki M, Bencherifa F, Berraho A (2005). Macular serous detachment revealing acute lymphoblastic leukemia. *J Fr Ophtalmol*, 28(1):39-44, ISSN 0181-5512.

Abdelouahed K, Laghmari M, Tachfouti S, Cherkaoui W, Khorassani M, M'Seffer FA, Mohcine Z (2005). Leucémie aiguë lymphoblastique T/Lymphome lymphoblastique orbitaire chez l'enfant. *J Fr Ophtalmol,* 28(2):197-200, ISSN 0181-5512.

Alemayehu W, Shamebo M, Bedri A, Mengistu Z (1996). Ocular manifestations of leukaemia in Ethiopians. *Ethiop Med J,* 34:217–224, ISSN 0014-1755.

Al-Rashid RA, Cress C (1977). Mumps uveitis complicating the course of leukaemia. *J Pediatr Ophthalmol,* 14:100–102, ISSN 0022-345X.

Arruga J (2000). Lesiones metastáticos y paraneoplásicas del nervio óptico. Rev Neurol 31:1256-1258. ISSN 0210-0010.

Ayliffe W, Foster CS, Marcoux P, Upton M, Finkelstein M, Legmann A (1995). Relapsing acute myeloid leukaemia manifesting as hypopyon uveitis. *Am J Ophthalmol,* 119:361–364, ISSN 0002-9394.

Ballantyne AJ, Michaelson IC (1970). *Textbook of the Fundus of the Eye.* Pp 290-292. Williams and Wilkins, ISBN 0443006598 Baltimore.

Bhatt UK, Gregory ME, Madi MS, Fraser M, Woodruff HA (2008). Sequential leukemic infiltration and human herpervirus optic neuropathy in acute lymphoblastic leukemia. *Journal of AAPOS* 12:200-202. ISSN 1528-3933.

Bandyopadhyay S, Das D, Das G, Gayen S (2010). Unilateral optic nerve infiltration as an initial site of relapse of acute lymphoblastic leukemia in remission. *Oman J Ophthalmol* 3:153-154. ISSN 0974-7842.

Burton BJ, Cunningham ET, Cree IA, Pavesio CE (2005). Eye involvement mimicking scleritis in a patient with chronic lymphocytic leukaemia. *Br J Ophthalmol,* 89(6):775-776, ISSN 0007-1161.

Campbell RA, Bouldin TW, Peiffer RL (1990). Large histiocytes in the choroid of leukemic patients. *Arch Pathol Lab Med,* 114(2):210-211, ISSN 0003-9985.

Campos-Campos LE, Mendoza-Altamirano L, Pérez RX, Beauregard-Escobar AM, Calderón LM (2004). Alteraciones oculares en pacientes pediátricos con leucemia aguda. Rev Mex Oftalmol 14:287-290, ISSN 01874519.

Cardone S, Yen MT, Chévez-Barrios P, Foroozan R, Yen KG (2006). Recurrent Acute Lymphoblastic Leukemia Presenting in the Lacrimal Gland. *Ophthal Plast Reconstr Surg,* 22(1):56-57, ISSN 1537-2677.

Cleveland KO, Gelfand MS (2009). Optic neuropathy following linezolid use in a patient with acute lymphocytic leukemia. *Clin Infect Dis* 49(4):645-646. ISSN 1537-6591.

Cogan DG (1977). Immunosuppression and eye disease. *Am J Ophthalmol,* 83:777–788, ISSN 0002-9394.

Cook BE, Bartley GB (1997). Acute lymphoblastic leukemia manifesting in an adult as a conjunctival mass. *Am J Ophthalmology* 124:104-105, ISSN 0002-9394.

Coskuncan N, Jabs D, Dunn JP, Haller JA, Green WR, Vogelsang GB, Santos GW (1994). The eye in bone marrow transplantation. *Arch Ophthalmology,* 112:372-379, ISSN 0096-6339.

Dahreddine M, Karim A, Moussaif H, Essakali NH, Mohcine Z (2004). White-centered retinal hemorrhage revealing acute lymphoblastic leukemia. *J Fr Ophtalmol,* 27(5):506-509, ISSN 0181-5512.

Decker EB, Burnstine RA (1993). Leukemic relapse presenting as acute unilateral hypopyon in acute lymphocyticleukemia. *Ann Ophthalmol*, 25:346-349, ISSN 1530-4086.

De Laey JJ, De Gersem R (1989). Clinical aspects of leukemic infiltration of the choroid and the optic nerve. *J Fr Ophtalmol*, 12(11):819-825, ISSN 0181-5512.

Eiferman R, Levartovsky S, Schultz (1988). Leukemic corneal infiltrates. *Am J Ophthalmology*, 105:319-320, ISSN 0002-9394.

Elliott AJ, Oakhill A, Goodman S (1985). Cataracts in childhood leukaemia. *Br J Ophthalmol* 69:459-461, ISSN 0007-1161.

Ellis W, Little HL (1973). Leukaemic infiltration of the optic nerve head. *Am J Ophthalmol*,75:867–871, ISSN 0002-9394.

Fernandez MC, Serrano JC, Jimenez S (1999). Valoración oftalmológica de los pacientes pediátricos con diagnóstico de leucemia. *Medunab* 2(6):149-154, ISSN 0123-7047.

Florensa L, Pérez-Vila E, Woessner S. (2006) Introducción al estudio de las leucemias agudas. Clasificación. Descripción de las diferentes variedades. Formas especiales. In: *Hematología clínica 5ª ed.* Sans-Sabrafen S, Besses C, Vives JL. pp 409-436. Elsevier, ISBN 84-8174-779-3 Madrid.

Fonken HA, Ellis PP (1966). Leukaemic infiltrates in the iris. *Arch Ophthalmol*, 76:32–36, ISSN 0003-9950.

Giagounidis AA, Meckenstock G, Flacke S, Burk M, Wehmeier A, Aul C (1997). Pseudomonas aeruginosa blepharoconjunctivitis during cytoreductive chemotherapy in a woman with acute lymphocytic leukaemia. *Ann Hematol*, 75:121–123, ISSN 0939-5555.

Goto K, Sugita M, Okada K, Hatano H, Ishiguro N, Yoshiki T, Ohno S (1993). Recurrent episcleritis associated with adult T cell leukaemia. *Br J Ophthalmol*, 77(11):743-744. ISSN 0007-1161.

Guyer DR, Sch, Schachat AP, Vitale S, Markowitz JA, Braine H, Burke PJ, Karp JE, Graham M. (1989) Leukemic retinopathy. Relationship between fundus lesions and hematologic parameters at diagnosis. *Ophthalmology*, 96:860-864, ISSN 0161-6420.

Hine JE, Kingham JD (1979). Myelogenous leukemia and bilateral exudative retinal detachment. *Ann Ophthalmol*, 11:1867-1872, ISSN 1530-4086.

Im SK, Yoon KC (2010). Corneal perforation with preseptal cellulitis in a patient with acute lymphocytic leukemia. *J Korean Med Sci* 25(8):1251-1252, ISSN 1598-6357.

Jabs DA, Wingard J, Green WR, Farmer ER, Vogelsang G, Saral R (1989). The eye in bone marrow transplantation. III. Conjunctival graft-versus-host disease. *Arch Ophthalmol*, 107:1343-1348, ISSN 0096-6339.

Jampol LM, Goldberg MF, Busse B (1975). Peripheral retinal micro aneurysms in chronic leukaemia. *Am J Ophthalmol*, 80:242–248, ISSN 0002-9394. - Jankovic M, Conter V, Pretto G, Placa F, D'Incalci M, Masera G (1995). Isolated bilateral anterior chamber eye relapse in a child with acute lymphoblastic leukaemia. *Med Pediatr Oncol*, 25:109–112, ISSN 0098-1532.

Joshi L, Taylor SRJ, Large O, Yacoub S, Lightman S (2009). A case of optic neuropathy after short-term linezolid use in a patient with acute lymphocytic leukemia. *Clin Infect Dis* 48:73-74. ISSN 1537-6591.

Kato Y, Takano Y, Kobayashi M, Ito F, Hara T, Yanagisawa T, Hoshi Y, Eto Y (2006). Retinochoroidal infarction during the treatment of acute lymphoblastic leukemia. *Pediatr Int*, 48(5):495-497, ISSN 1442-200X.

Kase S, Saito W, Saito A, Ohno S (2010). Uveal effusion syndrome caused by choroidal invasion of malignant lymphoma. *Jpn J Ophthalmol*, 54(1):109-110, ISSN 1613-2246.

Kim J, Chang W, Sagong M (2010). Bilateral serous retinal detachment as a presenting sign of acute lymphoblastic leukemia. *Korean J Ophthalmol*, 24(4):245-248, ISSN 1011-8942.

Kincaid MC, Green WR (1983). Ocular and orbital involvement in leukemia. *Surv Ophthalmol*, 27:211-232, ISSN 0039-6257.

Kuwabara T, Aiello L (1964). Leukaemic military nodule in retina. *Arch Ophthalmol*, 72:494–497, ISSN 0003-9950.

Lavid Jj, Herreras JM, Calonge M, Saornil MA, Aguirre C (1995). Calcareous corneal degeneration: report of two cases. *Cornea*, 14:97-102, ISSN 0277-3740.

Lin YC, Wang AG, Yen MY, Hsu WM (2004). Leukaemic infiltration of the optic nerve as the initial manifestation of leukaemic relapse. *Eye* 18:546-550, ISSN 0950-222X.

Lo Curto M, D'angelo P, Jankovik M, Fugardi MG, Ziino O, Casale F (1996). Isolated ocular relapse in childhood acute lymphoblastic leucemia during complete remission. *Haematologica* 81:47-50, ISSN 0390-6078.

MacLean H, Clarke MP, Strong NP, Kernahan J (1995). Primary relapse of acute leukaemia in anterior segment of the eye. *Lancet* 346:500, ISSN 0140-6736.

Malik R, Shah A, Greaney MJ, et al (2005). Bilateral serous macular detachment as a presenting feature of acute lymphoblastic leukemia. *Eur J Ophthalmol*, 15:284-286, ISSN 1120-6721.

Martin B (1968). Infiltration of the iris in chronic lymphatic leukaemia. *Br J Ophthalmol* 52:781–785, ISSN 0007-1161.

Mateo J, Abarzuza R, Núñez E, Cristóbal JA (2007). Infiltración bilateral del nervio óptico en un caso de leucemia aguda linfoblástica de células T en remisión. *Arch Soc Esp Oftalmol* 82:167-170, ISSN 0365-6691.

Mayo GL, Carter JE, McKinnon SJ (2002). Bilateral optic disk edema and blindness as inicial presentation of acute lymphocytic leukemia. *Am J Ophthalmol* 134:141-142, ISSN 0002-9394.

McManaway JW, Neely JE (1994). Choroidal and orbital leukemic infiltrate mimicking advanced retinoblastoma. *J Pediatr Ophthalmol Strabismus*, 31(6):394-296, ISSN: 0191-3913.

Meredith TA, Aaberg TM, Reeser FH (1979). Rhegmatogenous retinal detachment complicating CMV retinitis. *Am J Ophthalmol* 87: 793–796, ISSN 0002-9394.

Mesa F, Cordovés L, García M, Losada MJ, Martín F (2003). Manifestaciones oculares como presentación de recaída de leucemia aguda linfoblástica de células T. *Arch Soc Canar Oftal* 14:91-94, ISSN 0211-2698.

Mittelviefhaus H, Auw-Hadrich C (2003). Corneal complications after hematopoietic stem cell transplantation. *Ophthalmologe*, 100:222-229, ISSN 1433-0423.

Miyamoto K, Kashii S, Honda Y (2000). Serous retinal detachment caused by leukemic choroidal infiltration during complete remission. *Br J Ophthalmol*, 84:1318-9, ISSN 0007-1161.

Mondejar J, Navea A, Diaz-Llopis M (2001). Trasplante de médula ósea. Enfermedad del injerto contra el huésped. In: *Manifestaciones oftalmológicas de las enfermedades generales*. Sánchez-Salorio M, Díaz-Llopis M, Benítez del Castillo JM, Rodríguez T, pp 228-230, Mac Line, ISBN 84-89085-16-1, Madrid.

Nikaido H, Mishima H, Ono H, Choshi K, Dohy H (1988). Leukemic involvemet of the optic nerve. *Am J Ophthalmol* 105:294-298, ISSN 0002-9394.

Ninane J, Taylor D, Day S (1979). Leukaemic hypopyon in acute lymphoblastic leukaemia after interruption of treatment. *Arch Dis Child* 54:73–74, ISSN 0003-9888.

Ogawa Y, Kuwana M (2003). Dry eye as a major complication associated with chronic graft-versus-host disease after hematopoietic stem cell transplantation. *Cornea*, 22(Supl 1):S19-S27, ISSN 0277-3740.

Ohkoshi K, Tsiaras WG (1992). Prognostic importance of ophthalmic manifestations in childhood leukaemia. *Br J Ophthalmol*, 1992, 76: 651–655, ISSN 0007-1161.

O'Rourke JF, O'Connor GR (1980). The eye as a sanctuary in acute lymphoblastic leukaemia. *Lancet*, 1:452–453, ISSN 0140-6736.

Ortega JJ. (2006) Leucemias agudas infantiles. In: *Hematología clínica 5ª ed.* Sans-Sabrafen S, Besses C, Vives JL. pp 437-450. Elsevier, ISBN 84-8174-779-3 Madrid.

Park YK, Jun RM, Ahn CS (2000). A case of optic nerve infiltration of acute lymphocytic leukemia. *J Korean Ophthalmol Soc*, 41:2008-2012, ISSN 1011-8942.

Perry HD, Mallen FJ (1979). Iris involvement in granulocytic sarcoma. *Am J Ophthalmol*, 87:530–532, ISSN 0002-9394.

Primack JD, Smith ME, Tychsen L et al (1995). Retinal detachment in a child as the first sign of leukemic relapse. *J Pediatr Ophthalmol Strabismus*, 32:253–256, ISSN 0191-3913.

Ramsay A, Lightman S (2001). Hypopyon uveitis. *Surv Ophthalmol*, 46:1-18, ISSN 0039-6257.

Reddy SC, Menon BS (1998). A prospective study of ocular manifestations in childhood acute leukaemia. *Acta Ophthalmol Scand* 76:700-703, ISSN 1395-3907.

Reese AB, Guy L (1993). Exophthalmos in leukaemia. *Am J Ophthalmol*, 16:718–720, ISSN 0002-9394.

Ribera JM (2006). Tratamiento de la leucemia aguda linfoblástica del adulto, In: *Hematología clínica 5ª ed.* Sans-Sabrafen S, Besses C, Vives JL. pp 451-460. Elsevier, ISBN 84-8174-779-3 Madrid.

Ribera JM, Ortega JJ. (2003) Leucemia linfoide aguda. In: *Hematología*. García-Conde J, San Miguel JF, Sierra J, Urbano-Ispizua A, Vicente V, Vives JL. pp 1029-1042. Aran, ISBN 84-95913-23-2 Madrid.

Rosenthal AR (1983). Ocular manifestations of leukemia: a review. *Ophthalmology*, 90:899-905, ISSN 0161-6420.

Rowan PJ, Sloan JB (1976). Iris and Anterior chamber involvement in leukaemia. *Ann Ophthalmol*, 8:1081–1085, ISSN 1530-4086.

Sanders JE (2002). Chronic graft-versus-host disease and late effect after hematopoietic stem cell transplantation. *Int J Hematol*, 76:15-28, ISSN 0925-5710.

Schmiegelow K, Scherfig E, Prause JU, Jensen OA (1988). Isolated leukemic choroidal relapse in a child with acute lymphoblastic leukemia one year off therapy, diagnosed through transvitreal retino-choroidal biopsy. *Acta Ophthalmol Scand*, 66(1):33-37, ISSN 1395-3907.

Schocket LS, Massaro-Giordano M, Volpe NJ, Galetta SL (2003). Bilateral optic nerve infiltration in central nervous system leukemia. *Am J Ophthalmol* 135:94-96. ISSN ISSN 0002-9394.

Schworm HD, Nasemann JE, Schriever S (1995). Subretinal hypopyon in prolymphocytic leukaemia. *Br J Ophthalmol*, 79:863–864, ISSN 0007-1161.

Swartz M, Schumann GB (1980). Acute leukaemic infiltration of the vitreous diagnosed by pars plana aspiration. *Am J Ophthalmol*, 90:326–330, ISSN 0002-9394.

Sharma T, Grewal J, Gupta S, Murray PI. (2004) Ophthalmic manifestations of acute leukaemias: the ophthalmologist's role. *Eye*, 18,pp 663-672, ISSN 0950-222X.

Shibata K, Shimamoto Y, Nishimura T, Okinami S, Yamada H, Miyahara M (1997). Ocular manifestation in adult T cell leukaemia/lymphoma. *Ann Hematol*, 74:163–168, ISSN 0939-5555.

Soylu M, Ozdemir G, Anli A (1997). Pediatric uveitis in southern Turkey. *Ocul Immunol Inflamm*, 5:197–202, ISSN 0927-3948.

Stewart MW, Gitter KA, Cohen G (1989). Acute leukemia presenting as a unilateral exudative retinal detachment. *Retina*, 9:110-114, ISSN 0275-004X.

Swartz M, Jampol LM (1975). Comma shaped venular segment of conjunctiva chronic granulocytic leukemia. *Can J Ophthalmology*, 110:458-461, ISSN 0008-4182.

Taha R, Al Hijji I, El Omri H, Al-Laftah F, Negm R, Yassin M, El Ayoubi H (2010). Two Ocular Infections during Conventional Chemotherapy in a Patient with Acute Lymphoblastic Leukemia: A Case Report. *Case Rep Oncol*, 3(2):234-239, ISSN 1662-6575.

Tang RA, Vila-Coro AA, Wall S, et al (1988). Acute leukemia presenting as a retinal pigment epithelium detachment. *Arch Ophthalmol*, 106:21-22, ISSN 0003-9950.

Taylor D (1997). Leukaemia, In: *Paedriatic Ophthalmology 2nd ed*, Taylor D. pp 816-817. Blackwell Science, ISBN 086542831X Orford.

Uchino M, Ogawa Y, Kawai M, Shimada H, Kameyama K, Okamoto S, Dogru M, Tsubota K (2006). Ocular complications in a child with acute graft-versus-host disease following cord blood stem cell transplantation: therapeutic challenges. *Acta Ophthalmol Scand*, 84(4):545-548, ISSN 1600-0420.

Walton RC, Reed KL (1999). Herpes zoster ophthalmicus following bone marrow transplantation in children. *Bone Marrow Transplant*, 23: 1317–1320, ISSN 0268-3369.

Wetzler M, Lincoff N (2000). Unusual manifestation of acute leukemia. Case 3 -Unilateral leukemic hypopyon. *J Clin Oncol*, 18: 3439-3440, ISSN 1527-7755.

Wirostko WJ, Garcia GH, Cory S, Harris GJ (1999). Acute dacryocystitis as a presenting sign of pediatric leukemia. *Am J Ophthalmol*, 127:734-736, ISSN 0002-9394.

Wolintz AH, Goldstein JH, Seligman BR, Rosner F, Wesely AC, Lee SL (1971). Secondary glaucoma in leukaemia. *Ann Ophthalmol*, 3:1211–1213, ISSN 0939-5555.

Wu L, Calderon M, Hernandez G, et al (2006). Bilateral exudative retinal detachment as the first sign of relapsing acute myelogenous leukaemia. *Clin Exp Ophthalmol*, 34:623-625, ISSN 1442-9071.

Yang HK, Yu HG (2009). Acute lymphoblastic leukemia manifesting as acute Vogt-Koyanagi-Harada disease. *Korean J Ophthalmol*. 23(4):325-328, ISSN 1011-8942.

Yi DH, Rashid S, Cibas ES, Arrigg PG, Dana MR (2005). Acute unilateral leukemic hypopyon in an adult with relapsing acute lymphoblastic leukemia. *Am J Ophthalmol*, 139:719-721, ISSN 0002-9394.

Yoken J, Forbes B, Maguire AM, Prenner JL, Carpentieri D (2002). Microsporidial endophthalmitis in a patient with acute myelogenous leukaemia. *Retina*, 22:123–125, ISSN 0275-004X.

Zhioua R, Boussen I, Malek I, Ouertani A (2001). Acute lymphoblastic leukaemia and vitreous infiltration. A case study. *J Fr Ophtalmol*, 24:180–182, ISSN 0181-5512.

4

Acute Lymphoblastic Leukemia: What Have We Learned About the Effects of This Disease and Its Treatment on the Nervous System?

Van Huynh, Leonard Sender and Daniela A. Bota
University of California Irvine and Children Hospital of Orange County
USA

1. Introduction

The treatment of leukemia remains the success story of cancer. The patients with acute lymphoblastic leukemia survive longer and longer, with the rates of long time remission of over 80% in children and 30-40% in adults. Therefore, increased attention is given to diagnose and prevent central nervous system (CNS) complications, not only in order to increase the survival, but also in order to prevent neurologic deterioration and the resulting decreased quality of life.

CNS disease is relatively rare at diagnosis, with less than 10% of the patients being diagnosed with his condition. However, the rate of CNS involvement escalates to up to 75% in the first year, if no effective brain-targeted treatments are used- which justifies the need for CNS prophylaxis even in the absence of frank metastatic involvement.

Classically, patients received cranial radiation. However, a significant percentage of ALL survivors that received cranial radiation now present with a discouraging array of complications, including neurodevelopmental sequelae, strokes, seizures and increased rate of secondary CNS malignancies. More recent, it was suggested that effective CNS prophylaxis can be achieved with a combination of high dose systemic chemotherapy and intrathecal chemotherapy. Though less toxic, some survivors of this approach are still plagued by neurological complications, including cognitive deficits due to the effects of chemotherapy on the developing brain.

More research needs to be conducted on further decreasing the rate on CNS relapse, while minimizing the therapy effects of the brain. Our knowledge of the biological mechanisms involved in radiation and chemotherapy effects of different cerebral structures has to improve. For the ALL survivors, therapies to repair the cognitive damage caused by cancer treatments are still in infancy.

2. CNS Involvement in Acute Lymphoblastic Leukemia (ALL)

2.1 Diagnosis and Incidence

ALL is the most common malignancy in children. It follows a bimodal distribution, with a peak between the ages of 4 and 10, and a second peak after the age of 50 (M.J. Horner, 2009). It accounts for approximately 25% of all childhood cancers occurring in those younger than

20 years of age (Ries et al., 1999). In the United States, there are approximately 3000 cases of childhood ALL diagnosed each year, with an incidence of 3-4 cases per 100,000 children (Jemal et al., 2004). This incidence is similar worldwide. The incidence of ALL varies considerably with age. There is a sharp peak in ALL incidence among children 2-5 years of age, and this trend subsequently decreases with age. The median age at diagnosis is 4 years. Sex differences have been reported with the incidence greater in boys (Smith, et al., 1999). Race differences in incidence have also been observed. African Americans have a much lower incidence of childhood ALL compared to Whites. The incidence of ALL appears to be highest in Hispanic children (Ries et al., 1999).

At presentation, a bone marrow evaluation and lumbar puncture are performed. The bone marrow is the diagnostic test to establish the diagnosis of leukemia and determine the subtype. The lumbar puncture is required for cytologic examination to determine whether there are leukemic cells in the cerebrospinal fluid (CSF) - CNS leukemia. CNS leukemia can occur through several mechanisms. The presence of leukemic cells in the CSF can arise from hematogenous spread of lymphoblasts in the peripheral blood or by direct extension from involved bone marrow into the CSF (Bleyer, 1989; Pinkel & Woo, 1977; Azzarelli & Roessmann, 1977). Bleyer reports that the hematogenous migration through venous endothelium into the CNS is influenced by factors such as lymphoblast count, thrombocytopenia and maturity of the blood-brain barrier. Direct extension occurs by the migration of leukemic cells from the involved skull bone marrow through the choroid plexus into the CSF. The lymphoblasts subsequently invade the cerebral parenchyma or enter the leptomeninges.

Examination of CSF to determine the presence of leukemic cells is an important factor in assigning CNS directed therapy for children with leukemia (Figure 1). The cells are spun in a process called cytocentrifugation which allows for the leukemic cells to be concentrated, increasing the sensitivity of diagnosis of CNS leukemia (Lauer et al., 1989). Table 1 outlines the National Cancer Institute (NCI) derived criteria for grading CNS involvement at diagnosis. CNS 1 status is defined as having no leukemic lymphoblasts in the CSF. CNS 2 is defined as having less than 5 WBC per mL and blasts on CSF cystopin. CNS 3 or overt CNS disease is defined as having more than 5 WBC per mL and CSF lymphoblasts (or with cranial nerve palsy). Approximately 3% of children have overt CNS leukemia (CNS 3) at presentation. Another 15% are CNS 2 status at diagnosis (Mahmoud et al., 1993; Burger et al., 2003). The NCI criteria for grading CNS involvement assumes that the CSF is not contaminated with peripheral blood contents by a traumatic or "bloody tap". However, if a patient has leukemic cells in the peripheral blood and the lumbar puncture is traumatic and contains ≥5/mL WBCs (white blood cells) and blasts, many protocols employ the Steinherz/Bleyer algorithm to distinguish between CNS 2 and CNS 3 disease:

CSF WBC/CSF RBC > 2X Blood WBC/Blood RBC

Thus, if the patient has blasts in the peripheral blood and the lumbar puncture is traumatic (containing ≥5/mL WBCs and blasts), CNS disease (CNS 3) is present if the CSF WBC/RBC is is greater than 2 times the blood WBC/RBC. For example, if a patient has a traumatic tap with the following laboratory values: CSF WBC = 70/mL; CSF RBC = 1400/mL; blood WBC = 4300/mL; blood RBC = 3.5 X 10^6/mL:

$$\frac{70}{1400} = 0.05 > 2X \frac{43000}{3.5 \times 10^6} = 0.012$$

In this example, the CSF WBC/RBC is 0.05, which is 2X greater than the blood WBC/RBC of 0.012. Thus, this patient would have CNS 3 status.

A study by Mahmoud, et al. noted specific characteristics in patients who presented at diagnosis with CNS leukemia. They found that patients with CNS leukemia at diagnosis were more likely to be less than one year of age and had a leukocyte count greater than 100 X 10^6/mL, an anterior mediastinal mass, a T-cell phenotype, or blast cells not expressing CD10 antigen (Mahmoud, 1993). Symptoms of CNS leukemia can vary. The majority of children with leukemia in the CSF are asymptomatic. The CSF pressure may be normal with no abnormalities of CSF chemistry. With overt CNS leukemia (CNS 3) or advanced disease, symptomatic patients can present with elevated CSF pressure and symptoms which include headache, vomiting, seizures, and irritability (Laningham et al., 2007). Patients with overt CNS disease can also experience cranial nerve palsies, which typically involve unilateral facial nerve (VII) palsy (Paryani et al., 1983).

Overt CNS leukemia (CNS 3) is present in about 3% of children at initial presentation (Mahmoud et al., 1993; Burger et al., 2003). CNS 3 is considered high risk and associated with a poorer event-free survival (Smith et al., 1996; Pui & Crist, 1994; Hammond et al., 1986). In one study, CNS 3 leukemia at diagnosis was an independent predictor of inferior event free survival (Pui et al., 2009). Approximately 15-20% patients with ALL have CNS 2 status. Controversy exists as to the significance of CNS 2 disease, in which the CSF WBC count is low (less than 5 WBCs per mL) with the presences of CSF blasts. The Children's Cancer Group found that CNS 2 status is of no prognostic significance (Gilchrist et al., 1994; Tubergen et al., 1994). However, other investigators contend that CNS 2 disease was associated with a higher rate of CNS relapse when compared to those with undetectable CSF lymphoblasts (CNS 1) (Mahmoud et al., 1993; Lauer et al., 1994).

2.2 Therapy for ALL

The treatment of childhood ALL begins with risk stratification based on clinical and laboratory features. Risk-based therapy is utilized so that children who have favorable features and more likely to have good outcome are spared the more intensive and potentially toxic therapy reserved for patients who are higher risk, who would otherwise have a poorer outcome without the aggressive treatment. Age and leukocyte count at diagnosis are the most important prognostic factors (Margolin & Poplack, 2006). Hyperleukocytosis is associated with a worse outcome. Approximately 20% of children with ALL have a leukocyte count of > 50 X 10^6/mL, which has been noted to have a poorer prognosis (Margolin & Poplack, 2006). Age at diagnosis also influences outcome: children whose age at diagnosis is < 2 years or older than 10 years have a worse prognosis than those in the intermediate age group (Sather, 1986). In particular, infants with ALL aged < 12 months fared the worst (Kosaka et al., 2004). The identification of cytogenetic abnormalities also has important prognostic implications. In general, for patients with B-cell precursor ALL, favorable cytogenetic prognostic factors include hyperdiploidy (having more than 50 chromosomes per leukemia cells), TEL-AML1 fusion gene, and double trisomies 4 and 10. Cytogenetic prognostic markers which confer a less favorable outcome include hypodiploidy (fewer than 45 chromosomes, t(4;11) with the MLL-Af4 fusion gene which is seen 50% of cases of infant ALL, and t(9;22) with BCR-ABL fusion, also known as the Philadelphia chromosome (Margolin & Poplack, 2006). In recent years, minimal residual disease (MRD), which allows for detection of the smallest amount of leukemic cells during treatment, has also been recognized as an important prognostic factor (Borowitz et al., 2003). MRD assays which are most useful are those based on polymerase chain reaction (PCR) amplification of antigen-receptor genes, and on flow cytometric detection of abnormal immunophenotypes. Higher levels of MRD have been associated with greater risk for relapse.

Specific treatment regimens for ALL vary, but all essentially emphasize several components: remission induction, CNS preventive therapy, consolidation, and maintenance or continuation therapy. CNS preventative therapy starts early and will be discussed in a different section in this chapter. All treatment starts with induction therapy over 4 to 6 weeks. The goal of induction is to achieve remission by eliminating more than 99% of the initial leukemic burden and restoring normal hematopoiesis. Approximate 98% of patients achieve remission by the end of induction (Pui & Evans, 2006). During induction, patients receive a three-drug therapy which includes vincristine, corticosteroids (prednisone or dexamethasone), and L-asparaginase in conjunction with intrathecal chemotherapy. Children with high risk features receive daunorubicin in addition to the three-drug combination. This four-drug induction chemotherapy, along with intensive consolidation and maintenance has improved survival for even high-risk patients (Gaynon et al., 1988). Current regimens favor the use of dexamethasone over the use of prednisone during induction and later phases of therapy. Various trials have demonstrated that dexamethasone is associated with better overall survival when compared to prednisone or prednisolone (Bostrom et al., 2003; Mitchell et al., 2005). Due to its longer half-life and better CNS penetration, dexamethasone appears to provide better CNS and systemic control than prednisone (Bostrom et al., 2003).

Consolidation is a course of intensified treatment that follows remission induction. High-dose methotrexate with mercaptopurine, high dose asparaginase and reinduction treatment are some commonly used regimens during consolidation (Pui & Evans, 2006). Intensive post-induction treatment with L-asparaginase has led to improved outcome (Margolin & Poplack, 2006). Several forms of L-asparaginase are available for use in the treatment of ALL, however, the dose and duration of treatment is more important than the form of L-asparaginase used (Pui & Evans, 2006). Maintenance or continuation therapy is the last phase of treatment. Maintenance entails a combination of monthly vincristine in combination with corticosteroids, oral Mercaptopurine (6-MP) and methotrexate (MTX) and intrathecal methotrexate every 3 months. The combination of 6-MP and MTX administered continuously in varying schedules is the principal component of maintenance therapy. MTX has been found to have optimal effect when it is administered weekly, whereas 6-MP is most efficacious when administered daily in the evening.

The adaptation of pediatric protocols to the treatment of adult ALL has led to improved outcomes, but there is still a significant gap in the success rate between the two age groups. Treatment of ALL in adults remains a major challenge with overall survival rates limited to 30–40% (Narayanan, 2011).

2.3 Therapy for CNS involvement

2.3.1 Systemic chemotherapy

Effective systemic chemotherapy has shown to improve control of CNS leukemia. Many current trials use high dose methotrexate (5 gram/m^2) as compared to the lower dose (0.5 to 1 gram/m^2) administered in the past. Other agents able to penetrate the blood brain barrier and hence provide good CNS control include dexamethasone due to its longer half-life and low protein binding as previously mentioned. Results from the Children's Oncology Group (COG) have also shown that thioguanine at high doses provides effective systemic and CNS therapy (Stork et al., 2002).

2.3.2 Intrathecal chemotherapy

Intrathecal chemotherapy is an essential component of therapy for patients with clinically evident CNS disease (CNS 3). The three chemotherapeutic agents used most commonly through the intrathecal route are methotrexate, cytarabine and hydrocortisone. Methotrexate was the first to be administered through the intrathecal method. It is dosed by age, rather than weight. Some trials use triple intrathecals (methotrexate, cytarabine and hydrocortisone) or "IT triples". This arose from a study by the Pediatric Oncology Group which reported that the outcome for standard risk patients given IT triples was equivalent to those who received cranial radiation (Sullivan et al., 1982). Regardless of the chemotherapeutic agent selected for the intrathecal route, attention should be given to the dose to maximize therapeutic concentrations. Due to the anatomy of the brain and ventricles, only a small percentage of chemotherapy actually reaches the lateral ventricles. Several steps can optimize the therapeutic concentrations of chemotherapy in the ventricles. After a patient is infused with intrathecal chemotherapy, they should remain in the prone position for at least 30 minutes. This assists gravity in moving the chemotherapy to ventricles. Although intrathecal chemotherapy, particularly methotrexate, has improved outcome, it has produced a wide spectrum of acute and chronic neurotoxic sequelae, which will be discussed further in this chapter.

2.3.3 Cranial Irradiation

Aside from systemic and intrathecal chemotherapy, cranial irradiation is still recommended for patients who are CNS 3 at diagnosis. Cranial irradiation has replaced craniospinal irradiation. This shift is due to the fact that there is lack of evidence of the superior efficacy with craniospinal irradiation, along with the increased toxicity associated with spinal irradiation, including excessive myelosuppression, retardation of spinal growth and cardiac toxicity (Margolin & Poplack, 2006). In the COG trials (AALL0232, AALL0932, AALL0331) for patients who are CNS 3 at diagnosis, cranial radiation is given after successful induction of bone marrow remission. The dose of cranial irradiation is 18Gy (1800 cGy), which is administered in 10 daily fractions of 180 cGy per fraction to equal a total dose of 1800 cGy. The target volume consists of the entire brain and meninges. Although cranial irradiation is less toxic than craniospinal irradiation, its administration is not without short and long-term side effects. Many of these complications, which will be discussed in detail, include second malignancies, endocrinopathies, and neurocognitive deficits.

2.4 CNS relapse and risk factors

Decades ago, during the early years of treatment, survival was poor. However, in the 1960's, CNS relapse rose dramatically. Several investigators, including the Children's Cancer Group concluded that this rise was due to improved therapy leading to longer periods of remission and survival (Evans et al., 1970). Additionally, the CNS was the most common site of extramedullary relapse. With current treatment regimens, isolated CNS relapse has been reduced to <5% of pediatric cases of ALL (Laningham et al., 2007; Reiter et al., 1994). CNS relapse accounts for approximately 30-40% initial relapses (Henze et al., 1991; Roy et al., 2005; Gaynon et al., 1998). CNS relapses can occur isolated, or in combination with bone marrow relapse.

The clinical impact and prognosis of CNS relapse is significant due to two factors. CNS leukemia is challenging to treat and CNS relapse eventually leads to bone marrow relapse. The Children's Oncology Group found that children with standard risk ALL who relapsed had better overall survival (OS) if they had isolated CNS relapse rather than combined relapse of CNS and bone marrow involvement (Malempati et al., 2007). Current protocols incorporate therapy to prevent CNS relapse. Intrathecal chemotherapy and intensification of systemic chemotherapy has largely replaced cranial radiation for prophylaxis of CNS relapse. These measures have successfully reduced the rate of CNS relapse. For the <5% of CNS relapses that occur, it is not completely clear why such relapses occur.

There are, however, several factors that can increase the risk of CNS relapse. Patients with hyperleukocytosis, T- cell ALL, Philadelphia chromosome, t(4,11) and the presence of leukemic cells in the CSF have been noted to have a greater risk of CNS relapse. Those with hyperleukocytosis in which the presenting white blood cell (WBC) is greater than 100 X 10^6/L and patients diagnosed with T-cell ALL were found to have the highest risk for CNS relapse. These subgroups of patients receive CNS-directed therapy which includes cranial radiation, along with intrathecal and systemic chemotherapy. High risk groups with cytogenetic abnormalities who are also at a greater risk for CNS relapse include ALL patients positive for Philadelphia chromosome (which produces a translation in chromosome 9 and 22) and those with t(4,11) (Pui, 2006). Approximately 50% of infants with ALL have the translocation in chromosome 4 and 11, also referred to as MLL gene rearrangement. Infant ALL with t(4,11) carries a poor prognosis. Iatrogenic introduction of peripheral blasts into the CSF also has the potential to increase CNS relapse. Thus, it is especially important to prevent a traumatic lumbar puncture at diagnosis, when circulating leukemic blasts are most abundant (Figure 2). Various studies have shown that a traumatic lumbar puncture is a risk factor for later CNS relapse and results in worse event-free survival due to iatrogenic introduction of blasts from the peripheral blood into the CSF (Burger et al., 2003; Gajjar et al., 2000; te Loo et al., 2006). Thus, lumbar punctures should be routinely performed by the most experienced clinician in the center. Other measures to minimize "bloody taps" include effective sedation/anesthesia to keep the patient still during the procedure and adequate correction of thrombocytopenia and coagulopathy prior to the diagnostic lumbar puncture.

3. Arguments for CNS prophylaxis in ALL

CNS prophylaxis therapy is based on the premises that the CNS is a sanctuary for leukemic cells, which are undetected at diagnosis and are protected by the blood brain barrier from systemically administered chemotherapy (Margolin & Poplack, 2006). The overall survival of pediatric ALL has significantly improved due to risk based therapy and CNS-directly therapy, with standard-risk ALL patients having a disease free survival rate of more than 90% in the United States and other developed nations (Schrappe et al., 2010). Though the CNS remains the most common site of extramedullary relapse, after intensive treatment less than 5% of patients with ALL will have CNS relapse (Laningham, 2007; Reiter, 1994).

CNS leukemia poses a challenge for treatment success and has a far worse prognosis. Thus, current treatment regimens continue to incorporate therapy directed at preventing CNS relapse. CNS prophylaxis can be achieved by combinations of high dose systemic chemotherapy, intrathecal chemotherapy, and cranial or craniospinal radiation (Schrappe et al., 2010).

Effective CNS prophylactic regimens have resulted in a significant reduction in the incidence of CNS leukemia. In the 1970's, the first report was published which showed that the administration of intrathecal methotrexate with high dose cranial or cranial spinal radiation alone could improve the rate of CNS relapse from 50% to close to 10% (Aur et al., 1972). Investigators used either 24 Gy of cranial irradiation with serial doses of intrathecal methotrexate, or administered 24 Gy of cranial spinal irradiation alone. By the late 1970's , it became clear that although effective in improving CNS relapse, the intensive dose given in CNS-directed therapy caused significant acute and long term complications (Pizzo et al., 1979). This led to changes in therapy which eventually omitted craniospinal radiation altogether and reduced the prophylactic dose of cranial radiation from 24 Gy to 18 Gy as such changes were shown to be just as efficacious in preventing CNS relapse (Nesbit et al., 1981). In the mid -1990's, a trial conducted by BFM group showed that a reduced prophylactic dose of 12 Gy rather than 18 Gy provided effective CNS prophylaxis for high risk ALL (Schrappe et al., 2000). Despite the reduction in prophylactic cranial irradiation in contemporary regimens, the lower 12 Gy dose still results in substantial acute and subacute toxicities such as seizures, strokes, encephalopathies and late complications such as neurocognitive changes and second neoplasms. This has led to trials that have omitted cranial radiation for all patients. Trials by the St. Jude Children's Research Hospital and the Dutch Childhood Oncology Group report a good outcome for patients treated with high doses of intrathecal methotrexate post induction and increased frequency of triple intrathecal chemotherapy (methotrexate, cytarabine, hydrocortisone) with frequent vincristine/dexamethasone pulses (Pui et al., 2009 ; Verman, et al., 2009). It is important to mention that the prognosis of children with ALL living in less affluent nations-such as India (Arya et al., 2010) is different, even when the same radiation and chemotherapy protocols are used-with a CNS relapse rate of approximate 4%. Though much of the difference is probably attributable to the local conditions-such as poverty, illiteracy, inadequate facilities and therapy abandon, the remaining questions of different biological characteristics in different ethnic populations remains to be answered.

4. Cranial Irradiation for CNS prophylaxis

Although cranial radiation is an effective means of preventing CNS relapse for childhood ALL, its toxicity limits its use to a select group of patients. Only those who are considered high risk receive cranial irradiation for CNS prophylaxis. This subgroup of high risk patients include those who have T-cell ALL, have a high WBC at diagnosis (WBC ≥ 50,000/mL), were pre-treated with steroids within the week of diagnosis, and patients with certain cytogenetic abnormalities such as MLL rearrangements. Most current regimens do not administer cranial irradiation to infants or very young children, even if they are high risk (Pieters et al., 2007). Further, a review of 43 randomized trials reported that cranial irradiation is also not a necessary component of therapy for standard risk ALL (Clarke et al., 2003). For the high risk patients receiving CNS-directed therapy, cranial irradiation is initiated after patients have achieved bone marrow remission. It is generally administered during intensified consolidation. The prophylactic dose of cranial irradiation is 12 Gy (1200 cGy), given in 8 daily fractions of 150 cGy per fraction. The area that is targeted consists of the entire brain and meninges, including frontal lobe as well as the posterior halves of the globes of eyes, optic disk and optic nerve.

5. Chemotherapy for CNS prophylaxis

Chemotherapy for CNS prophylaxis is delivered both systemically and intrathecally. All regimens for childhood ALL include either intrathecal methotrexate or triple IT (methotrexate with cytarabine and hydrocortisone). The dose of intrathecal methotrexate is based on age. For example, in the COG trials for ALL, the dose of intrathecal methotrexate is 8 mg, 10 mg, 12 mg, and 15 mg for children ages 1 to 1.99, 2 to 2.99, 3 to 8.99, and 9 years or greater, respectively. Similarly, the dose for intrathecal cytarabine is also age based: 30 mg, 50 mg, and 70 mg are administered for children ages 1 to 1.99, 2 to 2.99, 3 years or older, respectively. Intrathecal chemotherapy is initiated on the first day of induction therapy, in which three doses are given during the first four weeks of induction. Intrathecal chemotherapy is intensified during consolidation (approximately four to eight doses every two to three weeks). It is continued during maintenance, in which one dose of intrathecal chemotherapy is given every three months.

Systemic chemotherapy is also an important component of CNS prophylaxis. Systemically administered chemotherapy agents which provide effective CNS prophylaxis include dexamethasone, L-asparaginase, and high dose methotrexate with leucovorin rescue. All patients receive corticosteroid and L-asparaginase. Dexamethasone has become the corticosteroid of choice and is initiated during induction chemotherapy and continued during consolidation and maintenance. Depending on the regimen and the phase of treatment, the dose of dexamethasone varies. For example, during induction, the dose of dexamethasone can range as high as 10 mg/m2/day for high risk patients to a lower dose of 6mg/m2/day for standard risk patients. L-asparaginase is also initiated with induction chemotherapy and continues during intensified consolidation, although it is not included in most maintenance regimens. The dose is 2500 International units/m2/dose and it can be given intramuscularly or intravenously. High dose methotrexate is recommended for patients who are considered high risk. This includes patients with T-cell ALL, hyperleukocytosis with WBC ≥ 50,000/mL, aged 10 or older, received prior steroid therapy, or have testicular leukemia involvement at diagnosis. The dose of high dose methotrexate is 5 gm/m2/dose and is administered in conjunction with leucovorin rescue. It is administered during intensified consolidation in which four doses are given biweekly.

CNS Status	Lymphoblasts in CSF	WBC count (cells/mL)
CNS 1:	0	
CNS 2:	Present	<5
CNS 3:	Present	>/5 (or cranial nerve palsy)

Table 1. Definitions of CNS Disease at Diagnosis

Targeted therapies have not been used until recently in the treatment of ALL. However, most of the small-molecule tyrosine kinase inhibitors have excellent CNS entrance and a better safety profile, which makes them excellent candidates for CNS prophylaxis. The Children Oncology Group study of Imatinib treatment in children with Philadelphia chromosome-positive ALL reports outstanding early outcomes for patients treated with Imatinib and intensive chemotherapy (Schultz, 2009). Longer follow-up is needed to confirm if this treatment also improves overall survival in these children who usually have poor outcomes.

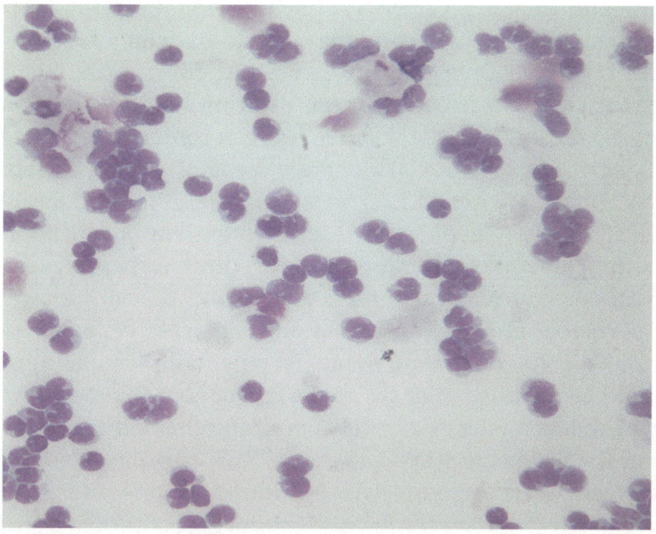

Fig. 1. CSF involvement in acute lymphoblastic leukemia. There are five or more white blood cells/mL with lymphoblasts. This appearance indicates CN S3 status (Wright-Giemsa stain; original magnification × 40, oil immersion) (Courtesy of Sachiv Sheth MD, CHOC Children's Hospital)

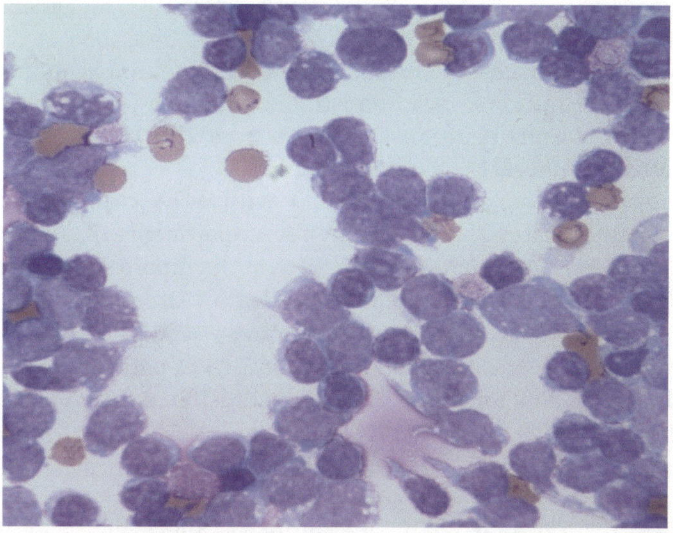

Fig. 2. CSF with lymphoblasts and RBC's due to a traumatic lumbar puncture (Wright-Giemsa stain; original magnification × 100, oil immersion) (Courtesy of Aaron Sasson MD, CHOC Children's Hospital)

6. Acute and sub-acute CNS complications after ALL treatment

6.1 Posterior Reversible Encephalopathy Syndrome (PRES)

PRES is defined by the clinical presentation of seizures, headaches, altered mental status and visual impairment. The imaging correlative is transient, bilateral lesions on T2/FLAIR sequences of MRI, predominantly affecting the occipito-parietal lobes. More than 40 cases of children with ALL who have developed PRES are described in the literature (Panis et al., 2010). Majority of the cases described happened during the induction phase (Gupta et al., 2008). Hypertension was one of the factors most commonly associated with PRES in children with ALL, however, in about 20% of the patients the blood pressure stayed normal.

PRES treatment in children with ALL is mostly supportive, and includes anti-epileptic medications (AEDs) for seizures, and antihypertensive medications (beta-blockers, angiotensin converting enzyme inhibitors and/or diuretics). (Panis et al., 2010). Most patients recover without neurological complications, and do not require long-term AEDs, but rare cases of persistent epilepsy and even only one case of death have been reported (Hourani et al., 2008). As treatment delay is potentially lethal in ALL patients, the chemotherapy should be resumed after the resolution of neurological symptoms.

Since the majority of children with ALL receive multiple chemotherapeutic agents, it is hard to identify which of the drugs are responsible for PRES. However, multiple reports suggest an association between L-asparaginase (ASP) administrations and PRES (Kieslich et al., 2003). ASP is well-known to inhibit the hepatic production of proteins such as antithrombin and fibrinogen, and hence has the potential to induce transient thrombotic events which might contribute to the PRES etiology (Pound 2007).

6.2 Methotrexate toxicity: Leukoencephalopathy (Acute confusion, Seizures, Encephalopathy)

Methtrexate (MTX) is a folate antagonist widely used in the treatment of ALL . It inhibits methionine synthesis, an important metabolite necessary for CNS myelination (Linnebank et al., 2005), (Winick et al., 1992). CNS complications were described at different stages of treatment (such as acute, subacute or chronic). Acute MTX neurotoxicity ranges from 3–10% and varies with the dose and route of administration (Mahoney et al., 1998). The time from induction to the onset of acute neurotoxicity varies from 2 to 127 weeks and is more often seen 10–11 days after intrathecal MTX induction therapy.

Some of the neurological symptoms associated with MTX include headaches, nausea, emesis, lethargy, mental status changes, cognitive impairments, Kluver- Bucy syndrome, blurred vision, aphasia, transient or persistent hemiparesis, seizures, choreiform movements, arachnoiditis, encephalomyelitis, and death (Atra et al., 2004), (Antunes et al., 2002), (Asato et al., 1992), (Brock and Jennings, 2004), (Rubnitz et al., 1998). Leukoencephalopathy has been observed in less than 10% of patients after intravenous MTX administration, and up to 40% following intrathecal infusion (Atra et al., 2004), (Mahoney et al., 1998), (Rubnitz et al., 1998), (Lai et al., 2004).

The biological bases of MTX-induced neurotoxicity remain unclear. Various factors have been suggested for the effects of MTX such as: direct toxic effect on myelin, inhibition of glucose metabolism (Quinn et al., 2004), (Quinn et al., 1997), injury to oligodendrocytes, with disruption of myelin synthesis, disruption of mitochondrial energy metabolism resulting in oxidative stress and increased vulnerability of neurons to physiological glutamate concentrations (Rzeski et al., 2004), breakdown of the blood–brain barrier (Lai et al., 2004) and inhibition of the enzyme dihydrofolate reductase, preventing the conversion of folic acid to tetrahydrofolic acid, thereby increasing the levels of homocysteine and excitotoxic neurotransmitters and inhibiting cell replication (Quinn et al., 2004), (Quinn et al., 1997).

Diagnostic Tests	**Reported Results**
CSF Analysis	Normal or sterile pleocytosis
MRI	White matter abnormalities (usually transient) Microcalcifications
EEG	Focal or diffuse slowing Epileptiform activities
Magnetic Resonance Spectroscopy	Metabolite changes

Table 2. Diagnostic Tests in Suspected Cases of Methotrexate Neurotoxicity

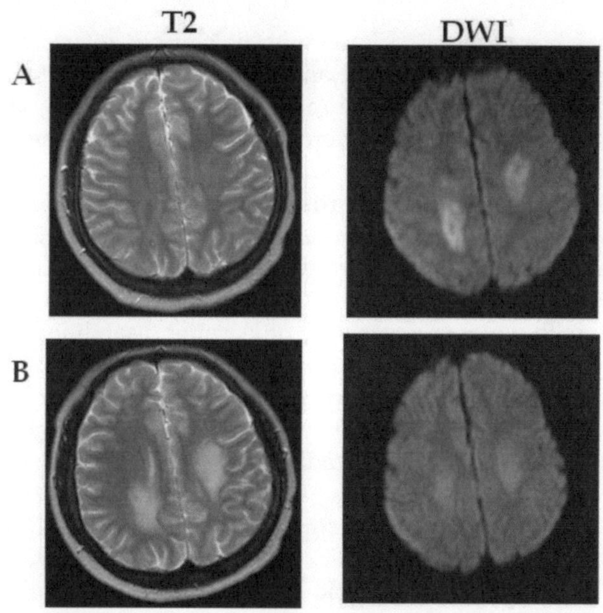

Fig. 3. Brain MRI in a patient with acute MTX toxicity. A. At time of initial diagnosis, hyperdense lesions are noted bilaterally on DWI in the centrum semiovale. B. Two months later. The patient's symptoms (seizures, paralysis) resolved.

MTX neurotoxicity is in the differential diagnosis for any ALL patient with acute neurologic findings and previously treated with the folate antagonist (see Table 2). In this population, CSF analysis is usually unremarkable (Table 3). Electroencephalographic findings are usually non-specific. Acutely, MRI-DW studies show white matter changes that are probably due to demyelination (Rollins et al., 2004), (Ebner et al., 1989), (Sandoval et al., 2003). Magnetic resonance spectroscopy may demonstrate metabolite changes in the absence of structural white matter abnormalities (Davidson et al., 2000).

The treatment of acute MTX toxicity is still under research (Bota and Dafer, 2009). MTX neurotoxicity was reported to be reversible with administration of dexamethasone and leucovorin (Shuper et al., 2000), (Cohen, 2004). Leucovorin antagonizes the effects of MTX on purine metabolism through maintenance of DNA/RNA synthesis, despite the blockade of dihydrofolatereductase. Significant improvement of neurological symptoms has also been achieved with combined administration of aminophylline - an adenosine antagonist - and high-dose folinic acid (Jaksic et al., 2004). Whether glutamate antagonists could prevent neurotoxicity of MTX when given with cancer chemotherapy remains to be determined (Murphy et al., 1999).

7. Long-term CNS complications after ALL treatment

7.1 Neurocognitive complications

As the number of long-term ALL survivors is progressively increasing, more and more attention is drawn to their long-term cognitive effects and to the quality of life. As majority of the patients are diagnoses during early childhood, the neurodevelopmental sequelae are mostly the effects of CNS-directed therapies on the developing brain (Temming and Jenney, 2010).

Cranial radiation has been long associated with deleterious effects on cognitive function-especially on verbal intelligence quotient and achievement tests of reading, spelling, and arithmetic, directly proportional with the radiation dose (Moore et al., 1991). Though the results of neurocognitive outcomes are heterogenous, a large meta-analysis has shown that, when measured across 30 comparisons in 20 different studies, an average intellectual quotient (IQ) decrement of about two-thirds of a standard deviation, or about 10 points, follows CNS prophylaxis that includes cranial irradiation (Cousens, 2006). The results of the meta-analysis also showed that children irradiated at a younger age (younger than four) are more seriously affected than older children. Girls also tend to be more affected by the CNS radiation treatment, with a higher prevalence of learning disabilities and lower IQs (Waber et al., 1990). Usually, cranial radiation is administered in combination with intrathecal MTX, which has potential additional neurotoxicities, especially in girls-with a demonstrated decreased intelligence quotient (IQ estimate, 9.3 points) when high-dose MTX (4 g/m^2) during induction was followed by cranial radiation (Waber 1995).

Chemotherapeutic prophylaxis has less deleterious effects in absence of radiation (Krappmann et al., 2007), with a slight but significant decline of the IQ score only in younger children and girls.

Another potential risk factor is allogeneic hematopoietic stem cell transplantation-with significant deficits immediately after transplantation (Syrjala 2011). Although neurocognitive function improved from 1 to 5 years after transplantation, deficits remained for more than 40% of survivors, especially in motor dexterity and verbal learning and retention.

Neuroimaging structural changes in the executive areas of the brains of ALL survivors are also well described-and between 16% and 52% of those who have received treatment for ALL experience at least one brain abnormality (Porto 2004). Additionally, ALL survivors displayed significant abnormalities in functional imaging, with greater activation in areas underlying working memory (dorsolateral and ventrolateral prefrontal cortex) and error monitoring (dorsal and ventral anterior cingulate cortex), which correlate with poor performance on working memory tasks (Fuller et al., 2009).

7.2 Behavioral disturbances and Attention deficit syndromes

As mentioned in the previous paragraphs, neuro-cognitive impairments are widely present in the ALL survivors. In addition, many survivors also have multiple behavioral symptoms suggestive of attention deficit/hyperactivity disorder (ADHD) (Krull et al., 2011). These abnormalities are assessed by behavioral ratings- especially from the family and classroom teachers. A recent survey of the parents of adolescent cancer survivors (almost 50% of them had leukemia) and their healthy siblings identified that the ALL survivors had significantly higher rates of parent- reported attention deficits, as well as of depression/anxiety and antisocial domains (Schultz, JCO 2007). More than one half of survivors (54%) received intrathecal methotrexate, cranial radiation, or both and treatments with cranial radiation and/or intrathecal methotrexate were specific risk factors for depression/anxiety, attention deficit, antisocial behaviors, and diminished social competence.

Attention problems are commonly reported in these patients (up to 25.5% of the survivors), but the rate of patients meeting the full criteria for ADHD is only of 10.5%- just slightly higher than the reported rate in the general population (Krull et al., 2011). Also, similar rates of ADHD were seen in boys and girls, and especially in the patients that have received cranial radiation therapy. Most of the patients had more inattention as compared with the general population (where hyperactive and impulsive behaviors are more common) which suggests that the cancer survivors might have a different phenotypic ADHD. One hypothesis is that attention difficulties in ALL survivors may be related to genetic variations such as polymorphisms of the folate pathway rather than dopamine transport or reuptake, as suspected in developmental ADHD (Krull et al., 2008).

The treatment of attention problems encountered by survivors of ALL is open for debate. A prospective, placebo-controlled, crossover trial of medications (methylphenidate) was successful in a significant number of the patients (45%) (Conklin et al., 2010), however the percentage of responders is much lower than the one reported in general ADHD population (75%) (Greenhill et al., 2001). Alternatively, a pilot study of computerized cognitive treatment suggests some benefit, but larger studies are needed to confirm clinical value (Hardy et al., 2011).

7.3 Cerebrovascular disease

As previously mentioned, radiation therapy had a major effect in improving the survival of ALL patients. However, the normal tissue damage associated with CNS radiation can be profound, and is not limited to the neural cells. The vascular response to radiation includes arteries of all calibers (small, medium and large), and can occur either acutely or as late as many years after the initial treatment (Morris et al., 2009). As such, the ALL survivors have a high risk of developing intracranial steno-occlusive disease (moyamoya disease) as well as vascular malformations (telengiectasias, cavernomas and rarely aneurysms).

Moyamoya disease is commonly seen in Asian populations and children. The Tokyo Children's Cancer Study Group reported the largest series of ALL patients evaluated for moyamoya, and found a cumulative incidence of moyamoya disease of 0.46% at 8 years-20 fold higher that the incidence in general Japanese population. None of the six patients with moyamoya had CNS involvement at the initial ALL diagnosis, and all of them received prophylactic cranial irradiation (Kikuchi et al., 2007). Majority of the children (4/6) improved after surgical revascularization, while one child died of extensive strokes before the procedure could be attempted.

Telengiectasias are the most commonly described vascular malformations in ALL survivors (Morris et al., 2009). The rate of telengiectasia was reported for the leukemia survivors to be 16%, in spite of the fact that almost all patients received only 18 Grays. The majority of the lesions were small, and the patients tended to remain asymptomatic during the duration of the study (five years) (Koike, 2003).

A study of long-term survivors of childhood tumors reported that the rate of strokes for leukemia survivors was 57.9 per 100,000 person-years (95% CI, 41.2 to 78.7), and the relative risk rate of stroke for leukemia survivors compared with the sibling comparison group was 6.4 (95% CI, 3.0 to 13.8; P < .0001) (Bowers 2006). Mean cranial radiation therapy dose of > or = 30 Gy was associated with an increased risk of stokes in a dose-dependent fashion. This increased incidence of strokes might be caused not only by the radiation-induced vascular damage but also by the high rate of metabolic abnormalities such as obesity, insulin resistance and low high-density lipoprotein levels seen in adult survivors of childhood leukemia (Talvensaari et al., 1996). The highest at-risk population is represented by the patients that have received hematopoietic stem cell transplantation with total body irradiation, and who had a very high rate of hypertriglyceridemia, low level of high-density lipoprotein cholesterol, and elevated fasting glucose (Oudin, 2011).

7.4 Secondary CNS malignancies: Meningiomas and gliomas

Cranial tumors following high-dose CNS radiation for childhood ALL have been reported initially (Tiberin et al, 1984a; Tiberin et al. 1984b). The cumulative rate of a secondary brain tumor is about 18-20% (Pui, Goshen), with the most common tumors being overwhelmingly meningioma, and less commonly gliomas.

A retrospective study of the ALL patients treated with radiation between 1974 -1989 at the Schneider Children's Medical Center of Israel determined that 18 out of 88 survivors developed meningiomas (Goshen et al., 2007). The initial diagnosis of ALL was made 10-29 years earlier, with a median interval of 21 years, and the rate of meningiomas considerably increased after 15 years from therapy. There was no female predominance- as is usually seen in the general population, and all of the meningiomas discovered were WHO grade I. One additional case of low-grade glioma was also identified.

Though the gliomas are rarer, they are a serious cause of concern in survivors of childhood cancer. The results from the British Childhood Cancer indicate that the 5 year relative survival for these patients is very poor-only 19.5%. The interval between the childhood cancer and glioma development was 15.5 years for the low-grade gliomas, 18.7 years for the anaplastic gliomas and 21 years for glioblastoma multiforme (Taylor et al., 2009). The long-term results of the Tokyo Children's Cancer Study group trials for ALL identified secondary brain tumors (gliomas) in 12 out of 1846 patients (Tsuchida et al., 2010). All the patients received cranial radiotherapy as part of their treatment, and the secondary tumors developed after 8-22 years after the initial treatment. There was an equal sex distribution. The cumulative incidence was 1.9% at 15 years, and 2.8% at 20 years. These numbers are very similar with the St Jude report of a cumulative incidence of brain tumors except meningioma of 3% at 30 years (Hijiya et al., 2007). Majority of radiation-induced gliomas are of astrocytic origin (Walter et al., 1998), however a few low grade and anaplastic oligodendrogliomas are also reported (Alexiou et al., 2010). These patients received standard treatment with focal brain radiation (50 Gray), followed by PCV chemotherapy. In patients with relapsed ALL, the rate of secondary CNS malignancies (glial in origin) was very low-2 out of 1376 patients, in spite of intensive second-line treatment. In general, the rate of secondary malignancy was found to be significantly associated with stem cell transplantation, and high cumulative doses of cranial irradiation, etoposide and cyclophosphamide-however the numbers are too small to conclude for CNS malignancies (Borgmann et al., 2008).

The use of intrathecal and systemic chemotherapy instead of cranial radiation has led to a reduced rate of secondary CNS tumors. The just-published results of the EORTC 58881 trial which did not include cranial radiotherapy showed a very low rate of secondary malignancies, with only one patient out of 2,261 enrolled being diagnosed with glioblastoma multiforme (Renard et al., 2011).

Our own experience at the UC Irvine Chao Cancer Center and the Children Hospital of Orange County is that often the secondary meningiomas in ALL survivors are atypical or anaplastic (see figure 4). The treatment of these patients is very difficult due to the fact that they have already received brain radiation, which is the standard of care and the only proven treatment for malignant meningiomas. Early diagnosis of secondary brain tumors allows for surgical approaches before the tumors become symptomatic. As the ALL patients live longer, a yearly neurological exam and periodic brain MRI's in search for intracranial lesions should be considered for those who received cranial or craniospinal radiation.

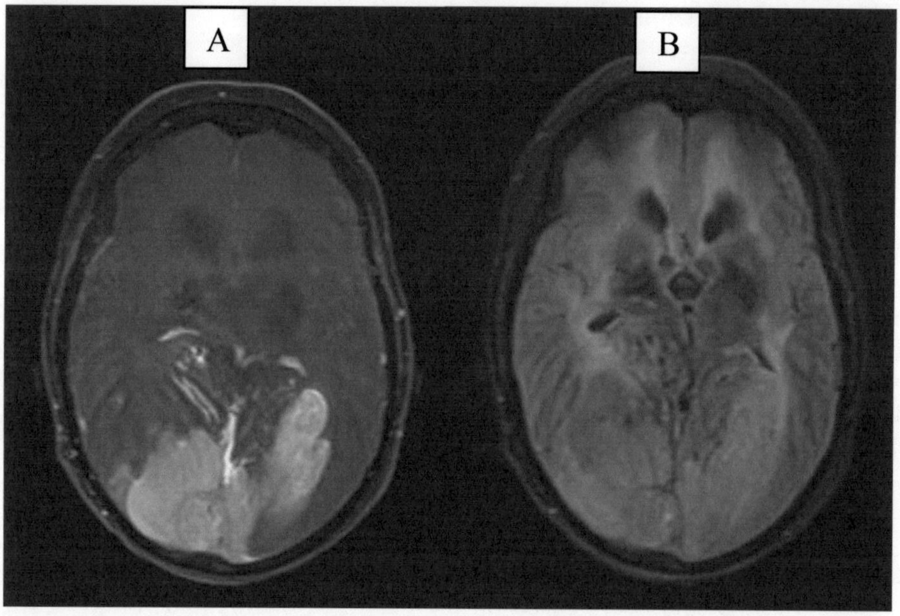

Fig. 4. Brain MRI in a patient with multiple malignant meningiomas and brain atrophy. The patient has received cranial radiation for ALL 18 years prior to the initial meningioma diagnosis.

8. Further directions: Neuroprotective and restorative treatments

The long-term implications of CNS-directed treatment in the life of ALL patients are very profound. A long-term study (twenty-five year follow-up) reported more adverse general and mental health, functional impairment, and activity limitations in ALL survivors compared with siblings. Rates of marriage, college graduation, employment, and health insurance were also all lower compared with sibling controls (Mody R, 2008). Hence, modalities to either limit the CNS toxicities or to restore the lost function have the potential to significantly improve the long-term outcome.

Radiation is well-known to affect different brain structures, including the neural stem cells as well as the glial and vascular (Sundgren and Cao, 2009), (Acharya et al., 2010). In addition, majority of the chemotherapeutics used for ALL treatments have numerous effects on the brain, increasing the oxidative stress, reducing neurogenesis, affecting the blood flow and generating white matter damage (Seigers and Fardell, 2011). Previous research has shown that some chemotherapy drugs including cytosine arabinoside as well as radiation (Monje et al., 2002) are toxic at therapeutic doses for the neural stem/progenitor cells (Seigers et al., 2008).

There are very few studies looking at the cognitive consequences of chemotherapeutic agents in animal models (Seigers et al., 2008), (Foley et al., 2008), (Winocur et al., 2006), (Reiriz et al., 2006), (Lee et al., 2006), (Macleod et al., 2007). Single dose administration of methotrexate impairs spatial memory, prolonging latency to finding the platform in the Morris water maze test, and impairing the novel object recognition (Seigers et al., 2008), hence suggesting hippocampal damage. Administration of multiple doses of methotrexate causes deficits in spatial and non-spatial memory, showing the importance of studying the effects of chronic chemotherapy (Winocur et al., 2006).

Hippocampal dedritic spine damage is found after single-dose administration of cyclophosphamide in hippocampal slices, and causes transient impairment of long-term potentiation (Lee et al., 2006). Clinically, reduced hippocampal volume and loss of neurogenesis have been found in chemotherapy treated colon cancer patients (Schneiderman, 2004) and brain tumor patients[37], respectively, though no clear changes were found in ALL survivors (Hill et al., 2004). However, the attention and memory deficits present in ALL patients might suggest a functional deficit even if no structural changes are clearly defined.

Limiting the toxicity of presently-used regimens is a subject of intense research. Elimination of radiation has played a significant role in limiting toxicity. Developing active chemotherapy agents that can limit CNS toxicity while still offering low-rates of CNS relapse will constitute the next step. Our recently-published work (Bota 2009) suggests that pathway targeted agents (such as tyrosine kinase inhibitors or proteasome inhibitors) might have *in vitro* a more favorable, neural stem-cell sparing profile than the classic DNA-targeted agents.

Reversal of neuropsychological late effects has been attempted through cognitive remediation, and ecological manipulations of the classroom environment (Mulhern and Butler, 2004). These methods are based on the treatment of traumatic brain injuries, and have moderate success in the treatment of ALL survivors (Butler et al., 2008). Specific modalities using computer-based cognitive training, which could be used at home by the patients in more remote communities, has the potential to improve working memory and decrease parent-rated attention problems and to bring further promise for ALL patients (Hardy et al., 2011).

Finally, medications that can either increase patient attention and concentration (based on the promising methylphenidate studies) or reverse the CAN damage (such as medication which can stimulate neurogenesis) should be further researched and better understood.

9. Acknowledgements

This book chapter is written in memory of our former patient and friend, Ms. Kimberly Hill who has survived childhood ALL, and played a major role in the building of the Ronald McDonald Houses. She has ultimately died this year due to the long-term neurologic complications of ALL treatment.

10. References

Acharya, M.M., Lan, M.L., Kan, V.H., Patel, N.H., Giedzinski, E., Tseng, B.P., and Limoli, C.L. (2010). Consequences of ionizing radiation-induced damage in human neural stem cells. Free Radic Biol Med *49*, 1846-1855.

Alexiou, G.A., Moschovi, M., Georgoulis, G., Neroutsou, R., Stefanaki, K., Sfakianos, G., and Prodromou, N. (2010). Anaplastic oligodendrogliomas after treatment of acute lymphoblastic leukemia in children: report of 2 cases. J Neurosurg Pediatr *5*, 179-183.

Antunes, N.L., Souweidane, M.M., Lis, E., Rosenblum, M.K., and Steinherz, P.G. (2002). Methotrexate leukoencephalopathy presenting as Kluver-Bucy syndrome and uncinate seizures. Pediatr Neurol *26*, 305-308.

Arya, L.S., Kotikanyadanam, S.P., Bhargava, M., Saxena, R., Sazawal, S., Bakhshi, S., Khattar, A., Kulkarni, K.P., Adde, M., Vats, T.S., *et al.* (2010). Pattern of relapse in childhood ALL: challenges and lessons from a uniform treatment protocol. J Pediatr Hematol Oncol *32*, 370-375.

Asato, R., Akiyama, Y., Ito, M., Kubota, M., Okumura, R., Miki, Y., Konishi, J., and Mikawa, H. (1992). Nuclear magnetic resonance abnormalities of the cerebral white matter in children with acute lymphoblastic leukemia and malignant lymphoma during and after central nervous system prophylactic treatment with intrathecal methotrexate. Cancer *70*, 1997-2004.

Atra, A., Pinkerton, C.R., Bouffet, E., Norton, A., Hobson, R., Imeson, J.D., and Gerrard, M. (2004). Acute neurotoxicity in children with advanced stage B-non-Hodgkin's lymphoma and B-acute lymphoblastic leukaemia treated with the United Kingdom children cancer study group 9002/9003 protocols. Eur J Cancer *40*, 1346-1350.

Azzarelli, V. & Roessmann, U. (1977). Pathogenesis of central nervous system infiltration in acute leukemia. *Archives of pathology & laboratory medicine* 101:203-5

Aur, R.; Simone J.; Hustu H & Verzosa, M. (1972). A comparative study of central nervous system irradiation and intensive chemotherapy early in remission of childhood acute lymphocytic leukemia. *Cancer* 29:381-91.

Bleyer, W. (1989). Biology and pathogenesis of CNS leukemia. *The American journal of pediatric hematology/oncology* 11:57-63

Borgmann, A., Zinn, C., Hartmann, R., Herold, R., Kaatsch, P., Escherich, G., Moricke, A., Henze, G., and von Stackelberg, A. (2008). Secondary malignant neoplasms after intensive treatment of relapsed acute lymphoblastic leukaemia in childhood. Eur J Cancer *44*, 257-268.

Borowitz, M.; Pullen, D.; Shuster, J. Viswanatha, D.; Montgomery, K.; Willman, C. & Camitta, B. (2003). Minimal residual disease detection in childhood precursor-B-cell acute lymphoblastic leukemia: relation to other risk factors. A Children's Oncology Group study. *Leukemia : official journal of the Leukemia Society of America*, Leukemia Research Fund, U.K 17:1566-72

Bostrom, B.; Sensel, M.; Sather, H.; Gaynon, P.; La, M.; Johnston, K.; Erdmann, G.; Gold, S.; Heerema, N.;

Bota, D.A., and Dafer, R.M. (2009). Acute methotrexate neurotoxicity with choreiform movements and focal neurological deficits: a case report. South Med J *102*, 1071-1074.

Bowers DC, Liu Y, Leisenring W, McNeil E, Stovall M, Gurney JG, Robison LL, Packer RJ, Oeffinger KC. Late-occurring stroke among long-term survivors of childhood leukemia and brain tumors: a report from the Childhood Cancer Survivor Study. J Clin Oncol. 2006 Nov 20;24(33):5277-82.

Brock, S., and Jennings, H.R. (2004). Fatal acute encephalomyelitis after a single dose of intrathecal methotrexate. Pharmacotherapy *24*, 673-676.

Burger, B.; Zimmermann, M.; Mann, G.; Kuhl, J.; Loning, L.; Riehm, H.; Reiter, A. & Schrappe, M. (2003) Diagnostic cerebrospinal fluid examination in children with acute lymphoblastic leukemia: significance of low leukocyte counts with blasts or traumatic lumbar puncture. *Journal of clinical oncology : official journal of the American Society of Clinical Oncology* 21:184-8

Butler, R.W., Copeland, D.R., Fairclough, D.L., Mulhern, R.K., Katz, E.R., Kazak, A.E., Noll, R.B., Patel, S.K., and Sahler, O.J. (2008). A multicenter, randomized clinical trial of a cognitive remediation program for childhood survivors of a pediatric malignancy. J Consult Clin Psychol *76*, 367-378.

Clarke, M.; Gaynon, P.; Hann, I.; Harrison, G.; Masera, G.; Peto, R. & Richards, S. (2003). CNS-directed therapy for childhood acute lymphoblastic leukemia: Childhood ALL Collaborative Group overview of 43 randomized trials. *Journal of clinical oncology : official journal of the American Society of Clinical Oncology* 21:1798-809

Cohen, I.J. (2004). Defining the appropriate dosage of folinic acid after high-dose methotrexate for childhood acute lymphatic leukemia that will prevent neurotoxicity without rescuing malignant cells in the central nervous system. J Pediatr Hematol Oncol *26*, 156-163.

Conklin, H.M., Helton, S., Ashford, J., Mulhern, R.K., Reddick, W.E., Brown, R., Bonner, M., Jasper, B.W., Wu, S., Xiong, X., *et al.* (2010). Predicting methylphenidate response in long-term survivors of childhood cancer: a randomized, double-blind, placebo-controlled, crossover trial. J Pediatr Psychol *35*, 144-155.

Cousens, P., Waters, B., Said, J. and Stevens, M. (1988), COGNITIVE EFFECTS OF CRANIAL IRRADIATION IN LEUKAEMIA: A SURVEY AND META-ANALYSIS. Journal of Child Psychology and Psychiatry, 29: 839–852. doi: 10.1111/j.1469-7610.1988.tb00757.x

Davidson, A., Payne, G., Leach, M.O., McVicar, D., Britton, J.M., Watson, M., and Tait, D.M. (2000). Proton magnetic resonance spectroscopy ((1)H-MRS) of the brain following high-dose methotrexate treatment for childhood cancer. Med Pediatr Oncol *35*, 28-34.

Ebner, F., Ranner, G., Slavc, I., Urban, C., Kleinert, R., Radner, H., Einspieler, R., and Justich, E. (1989). MR findings in methotrexate-induced CNS abnormalities. AJNR Am J Neuroradiol *10*, 959-964.

Evans, A.; Gilbert, E. & Zandstra, R. (1970). The increasing incidence of central nervous system leukemia in children. (Children's Cancer Study Group A). *Cancer* 26:404-9

Foley JJ, Raffa RB, Walker EA. Effects of chemotherapeutic agents 5-fluorouracil and methotrexate alone and combined in a mouse model of learning and memory. *Psychopharmacology (Berl)* 2008;199:527-38.

Fuller, R.L., Luck, S.J., Braun, E.L., Robinson, B.M., McMahon, R.P., and Gold, J.M. (2009). Impaired visual working memory consolidation in schizophrenia. Neuropsychology *23*, 71-80.

Gajjar, A; Harrison, P.; Sandlund, J.; Rivera, G.; Ribeiro, R.; Rubnitz, J.; Razzouk, B.; Relling, M.; Evans, W.; Boyett, J. & Pui, C. (2000). Traumatic lumbar puncture at diagnosis adversely affects outcome in childhood acute lymphoblastic leukemia. *Blood* 96:3381-4

Gaynon, P.; Bleyer, W.; Steinherz, P.; Finklestein, J. ; Littman, P.; Miller, D.; Reaman, G.; Sather, H. & Hammond, G. (1988). Modified BFM therapy for children with previously untreated acute lymphoblastic leukemia and unfavorable prognostic features. Report of Children's Cancer Study Group Study CCG-193P. *The American journal of pediatric hematology/oncology* 10:42-50.

Gaynon, P.; Qu, R.; Chappell, R.; Willoughby, M.; Tubergen, D.; Steinherz, P. & Trigg, M. (1998). Survival after relapse in childhood acute lymphoblastic leukemia: impact of site and time to first relapse--the Children's Cancer Group Experience. *Cancer* 82:1387-95

Gilchrist, G.; Tubergen, D.; Sather, H.; Coccia, P.; O'Brien, R.; Waskerwitz, M. & Hammond, G. (1994) Low numbers of CSF blasts at diagnosis do not predict for the development of CNS leukemia in children with intermediate-risk acute lymphoblastic leukemia: a Childrens Cancer Group report. *Journal of clinical oncology : official journal of the American Society of Clinical Oncology* 12:2594-600

Goshen, Y., Stark, B., Kornreich, L., Michowiz, S., Feinmesser, M., and Yaniv, I. (2007). High incidence of meningioma in cranial irradiated survivors of childhood acute lymphoblastic leukemia. Pediatr Blood Cancer *49*, 294-297.

Greenhill, L.L., Swanson, J.M., Vitiello, B., Davies, M., Clevenger, W., Wu, M., Arnold, L.E., Abikoff, H.B., Bukstein, O.G., Conners, C.K., *et al.* (2001). Impairment and deportment responses to different methylphenidate doses in children with ADHD: the MTA titration trial. J Am Acad Child Adolesc Psychiatry *40*, 180-187.

Gupta, A., Swaroop, C., Rastogi, R., Garg, R., and Bakhshi, S. (2008). Simultaneous occurrence of posterior reversible leukoencephalopathy syndrome in two cases of childhood acute lymphoblastic leukemia induction chemotherapy. Pediatr Hematol Oncol *25*, 351-358.

Hammond, D.; Sather, H.; Nesbit, M.; Miller, D.; Coccia, P.; Bleyer, A.; Lukens, J. & Siegel, S. (1986). Analysis of prognostic factors in acute lymphoblastic leukemia. *Medical and pediatric oncology* 14:124-34

Hardy, K.K., Willard, V.W., and Bonner, M.J. (2011). Computerized cognitive training in survivors of childhood cancer: a pilot study. J Pediatr Oncol Nurs *28*, 27-33.

Hijiya, N., Hudson, M.M., Lensing, S., Zacher, M., Onciu, M., Behm, F.G., Razzouk, B.I., Ribeiro, R.C., Rubnitz, J.E., Sandlund, J.T., *et al.* (2007). Cumulative incidence of secondary neoplasms as a first event after childhood acute lymphoblastic leukemia. JAMA *297*, 1207-1215.

Hill, D.E., Ciesielski, K.T., Hart, B.L., and Jung, R.E. (2004). MRI morphometric and neuropsychological correlates of long-term memory in survivors of childhood leukemia. Pediatr Blood Cancer *42*, 611-617.

Henze, G.; Fengler, R.; Hartmann, R.; Kornhuber, B.; Janka-Schaub, G.; Niethammer, D. & Riehm, H. (1991). Six-year experience with a comprehensive approach to the treatment of recurrent childhood acute lymphoblastic leukemia (ALL-REZ BFM 85). A relapse study of the BFM group. *Blood* 78:1166-72

Hourani, R., Abboud, M., Hourani, M., Khalifeh, H., and Muwakkit, S. (2008). L-asparaginase-induced posterior reversible encephalopathy syndrome during acute lymphoblastic leukemia treatment in children. Neuropediatrics *39*, 46-50.

Hutchinson, R. ; Provisor, A. & Trigg, M. (2003). Dexamethasone versus prednisone and daily oral versus weekly intravenous mercaptopurine for patients with standard-risk acute lymphoblastic leukemia: a report from the Children's Cancer Group. *Blood* 101:3809-17

M.J. Horner, L.A.G.R., and M. Krapcho et al., Editors (2009). SEER Cancer Statistics Review 1975-2006.

Jaksic, W., Veljkovic, D., Pozza, C., and Lewis, I. (2004). Methotrexate-induced leukoencephalopathy reversed by aminophylline and high-dose folinic acid. Acta Haematol *111*, 230-232.

Jemal, A.; Tiwari, R.; Murray T.; Ghafoor, A.; Samuels, A.; Ward, E.; Feuer, E. & Thun, M. (2004) Cancer statistics. CA: a cancer journal for clinicians 54:8-29

Kieslich, M., Porto, L., Lanfermann, H., Jacobi, G., Schwabe, D., and Bohles, H. (2003). Cerebrovascular complications of L-asparaginase in the therapy of acute lymphoblastic leukemia. J Pediatr Hematol Oncol *25*, 484-487.

Kikuchi, A., Maeda, M., Hanada, R., Okimoto, Y., Ishimoto, K., Kaneko, T., Ikuta, K., and Tsuchida, M. (2007). Moyamoya syndrome following childhood acute lymphoblastic leukemia. Pediatr Blood Cancer *48*, 268-272.

Koike, S., Aida, N., Hata, M., Fujita, K., Ozawa, Y., and Inoue, T. (2004). Asymptomatic radiation-induced telangiectasia in children after cranial irradiation: frequency, latency, and dose relation. Radiology *230*, 93-99.

Kosaka, Y.; Koh, K.; Kinukawa, N.; Wakazono, Y.; Isoyama, K.; Oda, T.; Hayashi, Y.; Ohta, S.; Moritake, H.; Oda, M.; Nagatoshi, Y.; Kigasawa, H.; Ishida, Y.; Ohara, A.; Hanada, R.; Sako, M.; Sato, T.; Mizutani, S.; Horibe, K. & Ishii, E. (2004). Infant acute lymphoblastic leukemia with MLL gene rearrangements: outcome following intensive chemotherapy and hematopoietic stem cell transplantation. *Blood* 104:3527-34

Krappmann, P., Paulides, M., Stohr, W., Ittner, E., Plattig, B., Nickel, P., Lackner, H., Schrappe, M., Janka, G., Beck, J.D., *et al.* (2007). Almost normal cognitive function in patients during therapy for childhood acute lymphoblastic leukemia without cranial irradiation according to ALL-BFM 95 and COALL 06-97 protocols: results of an Austrian-German multicenter longitudinal study and implications for follow-up. Pediatr Hematol Oncol *24*, 101-109.

Krull KR, Brouwers P. Jain N, Zhang L, Bomgaars L, Dreye Z, et al. Folate pathway genetic polymorphisms are related to attention disorders in chidlhood leukemia survivors. Journal of Pediatrics 2008; 152:101-105.

Krull, K.R., Khan, R.B., Ness, K.K., Ledet, D., Zhu, L., Pui, C.H., Howard, S.C., Srivastava, D.K., Sabin, N.D., Hudson, M.M., *et al.* (2011). Symptoms of attention-deficit/ hyperactivity disorder in long-term survivors of childhood leukemia. Pediatr Blood Cancer.

Lai, R., Abrey, L.E., Rosenblum, M.K., and DeAngelis, L.M. (2004). Treatment-induced leukoencephalopathy in primary CNS lymphoma: a clinical and autopsy study. Neurology *62*, 451-456.

Laningham, F.; Kun, L.; Reddick, W.; Ogg, R.; Morris, E. & Pui, C. (2007) Childhood central nervous system leukemia: historical perspectives, current therapy, and acute neurological sequelae. *Neuroradiology* 49:873-88

Lauer, S.; Krichner, P.; Kiefer, G.; Pullen, J. & Camitta, B. (1994). Prognostic significance of cerebrospinal fluid (CSF) lymphoblasts (LB) at diagnosis (dx) in children with acute lymphoblastic leukemia (ALL). *Proc Am Soc Clin Oncol* 13:217

Lauer, S.; Kirchner, P. & Camitta, B. (1989). Identification of leukemic cells in the cerebrospinal fluid from children with acute lymphoblastic leukemia: advances and dilemmas. *The American journal of pediatric hematology/oncology* 11:64-73

Lee GD, Longo DL, Wang Y, Rifkind JM, Abdul-Raman L, Mamczarz JA, et al. Transient improvement in cognitive function and synaptic plasticity in rats following cancer chemotherapy. *Clin Cancer Res* 2006;12:198-205.

Linnebank, M., Pels, H., Kleczar, N., Farmand, S., Fliessbach, K., Urbach, H., Orlopp, K., Klockgether, T., Schmidt-Wolf, I.G., and Schlegel, U. (2005). MTX-induced white matter changes are associated with polymorphisms of methionine metabolism. Neurology *64*, 912-913.

Macleod JE, DeLeo JA, Hickey WF, Ahles TA, Saykin AJ, Bucci DJ. Cancer chemotherapy impairs contextual but not cue-specific fear memory. *Behav Brain Res* 2007;181:168-72.

Mahmoud, H.; Rivera, G.; Hancock, M.; Krance, R.; Kun, L.; Behm, F.; Ribeiro, R.; Sandlund, J.; Crist, W. & Pui, C. (1993) Low leukocyte counts with blast cells in cerebrospinal fluid of children with newly diagnosed acute lymphoblastic leukemia. *The New England journal of medicine* 329:314-9

Mahoney, D.H., Jr., Shuster, J.J., Nitschke, R., Lauer, S.J., Steuber, C.P., Winick, N., and Camitta, B. (1998). Acute neurotoxicity in children with B-precursor acute lymphoid leukemia: an association with intermediate-dose intravenous methotrexate and intrathecal triple therapy--a Pediatric Oncology Group study. J Clin Oncol *16*, 1712-1722.

Malempati, S.; Gaynon, P.; Sather, H.; La, M. & Stork, L. (2007) Outcome after relapse among children with standard-risk acute lymphoblastic leukemia: Children's Oncology Group study CCG-1952. *Journal of clinical oncology : official journal of the American Society of Clinical Oncology* 25:5800-7

Margolin, J.; Steuber, C. & Poplack, D. Acute lymphoblastic leukemia (ed 5th). Philadelphia, 2006 pp. 538-90

Mitchell, C.; Richards, S.; Kinsey, S.; Lilleyman, J.; Vora, A. & Eden, T. (2005) Benefit of dexamethasone compared with prednisolone for childhood acute lymphoblastic leukaemia: results of the UK Medical Research Council ALL97 randomized trial. *British journal of haematology* 129:734-45, 2005

Monje ML, Mizumatsu S, Fike JR, Palmer TD. Irradiation induces neural precursor-cell dysfunction. *Nat Med* 2002;8:955-62.

Mulhern, R.K., and Butler, R.W. (2004). Neurocognitive sequelae of childhood cancers and their treatment. Pediatr Rehabil *7*, 1-14; discussion 15-16.

Rajen Mody, Suwen Li, Douglas C. Dover, Stephen Sallan, Wendy Leisenring, Kevin C. Oeffinger, Yutaka Yasui, Leslie L. Robison, and Joseph P. Neglia. Twenty-five–year follow-up among survivors of childhood acute lymphoblastic leukemia: a report from the Childhood Cancer Survivor Study. Blood June 15, 2008 vol. 111 no. 12 5515-5523

Moore, I.M., Kramer, J.H., Wara, W., Halberg, F., and Ablin, A.R. (1991). Cognitive function in children with leukemia. Effect of radiation dose and time since irradiation. Cancer *68*, 1913-1917.

Morris, B., Partap, S., Yeom, K., Gibbs, I.C., Fisher, P.G., and King, A.A. (2009). Cerebrovascular disease in childhood cancer survivors: A Children's Oncology Group Report. Neurology *73*, 1906-1913.

Murphy, A.N., Fiskum, G., and Beal, M.F. (1999). Mitochondria in neurodegeneration: bioenergetic function in cell life and death. J Cereb Blood Flow Metab *19*, 231-245.

Murphy, S.; Pui, C.; Pullen, J.; Reamon, G.; Sallan, S.; Sather, H.; Shuster, J.; Simon, R.; Trigg, M.; Tubergen, D.; Uckun, F. & Ungerleider, R. (1996). Uniform approach to risk classification and treatment assignment for children with acute lymphoblastic leukemia. *Journal of clinical oncology : official journal of the American Society of Clinical Oncology* 14:18-24, 1996

Narayanan, S., and Shami, P.J. (2011). Treatment of acute lymphoblastic leukemia in adults. Crit Rev Oncol Hematol.

Nesbit, M.; Sather, H.; Robison, L.; Ortega, J.; Littman, P.; D'Angio, G. & Hammond, G. (1981) Presymptomatic central nervous system therapy in previously untreated childhood acute lymphoblastic leukaemia: comparison of 1800 rad and 2400 rad. A report for Children's Cancer Study Group. *Lancet* 1:461-6

Claire Oudin, Marie-Claude Simeoni, Nicolas Sirvent, Audrey Contet, Audrey Begu-Le Coroller, Pierre Bordigoni, Catherine Curtillet, Maryline Poirée, Isabelle Thuret, Barbara Play, Mara Carazza Massot, Pascal Chastagner, Hervé Chambost, Pascal Auquier, and Gérard Michel. Prevalence and risk factors of the metabolic syndrome in adult survivors of childhood leukemia. Blood April 28, 2011 vol. 117 no. 17 4442-4448.

Panis, B., Vlaar, A.M., van Well, G.T., Granzen, B., Weber, J.W., Postma, A.A., and Klinkenberg, S. (2010). Posterior reversible encephalopathy syndrome in paediatric leukaemia. Eur J Paediatr Neurol *14*, 539-545.

Paryani, S.; Donaldson, S.; Amylon, M. & Link, M. (1983) Cranial nerve involvement in children with leukemia and lymphoma. *Journal of clinical oncology : official journal of the American Society of Clinical Oncology* 1:542-5

Pieters, R.; Schrappe, M.; De Lorenzo, P.; Hann, I.; De Rossi, G.; Felice, M.; Hovi, L.; LeBlanc, T.; Szczepanski, T.; Ferster, A.; Janka, G.; Rubnitz, J.; Silverman, L.; Stary, J.; Campbell, M.; Li, C.; Mann, G.; Suppiah, R.; Biondi, A.; Vora, A. & Valsecchi, M. (2007) A treatment protocol for infants younger than 1 year with acute lymphoblastic leukaemia (Interfant-99): an observational study and a multicentre randomised trial. *Lancet* 370:240-50

Pinkel, D. & Woo, S. (1994). Prevention and treatment of meningeal leukemia in children. Blood 84:355-66

Pizzo, P.; Poplack, D. & Bleyer, W. (1979) Neurotoxicities of current leukemia therapy. *The American journal of pediatric hematology/oncology* 1:127-40

L. Porto, , a, M. Kieslichb, D. Schwabec, F. E. Zanellaa and H. Lanfermanna. Central nervous system imaging in childhood Leukemia. European Journal of Cancer Volume 40, Issue 14, September 2004, Pages 2082-2090.

Pui, C.; Campana, D.; Pei, D.; Bowman, W. ;Sandlund, J.; Kaste, S.; Ribeiro, R.; Rubnitz, J.; Raimondi, S.; Onciu, M.; Coustan-Smith, E.; Kun, L.; Jeha, S.; Cheng, C.; Howard, S.; Simmons, V.; Bayles, A.; Metzger, M.; Boyett, J.; Leung, W.; Handgretinger, R.; Downing, J.; Evans, W. & Relling, M. (2009). Treating childhood acute lymphoblastic leukemia without cranial irradiation. *The New England journal of medicine* 360:2730-41

Pui, C. & Crist, W. (1994). Biology and treatment of acute lymphoblastic leukemia. *The Journal of pediatrics* 124:491-503

Pui, C. & Evans, W. (2006). Treatment of acute lymphoblastic leukemia. *The New England journal of medicine* 354:166-78

Pui, C. (2006). Central nervous system disease in acute lymphoblastic leukemia: prophylaxis and treatment. Hematology / the Education Program of the American Society of Hematology. *American Society of Hematology Education Program*:142-6

Quinn, C.T., Griener, J.C., Bottiglieri, T., Arning, E., and Winick, N.J. (2004). Effects of intraventricular methotrexate on folate, adenosine, and homocysteine metabolism in cerebrospinal fluid. J Pediatr Hematol Oncol *26*, 386-388.

Quinn, C.T., Griener, J.C., Bottiglieri, T., Hyland, K., Farrow, A., and Kamen, B.A. (1997). Elevation of homocysteine and excitatory amino acid neurotransmitters in the CSF of children who receive methotrexate for the treatment of cancer. J Clin Oncol *15*, 2800-2806.

Reiriz AB, Reolon GK, Preissler T, Rosado JO, Henriques JA, Roesler R, et al. Cancer chemotherapy and cognitive function in rodent models: memory impairment induced by cyclophosphamide in mice. *Clin Cancer Res* 2006;12:5000.

Reiter, A.; Schrappe, M. Ludwig, W.; Hiddemann, W.; Sauter, S.; Henze, G.; Zimmermann, M.; Lampert, F.; Havers, W. & Niethammer (1994). Chemotherapy in 998 unselected childhood acute lymphoblastic leukemia patients. Results and conclusions of the multicenter trial ALL-BFM 86. *Blood* 84:3122-33

Renard, M., Suciu, S., Bertrand, Y., Uyttebroeck, A., Ferster, A., van der Werff Ten Bosch, J., Mazingue, F., Plouvier, E., Robert, A., Boutard, P., *et al.* (2011). Second neoplasm in children treated in EORTC 58881 trial for acute lymphoblastic malignancies: low incidence of CNS tumours. Pediatr Blood Cancer *57*, 119-125.

Ries, L.; Rosary, C.; Hankey, B. & et al. (1999) SEER Cancer Statistics Review, 1973-1996. Bethesda, MD: National Cancer Institute, 1999. Last accessed May 18, 2011.

Rollins, N., Winick, N., Bash, R., and Booth, T. (2004). Acute methotrexate neurotoxicity: findings on diffusion-weighted imaging and correlation with clinical outcome. AJNR Am J Neuroradiol *25*, 1688-1695.

Roy, A.; Cargill, A.; Love, S.; Moorman, A.; Stoneham, S.; Lim, A.; Darbyshire, P.; Lancaster, D.; Hann, I.; Eden, T. & Saha, V. (2005). Outcome after first relapse in childhood acute lymphoblastic leukaemia - lessons from the United Kingdom R2 trial. *British journal of haematology* 130:67-75

Rubnitz, J.E., Relling, M.V., Harrison, P.L., Sandlund, J.T., Ribeiro, R.C., Rivera, G.K., Thompson, S.J., Evans, W.E., and Pui, C.H. (1998). Transient encephalopathy following high-dose methotrexate treatment in childhood acute lymphoblastic leukemia. Leukemia *12*, 1176-1181.

Rzeski, W., Pruskil, S., Macke, A., Felderhoff-Mueser, U., Reiher, A.K., Hoerster, F., Jansma, C., Jarosz, B., Stefovska, V., Bittigau, P., *et al.* (2004). Anticancer agents are potent neurotoxins in vitro and in vivo. Ann Neurol *56*, 351-360.

Sandoval, C., Kutscher, M., Jayabose, S., and Tenner, M. (2003). Neurotoxicity of intrathecal methotrexate: MR imaging findings. AJNR Am J Neuroradiol *24*, 1887-1890.

Sather, H. (1986). Age at diagnosis in childhood acute lymphoblastic leukemia. *Medical and pediatric oncology* 14:166-72

Schneiderman, B. (2004). Hippocampal volumes smaller in chemotherapy patients. Lancet Oncol *5*, 202.

Schrappe, M., Nachman, J., Hunger, S., Schmiegelow, K., Conter, V., Masera, G., Pieters, R., and Pui, C.H. (2010). 'Educational symposium on long-term results of large prospective clinical trials for childhood acute lymphoblastic leukemia (1985-2000)'. Leukemia *24*, 253-254.

Schrappe, M.; Reiter, A.; Ludwig, W.; Harbott, J.; Zimmermann, M.; Hiddemann, W.; Niemeyer, C.; Henze, G.; Feldges, A.; Zintl, F.; Kornhuber, B.; Ritter, J.; Welte, K.; Gadner, H. & Riehm, H. (2000). Improved outcome in childhood acute lymphoblastic leukemia despite reduced use of anthracyclines and cranial radiotherapy: results of trial ALL-BFM 90. German-Austrian-Swiss ALL-BFM Study Group. *Blood* 95:3310-22

Schultz, K.R., Bowman, W.P., Aledo, A., Slayton, W.B., Sather, H., Devidas, M., Wang, C., Davies, S.M., Gaynon, P.S., Trigg, M., *et al.* (2009). Improved early event-free survival with imatinib in Philadelphia chromosome-positive acute lymphoblastic leukemia: a children's oncology group study. J Clin Oncol *27*, 5175-5181.

Seigers, R., and Fardell, J.E. (2011). Neurobiological basis of chemotherapy-induced cognitive impairment: a review of rodent research. Neurosci Biobehav Rev *35*, 729-741.

Seigers R, Schagen SB, Beerling W, Boogerd W, van Tellingen O, van Dam FSAM, et al. Long-lasting suppression of hippocampal cell proliferation and impaired cognitive performance by methotrexate in the rat. *Behav Brain Res* 2008;186:168-75.

Shuper, A., Stark, B., Kornreich, L., Cohen, I.J., Aviner, S., Steinmetz, A., Stein, J., Goshen, Y., and Yaniv, I. (2000). Methotrexate treatment protocols and the central nervous system: significant cure with significant neurotoxicity. J Child Neurol *15*, 573-580.

Smith, M.; Ries, L.; Gurney, J. & et al. (1999). Leukemia. In: Ries LA, Smith MA, Gurney JG, et al., eds.: Cancer incidence and survival among children and adolescents: United States SEER Program 1975-1995. Bethesda, Md: National Cancer Institute, SEER Program, 1999. NIH Pub.No. 99-4649., pp 17-34. Also available online. Last accessed May 18, 2011

Smith, M.; Arthur, D.; Camitta, B.; Carroll, A.; Crist, W.; Gaynon, P.; Gelber, R.; Heerema, N.; Korn, E.; Link, M.;

Stork, L.; Sather, H.; Hutchinson, R.; Broxson, E.; Matloub, Y.; Yanofsky, R.; Masterson, M.; Sorrell, A.; Wells, A.; Blake, M. & Gaynon, P. (2002). Comparison of mercaptopurine with thioguanine and IT methotrexate with IT "triples" in children with standard risk (SR) ALL: results of CCG-1952. *Blood* 100:156

Sullivan, M.; Chen, T.; Dyment, P. & et al. (1982) Equivalence of intrathecal chemotherapy and radiotherapy as central nervous system prophylaxis in children with acute lymphatic leukemia: a pediatric oncology group study. *Blood* 60:948-58

Sundgren, P.C., and Cao, Y. (2009). Brain irradiation: effects on normal brain parenchyma and radiation injury. Neuroimaging Clin N Am *19*, 657-668.

Karen L. Syrjala, Samantha B. Artherholt, Brenda F. Kurland, Shelby L. Langer, Sari Roth-Roemer, JoAnn Broeckel Elrod and Sureya Dikmen. Prospective Neurocognitive Function Over 5 Years After Allogeneic Hematopoietic Cell Transplantation for Cancer Survivors Compared with Matched Controls at 5 Years. Journal of Clinical Oncology, May 2, 2011.

Talvensaari, K.K., Lanning, M., Tapanainen, P., and Knip, M. (1996). Long-term survivors of childhood cancer have an increased risk of manifesting the metabolic syndrome. J Clin Endocrinol Metab *81*, 3051-3055.

Taylor, A.J., Frobisher, C., Ellison, D.W., Reulen, R.C., Winter, D.L., Taylor, R.E., Stiller, C.A., Lancashire, E.R., Tudor, E.C., Baggott, C., *et al.* (2009). Survival after second primary neoplasms of the brain or spinal cord in survivors of childhood cancer: results from the British Childhood Cancer Survivor Study. J Clin Oncol *27*, 5781-5787.

te Loo, D.; Kamps, W.; van der Does-van den Berg, A.; van Wering, E. & de Graaf, S. (2006). Prognostic significance of blasts in the cerebrospinal fluid without pleiocytosis or a traumatic lumbar puncture in children with acute lymphoblastic leukemia: experience of the Dutch Childhood Oncology Group. *Journal of clinical oncology : official journal of the American Society of Clinical Oncology* 24:2332-6.

Temming, P., and Jenney, M.E. (2010). The neurodevelopmental sequelae of childhood leukaemia and its treatment. Arch Dis Child *95*, 936-940.

Tiberin, P., Heilbronn, Y.D., Hirsch, M., and Barmeir, E. (1984a). Giant cerebral Echinococcus cyst with galactorrhea and amenorrhea. Surg Neurol *21*, 505-506.

Tiberin, P., Maor, E., Zaizov, R., Cohen, I.J., Hirsch, M., Yosefovich, T., Ronen, J., and Goldstein, J. (1984b). Brain sarcoma of meningeal origin after cranial irradiation in childhood acute lymphocytic leukemia. Case report. J Neurosurg *61*, 772-776.

Tsuchida, M., Ohara, A., Manabe, A., Kumagai, M., Shimada, H., Kikuchi, A., Mori, T., Saito, M., Akiyama, M., Fukushima, T., *et al.* (2010). Long-term results of Tokyo Children's Cancer Study Group trials for childhood acute lymphoblastic leukemia, 1984-1999. Leukemia *24*, 383-396.

Tubergen, D. ; Cullen, J.; Boyett, J.; Gilchrist, G.; O'Brien, R.; Coccia, P. & Waskerwitz, M. (1994) Blasts in CSF with a normal cell count do not justify alteration of therapy for acute lymphoblastic leukemia in remission: a Childrens Cancer Group study. *Journal of clinical oncology : official journal of the American Society of Clinical Oncology* 12:273-8

Veerman A.; Kamps W.; van den Berg H.; van den Berg, E.; Bokkerink, J. ;Bruin, M. ; van den Heuvel-Eibrink, M.; M.Korbijn, C.; Korthof, E.; van der Pal, K.; Stijnen, T.; van Weel Sipman, M.; H.van Weerden, J. ; van Wering, E. & van der Does-van den Berg, A. (2009). Dexamethasone-based therapy for childhood acute lymphoblastic leukaemia: results of the prospective Dutch Childhood Oncology Group (DCOG) protocol ALL-9 (1997-2004). *The lancet oncology* 10:957-66

Waber DP, Tarbell NJ, Fairclough D, Atmore K, Castro R, Isquith P, Lussier F, Romero I, Carpenter PJ, Schiller M, et al. Cognitive sequelae of treatment in childhood acute lymphoblastic leukemia: cranial radiation requires an accomplice. J Clin Oncol. 1995 Oct;13(10):2490-6.

Waber, D.P., Urion, D.K., Tarbell, N.J., Niemeyer, C., Gelber, R., and Sallan, S.E. (1990). Late effects of central nervous system treatment of acute lymphoblastic leukemia in childhood are sex-dependent. Dev Med Child Neurol *32*, 238-248.

Walter, A.W., Hancock, M.L., Pui, C.H., Hudson, M.M., Ochs, J.S., Rivera, G.K., Pratt, C.B., Boyett, J.M., and Kun, L.E. (1998). Secondary brain tumors in children treated for acute lymphoblastic leukemia at St Jude Children's Research Hospital. J Clin Oncol *16*, 3761-3767.

Winick, N.J., Bowman, W.P., Kamen, B.A., Roach, E.S., Rollins, N., Jacaruso, D., and Buchanan, G.R. (1992). Unexpected acute neurologic toxicity in the treatment of children with acute lymphoblastic leukemia. J Natl Cancer Inst *84*, 252-256.

Winocur G, Vardy J, Binns MA, Kerr L, Tannock I. The effects of the anti-cancer drugs, methotrexate and 5-fluorouracil, on cognitive function in mice. *Pharmacol Biochem Behav* 2006;85:66-75.

Part 4

Therapy of Acute Lymphoblastic Leukemia

5

Treatment of Pediatric Acute Lymphoblastic Leukemia and Recent Advances

Tai-Tsung Chang and Pei-Chin Lin
Kaohsiung Medical University Hospital, Kaohsiung Medical University
Taiwan

1. Introduction

Pediatric acute lymphoblastic leukemia (ALL) is the most prevalent cancer in children. Today in developed countries around 80% of children with ALL can achieve 10 year survival. This great improvement in treatment outcomes for pediatric ALL is due to several important advances which have taken place since the 1960s, including intensive induction/consolidation chemotherapy regimens, risk-adapted therapy, central nervous system prophylaxis, aggressive supportive care (especially prophylaxis and treatment for infections) and minimal residual disease detection. Rapid progress in molecular biology has helped to select patients with specific poor prognostic genetic factors and sensitive monitoring of minimal residual disease has also contributed significantly to the management of pediatric ALL. However, patients with extremely poor prognostic factors or delayed response to chemotherapy still experience disease relapse. Hematopoietic stem cell transplantation (HSCT), mainly using allogenic stem cells (bone marrow, peripheral blood or umbilical cord blood stem cells), has been proven to be an effective alternative and to ensure long-term survival for patients with relapsed ALL or with extremely poor prognostic factors. However, there are complications such as severe infections and chronic graft-versus-host disease (GVHD) that may be occurred. Recent advances in the development of new formulations of existing drugs, targeted therapy and immunotherapy provide new options in treatment of patients with refractory disease and promise to further improve of the cure rates of pediatric ALL.

2. Characteristics of pediatric acute lymphoblastic leukemia

Leukemia is the most common malignancy in the pediatric population, comprising 30% of malignant tumors in children (Chiang et al., 2010; Young and Miller, 1975). The most prevalent subtypes of pediatric leukemia are acute lymphoblastic leukemia (75~80%) and acute myelogenous leukemia (15~17%)(Feltbower et al., 2009).

Common presenting symptoms of pediatric ALL include fever, pallor, hepatosplenomegaly, lymph node swelling and hemorrhage. Bone pain or arthralgia is sometimes reported. The diagnosis of pediatric ALL is based on examination of cell morphology, cytochemistry and immunochemical analysis of bone marrow aspirates. Pediatric ALL can be classified according to different characteristics: L1, L2 or L3 by morphology, and B-cell, T-cell, co-expression of myeloid antigens or mixed type by immunophenotyping. Risk-adapted therapy is the main strategy for pediatric ALL treatment and has achieved a 5-year event-free survival rate of approximately 80% in recent years.

3. Chemotherapy

3.1 Basic treatment principles

Treatment for pediatric ALL comprises two major components: multi-drug combination chemotherapy and intrathecal (IT) chemotherapy for central nervous system (CNS) prophylaxis. Modern protocols have a number of design elements in common including a remission induction phase, a consolidation/intensification phase, and a CNS treatment and continuation (maintenance) phase, with or without delayed intensification (Provan et al., 2009). Multi-drug combination chemotherapy has been the mainstay of ALL management since the late 1960s and a major survival improvement was achieved when 8-week, 8-drug induction/consolidation regimens followed by maintenance therapy were introduced in the 1970s. CNS prophylaxis therapy with IT chemotherapy alone or with cranial radiation was added to the treatment regimen after the induction phase and markedly reduced CNS involvement in leukemia from around 80% to 4~6%(Evans et al., 1970; Moghrabi et al., 2007; Pui, C.H. et al., 2009). Following consolidation treatment, maintenance chemotherapy is initiated and continued for 2~3 years.

3.2 Evolution of regimens

During the late 1960s and early 1970s, patients with pediatric ALL were treated with a three-drug regimen (vincristine, prednisolone and asparaginase) to induce remission, CNS prophylaxis therapy with weekly IT methotrexate (MTX) and cranial radiation was performed during the intensification phase followed by continuation treatment consisting of daily oral mercaptopurine, weekly oral MTX and monthly pulses of prednisolone and vincristine (Schrappe et al., 2010). Later, an early multiple agent induction/consolidation regimen was developed by Dr Riehm (Riehm et al., 1977). This comprised 8-drug induction chemotherapy for 9 weeks (prednisolone, daunorubicin, vincristine, asparaginase, methotrexate, mercaptopurine, cyclophosphamide and cytarabine) and 4 cycles of high-dose methotrexate (HDMTX) with daily oral mercaptopurine for 8 weeks. This improved the cure rate to over 50%. The high remission rate was thought to be related to the intensified remission induction phase. The requirement for precise and robust supportive care in specialized hospitals undertaken by experienced medical staff was emphasized in order to control treatment-related complications (Riehm et al., 1977; Schrappe et al., 2010). This approach remains at the core of modern pediatric ALL regimens.

Risk-adapted therapy stratified by age and initial white blood cell count was demonstrated to increase the remission rate in poor risk groups and to decrease acute and chronic toxicities in good risk groups (Henze et al., 1981). The system of risk classification based on age and white blood cell count was extended by addition of other important prognostic factors for pediatric ALL (Table 1). The application of risk-adapted therapy in clinical trials has resulted in a steady improvement in the outcome of pediatric ALL, with a current overall survival rate of around 80% in developed countries (Jeha and Pui, 2009). The significance of early response to induction treatment , as measured by reduction in peripheral blood blast cells, was proposed in 1987 and used as an indicator to divide patients into different risk groups (Riehm et al., 1987). Since then, many more prognostic factors have been identified and integrated into risk-classification systems. With the advances in genome-wide screening techniques, pharmacogenomic studies, and development of molecular therapeutics an era of more refined personalized therapy is anticipated (Pui, C.H., 2010).

Risk group	Age (y)	Leukocyte count (/ul)	Immunophenotype	Chromosome	Genotype	Early response to chemotherapy#
Low	1-9	<50, 000	Precursor B-cell	Hyperdiploidy*	*TEL-AML1*	Good
High	<1 or ≧10	>50, 000	T-cell	Hypodiploidy*	*MLL-AF4* *BCR-ABL*	Poor

*hyperdiploidy: >50 chromosome; hypodiploidy: <44 chromosome
#defined as MRD at the end of induction chemotherapy (good response: MRD<0.01%; poor response: MRD≧1%)

Table 1. Prognostic factors used for risk classification in pediatric ALL (adapted from (Pui, C.H., 2010) with permission)

National and international treatment groups have been established worldwide with the objective of improving the management of childhood ALL. The long-term results of recently completed clinical trials are listed in Table 2 (Conter et al., 2010; Gaynon et al., 2010; Liang et al., 2010; Mitchell et al., 2010; Moricke et al., 2010; Pui, C.H. et al., 2010). In Taiwan, the Taiwan Pediatric Oncology Group was formed in 1988 and marked progress in ALL treatment has been achieved with overall survival increasing from 59% during 1988~1995 to 82% during 2003~2009.

Study group	Trial	Year	Case number	10-year EFS (%)	10-year OS (%)
CCG	CCG-1900	1996-2002	4464	72.6	82.1
AIEOP	AIEOP-ALL 95	1995-2000	1743	71.7	82.4
BFM	ALL-BFM 95	1995-2000	2169	78	85
SJCRH	Total 13B	1994-1998	247	80.1*	85.7*
SJCRH	Total 14	1998-1999	53	79.2	77.4
SJCRH	Total 15	2000-2007	498	85.6*	93.5*
UK-WPCL	UKALL 97	1997-2002	1948	74	83
TPOG	TPOG-2002	2002-2007	788	77.4*	83.5*

CCG: Children's Cancer Group; AIEOP: Associazione Italiana di ematologia ed Oncologia Pediatrica; BFM: Berlin-Frankfurt-Munster ALL Study Group; SJCRH: St Jude Children's Research Hospital; UK-WPCL: UK Medical Research Council Working Party on Childhood Leukemia; TPOG: Taiwan Pediatric Oncology group; EFS: event-free survival; OS: overall survival ; *5-year EFS and OS

Table 2. Treatment outcomes for selected pediatric ALL study groups

3.3 Central nervous system treatment

Early in the 1960s central nervous system(CNS) treatment was applied to the "total" therapy for pediatric ALL since it was found that better control of systemic leukemia was accompanied by increased frequency of CNS involvement (Aur, R.J. and Pinkel, 1973; Simone, J.V., 1973). Radiation therapy of the CNS and IT MTX administration were the two main strategies for preventing CNS disease (Glidewell and Holland, 1973; Kim et al., 1972; Rosner and Grunwald, 1973; Simone, J. and Pinkel, 1973). Dosage and treatment modalities of CNS radiation were studied in an attempt to reduce neurotoxicities while maintaining effectiveness (Simpson et al., 1973). The St. Jude leukemia group compared cranial radiation with IT MTX and craniospinal irradiation in clinical trials and suggested that combined cranial radiation and IT MTX treatment was as effective as craniospinal irradiation with fewer toxicities (leukopenia and interruption of treatment)(Aur, R.J.A. et al., 1973). Since then, combined cranial irradiation and IT MTX have become the standard treatment for preventing CNS disease. However, further studies revealed that survivors of pediatric ALL who received high doses of cranial irradiation (over 25 Gy) or who were treated at a young age (younger than 2 years) suffered from significant long-term sequelae, such as defective cognitive function and secondary malignancy (Moe and Holen, 2000; Spiegler et al., 2006). Therefore, some study groups suggested that the dose of radiation be decreased to less than 18 Gy (Henze et al., 1983) or that the extended IT MTX treatment be used as a replacement for cranial irradiation in low-risk patients (Conter et al., 1995). However, some treatment groups preferred to continue to employ cranial irradiation because of the poor prognosis with CNS leukemia (Gelber et al., 1993). After a lengthy debate regarding the role of cranial irradiation in pediatric ALL treatment, Pui CH et al. published their study results in this issue and suggested that 'with effective risk-adjusted chemotherapy, prophylactic cranial irradiation can be safely omitted from the treatment of childhood ALL'(Pui, C.H. et al., 2009).

4. Minimal residual disease

Complete remission of ALL has been defined as blastic cells less than 5% of nucleated cells on bone marrow smear. Before the introduction of molecular methods or multicolor flow cytometry techniques, the percentage of blastic cells was measured by morphology, with a sensitivity of 1%. During the last twenty years, rapid progress in molecular biology has greatly improved the sensitivity of residual blastic cell detection, especially in the range 1% to 0.01%, which is designated minimal residual disease (MRD) (Campana and Pui, 1995; Neale et al., 1994). A new definition of remission was then established on the basis of immunologic or molecular response. A better clinical outcome is predicted in patients who achieve 'immunologic' or 'molecular' remission (ie leukemic involvement of <0.01% of nucleated bone marrow cells after initial intensive chemotherapy) compared with patients whose remission is defined solely by morphologic criteria (Coustan-Smith et al., 2000; Pui, C.H. and Campana, 2000). Among the various methods using immunologic or molecular characteristics of blastic cells as markers, the most promising are flow cytometric detection of aberrant immunophenotypes, and polymerase chain reaction analysis of clonal antigen-receptor gene rearrangements or leukemia-specific fusion genes (Campana and Pui, 1995; Coustan-Smith et al., 1998; Ludwig et al., 1990; van Dongen et al., 1999). Taken together, almost all patients with pediatric ALL can be monitored for MRD during the course of treatment (Campana et al., 2001; Chen et al., 2001; Neale et al., 2004; Pui, C.H. and Campana, 2000). Recent studies indicated that monitoring of MRD constituted an essential prognostic marker, and that detection of MRD, particularly at the end of induction and after treatment completion, was significantly predictive for patient outcome (Katsibardi et al., 2010; Stow et al., 2010).

5. The role of hemopoietic stem cell transplantation in pediatric acute lymphoblastic leukemia

Hemopoietic stem cell transplantation was introduced for children with ALL in the 1970s. Along with the significant improvements in clinical outcome observed in patients receiving chemotherapy, HSCT became the treatment choice for relapsed cases and patients with poor prognostic factors (Gratwohl et al., 1990; Makipernaa et al., 1995; Uderzo et al., 1995). In early studies, 40 to 50% of relapsed patients achieved long remissions and were potentially cured by marrow transplantation. However, the effectiveness of the approach was diminished by the problems of acute and chronic GVHD, infection, and relapse(Johnson, 1990; Moussalem et al., 1995; Pinkel, 1994; Wingard et al., 1990). Currently, HSCT is only considered in patients with extremely poor prognostic factors (for example, Philadelphia chromosome positive [PH^+] ALL with poor response to induction therapy), with delayed response to chemotherapy (induction failure, MRD >1% on the end of remission date or MRD >0.01% prior to reinduction of chemotherapy) and in patients who experience early relapse (Arico et al., 2010; Burke et al., 2009; Davies and Mehta, 2010; Pulsipher et al., 2011).

6. Recent advances in therapy and research in pediatric ALL

Philadelphia chromosome-positive ALL has been found to be associated with a poor response to conventional chemotherapy and a high relapse rate, especially in patients older than 10 years (Arico et al., 2010). HSCT has been employed in patients with PH^+ ALL in an attempt to improve long-term outcomes. In the early 2000s, BCR-ABL targeted strategies started to be incorporated into the treatment for PH^+ ALL. Imatinib, a first generation tyrosine kinase inhibitor, showed its efficacy in improving the treatment outcome in PH^+ALL with or without HSCT (Alvarado et al., 2007; Carpenter et al., 2007; Champagne et al., 2004; Fuster et al., 2007; Jones, L.K. and Saha, 2005). Given the marked improvement in treatment results achieved with combinations of a tyrosine kinase inhibitor (imatinib) and intensive chemotherapy, transplantation is not recommended for the first remission of children with PH+ ALL, unless the early response to treatment was poor (Barr, 2010; Gruber et al., 2009; Koo, 2011; Liu et al., 2009; Milone and Enrico, 2009; Ottmann and Pfeifer, 2009; Schultz et al., 2009). Second generation tyrosine kinase inhibitors were developed because imatinib may induce specific resistance mainly due to ABL1 mutations. Dasatinib, a multi tyrosine kinase inhibitor targeted to BCR-ABL, SRC, C-KIT, PDGFR and ephrin A receptor kinase, and nilotinib, another BCR-ABL targeted agent similar to imatinib but with a higher affinity, are two novel agents with the potential to address PH+ALL resistance to imatinib (Alvarado et al., 2007; Aplenc et al., 2011; Kawaguchi et al., 2005; Kolb et al., 2008; Linger et al., 2009; Piccaluga et al., 2007; Porkka et al., 2008).

Mixed lineage leukemia (MLL) rearrangements occur in 80% of infants and 5% of older children with ALL. MLL-rearranged ALL patients have poor treatment outcomes with conventional chemotherapy. FLT3 (FMS-like tyrosine kinase receptor-3) is one of the unique gene expression profiles in MLL-rearranged ALL. Eighteen percent of MLL-rearranged ALL harbored activating mutations of FLT3 with high expression levels (Armstrong et al., 2003; Brown et al., 2005). *In vitro* studies have demonstrated that FLT3 inhibitor, CEP-701, effectively suppresses FLT3 driven leukemic cell survival (Brown et al., 2006; Brown et al., 2005).

Monoclonal antibodies, including rituximab (anti-CD20), epratuzumab (anti-CD22), inotuzumab (anti-CD22), recombinant immunotoxins and bispecific antibodies (blinatumomab) and radioimmunotherapy have already been incorporated into clinical trials or are undergoing investigation. (Attias and Weitzman, 2008; Christiansen and Rajasekaran, 2004; Dworzak et al., 2008; Oriuchi et al., 2005; Reichert and Valge- Archer, 2007; Topp et al., 2011)

The application of emerging DNA and RNA techniques, SNP arrays, DNA methylation arrays and genome-wide association studies has led to the discovery of further genetic and epigenetic alterations. IKZF1, JAK mutations, and CDKN2A/B are among several examples which have been shown to be related to leukemogenesis and drug resistance (Davidsson et al., 2009; Yang et al., 2009; Yu et al., 2011). MicroRNAs alterations and dysregulation of DNA methylation have also been found in children with ALL and are being assessed as new targets for treatment (Bachmann et al., 2010; Davidsson et al., 2009; Herman et al., 1996; Schotte et al., 2011). In the near future, more individualized treatment strategies will be established based on detailed genetic and epigenetic characteristics, response to early treatment and MRD monitoring Such strategies will require precise supportive care.

7. Supportive care

7.1 Tumor lysis syndrome

Tumor lysis syndrome (TLS) is a well-recognized complication of leukemia and lymphoma, especially in patients with B-cell or T-cell neoplasms and a large tumor burden (Alperin and Levin, 1964; Cohen et al., 1980; Jones, D.P. et al., 1990; Kedar et al., 1995; Kuhbock et al., 1968; Rieselbach et al., 1964). TLS may occur spontaneously or during the early phase of treatment and can lead to severe metabolic disturbances (hyperuricemia, hyperphosphatemia, hyperkalemia, and hypocalcemia) (Jones, D.P. et al., 1995). TLS-associated hyperuricemia may cause acute renal failure because of the rapid and dramatic increase of uricemia and renal burden of uric acid urate. Without appropriate management, precipitation of uric acid crystals can obstruct the tubules and collecting ducts, resulting in tubular necrosis and renal failure (Renyi et al., 2007). Allopurinol, which is an inhibitor of the enzyme xanthine oxidase, combined with hydration, osmotic diuretics and urinary alkalization has been the standard treatment for TLS since the late 1960s and remains an important part of leukemia treatment (Aviles, 1995; DeConti and Calabresi, 1966; Holland and Holland, 1968; Jones, D.P. et al., 1995; Rundles, 1966; Watts, 1966). Through blocking uric acid formation, allopurinol can effectively lower the serum uric acid level, but it increases the renal load of hypoxanthine and xanthine (both are uric acid precursors) (Andreoli et al., 1986; DeConti and Calabresi, 1966). Allopurinol treatment has been associated with xanthine nephropathy and calculi because xanthine is actually less soluble than uric acid in urine (Band et al., 1970; Wyngaarden, 1970). Moreover, allopurinol may interact with chemotherapy agents and affect drug metabolite concentrations (Rundles, 1966).

Urate oxidase, an endogenous enzyme in most mammals but not in humans, can act as a catalyst in the oxidation of uric acid to allantoin. Because allantoin is five to ten-fold more soluble than uric acid, urate oxidase can effectively decrease uric acid levels in patients with TLS (Brogard et al., 1972). Recombinant urate oxidase was introduced in France in 1975. During the 1980s and 1990s, non-recombinant urate oxidase (Uricozyme; Sanofi-Synthelabo,

Inc, Paris), purified from cultures of Aspergillus flavus, was used in the treatment of TLS in ALL patients (Masera et al., 1982). Although it improved the elimination of uric acid, however, this agent was found to be associated with allergic reactions (rashes, bronchospasm , urticaria and angioedema) in about 5% of patients, even in those without a history of allergy (Patte et al., 2001; Pui, C.H. et al., 1997). A new urate oxidase (rasburicase) was developed by use of a recombinant DNA technique in 1996 (Cammalleri and Malaguarnera, 2007). This approach allowed more rapid production of greater quantities of urate oxidase. Rasburicase is purer than non-recombinant urate oxidase, has greater activity and lower allergic reaction rates. Studies of the use of rasburicase in patients with ALL, have shown it to be a safe and effective alternative to allopurinol for the prevention and treatment of hyperuricemia (Cammalleri and Malaguarnera, 2007; Cheson and Dutcher, 2005; Lee et al., 2003; McNutt et al., 2006; Patte et al., 2001; Pui, C.H., 2001; Sood et al., 2006; Wang et al., 2006). The toxicity of rasburicase is negligible, although the presence of anti-rasburicase antibodies has been reported in some patients (Pui, C.-H. et al., 2001).

7.2 Infections

Neutropenia is usually found when ALL is newly diagnosed or during chemotherapy, especially induction therapy. Children with ALL and disease-induced or treatment-related neutropenia, (usually defined as absolute neutrophil count less than 500 per mm^3) are more prone to severe bacterial, fungal and viral infections (Freifeld et al., 2011). More febrile neutropenia episodes occur during induction of remission than during remission in children with ALL. The risk of severe infection is high with severe neutropenia (less than 200 per mm^3)(Jones, G.R. et al., 1996; Peng et al., 1981). Both the degree and duration of neutropenia affect the risk of infection. For the purpose of managing febrile neutropenia, patients have been categorized into different risk groups. Rackoff et al. classified patients with febrile neutropenia into three risk groups based on the absolute monocyte count and temperature at the time of admission. They found that the odds ratio of bacteremia for the high-risk versus the intermediate-risk group is 4.4 (no bacteremia episodes were found in the low-risk group)(Rackoff et al., 1996). The Infectious Disease Society of America (IDSA) started categorizing patients with febrile neutropenia in 2002 and the updated recommendation published in 2010 divided these patients into high-risk or low-risk groups according to the presenting symptoms and signs, neutrophil counts, underlying cancer, type of therapy, the anticipated length of neutropenia and medical comorbidities. The high-risk group was defined when any of the following criteria applied : profound neutropenia anticipated for longer than 7 days, evidence of hepatic or renal insufficiency, comorbidities with unstable vital signs, severe mucositis, gastrointestinal symptoms, neurological symptoms, catheter-related infections, new pulmonary infiltration or hypoxia (Freifeld et al., 2011). It was suggested that high-risk patients be admitted at once and that antibiotics should be administered on an empirical basis as soon as possible. Worldwide, the etiology of infections is now predominantly due to Gram-positive bacterial pathogens. In a study conducted in 1981, Gram-positive and Gram-negative bacteria were equally represented (Peng et al., 1981). In another study, Gram-negative bacteria accounted for the great majority of the etiologic agents (Escherichia coli, Klebsiella spp. and Pseudomonas aeruginosa were the three most common pathogens) (Bodey et al., 1978). Recent studies have showed that Gram-positive bacteria account for more than fifty percent of bacterial episodes with coagulase-negative staphylococci, viridans streptococci and Staphylococcus aureus being the most common pathogens (Hakim et al., 2009).

Systemic (invasive) fungal infections are another common infection in patients with febrile neutropenia. ALL was the second most common underlying disease associated with proven invasive fungal infections after acute myelogenous leukemia in children treated for cancers (Mor et al., 2011). In earlier studies, systemic fungal infections occurred in around 20% of cases of pediatric acute leukemia during induction chemotherapy and the duration of neutropenia was a significant risk factor (Wiley et al., 1990). In the late 1990s, when antifungal prophylaxis and early initiation of empirical antifungal therapy were introduced, the rate of invasive fungal infections decreased, although the rate of fungal colonization in children receiving remission induction therapy for acute leukemia was still high (Gozdasoglu et al., 1999). In a study conducted in 2007, the occurrence of invasive fungal infections was monitored after renovation of the ventilation system on a pediatric hematology/oncology unit and initiation of routine azole antifungal prophylaxis. The incidence of proven invasive fungal infection was 3.2% (1/31) in the allogenic stem cell transplant group, 0/26 in autologous stem cell transplant group and 1.6%(1/60) in the induction therapy group (Hovi et al., 2007). In 2010, IDSA guidelines proposed antifungal prophylaxis administration in high-risk groups, and empiric antifungal therapy or preemptive therapy in patients with febrile neutropenia 4-7 days after broad-spectrum antibiotics treatment (Freifeld et al., 2011). However, a shift of fungal pathogens from Candida sp. towards mold infections was observed along with the increasing use of antifungal prophylaxis. In a recent study which enrolled 1047 children with different malignancies, 20% of the proven invasive fungal infections had candidemia and 80% had mold infections. Non-albicans candida accounted for 60% of all candidemia and 55% of mold infections were non-Aspergillus (Mor et al., 2011). Although the incidence of and mortality due to invasive fungal infections were both lower than previously reported, the epidemiologic spectrum of fungus isolates has broadened and this should be considered in the selection of antifungal agents for prophylaxis or empirical treatment.

Granulocyte-colony stimulation factor (G-CSF) or granulocyte-monocyte colony stimulating factor (GM-CSF) have the potential benefits of reducing the duration of neutropenia and, in turn, the risk of infection. A meta-analysis of 16 randomized controlled trials concluded that prophylactic use of G-CSF or GM-CSF was associated with a 20% reduction in febrile neutropenia and a two-day decrease in duration of hospitalizations (Sung et al., 2004). IDSA 2010 guidelines recommend prophylactic use of G-CSF or GM-CSF for patients in whom the predicted risk of fever and neutropenia is over 20% (Freifeld et al., 2011).

8. Conclusion

Pediatric ALL is the most common malignancy in children. The cure rates of pediatric ALL have improved greatly through use of risk-adapted therapy and aggressive supportive care. Advances in molecular biology and high-throughput technology will allow further investigation of the mechanisms of leukemogenesis and disease relapse and will, in turn, lead to more sophisticated treatments in the future.

9. Acknowledgements

The authors thank the members of Taiwan Pediatric Oncology Group (TPOG) for their distinguished work and all of our colleagues at the Division of Hematology/Oncology, Department of Pediatrics, Kaohsiung Medical University Hospital.

10. References

Alperin, J. B. and Levin, W. C. (1964). "Extreme Hyperuricemia Associated with Prednisone Therapy for Acute Lymphoblastic Leukemia." Tex Med 60: 1001-4.

Alvarado, Y., et al. (2007). "Emerging therapeutic options for Philadelphia-positive acute lymphocytic leukemia." Expert Opin Emerg Drugs 12(1): 165-79.

Andreoli, S. P., et al. (1986). "Purine excretion during tumor lysis in children with acute lymphocytic leukemia receiving allopurinol: relationship to acute renal failure." J Pediatr 109(2): 292-8.

Aplenc, R., et al. (2011). "Pediatric phase I trial and pharmacokinetic study of dasatinib: a report from the children's oncology group phase I consortium." J Clin Oncol 29(7): 839-44.

Arico, M., et al. (2010). "Clinical outcome of children with newly diagnosed Philadelphia chromosome-positive acute lymphoblastic leukemia treated between 1995 and 2005." J Clin Oncol 28(31): 4755-61.

Armstrong, S. A., et al. (2003). "Inhibition of FLT3 in MLL. Validation of a therapeutic target identified by gene expression based classification." Cancer Cell 3(2): 173-83.

Attias, D. and Weitzman, S. (2008). "The efficacy of rituximab in high-grade pediatric B-cell lymphoma/leukemia: a review of available evidence." Curr Opin Pediatr 20(1): 17-22.

Aur, R. J. and Pinkel, D. (1973). "Total therapy of acute lymphocytic leukemia." Prog Clin Cancer 5: 155-70.

Aur, R. J. A., et al. (1973). "Comparison of Two Methods of Preventing Central Nervous System Leukemia." Blood 42(3): 349-357.

Aviles, A. (1995). "Acute tumor lysis syndrome and alkali therapy." Am J Med 98(4): 417-8.

Bachmann, P. S., et al. (2010). "Epigenetic silencing of BIM in glucocorticoid poor-responsive pediatric acute lymphoblastic leukemia, and its reversal by histone deacetylase inhibition." Blood 116(16): 3013-22.

Band, P. R., et al. (1970). "Xanthine nephropathy in a patient with lymphosarcoma treated with allopurinol." N Engl J Med 283(7): 354-7.

Barr, R. D. (2010). "Imatinib mesylate in children and adolescents with cancer." Pediatr Blood Cancer 55(1): 18-25.

Bodey, G. P., et al. (1978). "Fever and infection in leukemic patients: a study of 494 consecutive patients." Cancer 41(4): 1610-22.

Brogard, J. M., et al. (1972). "Enzymatic uricolysis: a study of the effect of a fungal urate-oxydase." Rev Eur Etud Clin Biol 17(9): 890-5.

Brown, P., et al. (2006). "Combinations of the FLT3 inhibitor CEP-701 and chemotherapy synergistically kill infant and childhood MLL-rearranged ALL cells in a sequence-dependent manner." Leukemia 20(8): 1368-76.

Brown, P., et al. (2005). "FLT3 inhibition selectively kills childhood acute lymphoblastic leukemia cells with high levels of FLT3 expression." Blood 105(2): 812-20.

Burke, M. J., et al. (2009). "Allogeneic hematopoietic cell transplantation (allogeneic HCT) for treatment of pediatric Philadelphia chromosome-positive acute lymphoblastic leukemia (ALL)." Pediatr Blood Cancer 53(7): 1289-94.

Cammalleri, L. and Malaguarnera, M. (2007). "Rasburicase represents a new tool for hyperuricemia in tumor lysis syndrome and in gout." Int J Med Sci 4(2): 83-93.

Campana, D., et al. (2001). "Detection of minimal residual disease in acute lymphoblastic leukemia: the St Jude experience." Leukemia 15(2): 278-9.

Campana, D. and Pui, C. H. (1995). "Detection of minimal residual disease in acute leukemia: methodologic advances and clinical significance." Blood 85(6): 1416-34.

Carpenter, P. A., et al. (2007). "Prophylactic administration of imatinib after hematopoietic cell transplantation for high-risk Philadelphia chromosome-positive leukemia." Blood 109(7): 2791-3.

Champagne, M. A., et al. (2004). "Imatinib mesylate (STI571) for treatment of children with Philadelphia chromosome-positive leukemia: results from a Children's Oncology Group phase 1 study." Blood 104(9): 2655-60.

Chen, X., et al. (2001). "Quantification of minimal residual disease in T-lineage acute lymphoblastic leukemia with the TAL-1 deletion using a standardized real-time PCR assay." Leukemia 15(1): 166-70.

Cheson, B. D. and Dutcher, B. S. (2005). "Managing malignancy-associated hyperuricemia with rasburicase." J Support Oncol 3(2): 117-24.

Chiang, C.-J., et al. (2010). "Cancer Trends in Taiwan." Japanese Journal of Clinical Oncology 40(10): 897-904.

Christiansen, J. and Rajasekaran, A. K. (2004). "Biological impediments to monoclonal antibody-based cancer immunotherapy." Mol Cancer Ther 3(11): 1493-501.

Cohen, L. F., et al. (1980). "Acute tumor lysis syndrome. A review of 37 patients with Burkitt's lymphoma." Am J Med 68(4): 486-91.

Conter, V., et al. (2010). "Long-term results of the Italian Association of Pediatric Hematology and Oncology (AIEOP) Studies 82, 87, 88, 91 and 95 for childhood acute lymphoblastic leukemia." Leukemia 24(2): 255-64.

Conter, V., et al. (1995). "Extended intrathecal methotrexate may replace cranial irradiation for prevention of CNS relapse in children with intermediate-risk acute lymphoblastic leukemia treated with Berlin-Frankfurt-Munster-based intensive chemotherapy. The Associazione Italiana di Ematologia ed Oncologia Pediatrica." J Clin Oncol 13(10): 2497-502.

Coustan-Smith, E., et al. (1998). "Immunological detection of minimal residual disease in children with acute lymphoblastic leukaemia." Lancet 351(9102): 550-4.

Coustan-Smith, E., et al. (2000). "Clinical importance of minimal residual disease in childhood acute lymphoblastic leukemia." Blood 96(8): 2691-6.

Davidsson, J., et al. (2009). "The DNA methylome of pediatric acute lymphoblastic leukemia." Hum Mol Genet 18(21): 4054-65.

Davies, S. M. and Mehta, P. A. (2010). "Pediatric acute lymphoblastic leukemia: is there still a role for transplant?" Hematology Am Soc Hematol Educ Program 2010: 363-7.

DeConti, R. C. and Calabresi, P. (1966). "Use of allopurinol for prevention and control of hyperuricemia in patients with neoplastic disease." N Engl J Med 274(9): 481-6.

Dworzak, M. N., et al. (2008). "CD20 up-regulation in pediatric B-cell precursor acute lymphoblastic leukemia during induction treatment: setting the stage for anti-CD20 directed immunotherapy." Blood 112(10): 3982-8.

Evans, A. E., et al. (1970). "The increasing incidence of central nervous system leukemia in children. (Children's Cancer Study Group A)." Cancer 26(2): 404-9.

Feltbower, R. G., et al. (2009). "Epidemiology of leukaemia and lymphoma in children and young adults from the north of England, 1990-2002." European Journal of Cancer 45(3): 420-427.

Freifeld, A. G., et al. (2011). "Clinical practice guideline for the use of antimicrobial agents in neutropenic patients with cancer: 2010 update by the infectious diseases society of america." Clin Infect Dis 52(4): e56-93.

Fuster, J. L., et al. (2007). "Imatinib mesylate in combination with chemotherapy in four children with de novo and advanced stage Philadelphia chromosome-positive acute lymphoblastic leukemia." Haematologica 92(12): 1723-4.

Gaynon, P. S., et al. (2010). "Long-term results of the children's cancer group studies for childhood acute lymphoblastic leukemia 1983-2002: a Children's Oncology Group Report." Leukemia 24(2): 285-97.

Gelber, R. D., et al. (1993). "Central nervous system treatment in childhood acute lymphoblastic leukemia. Long-term follow-up of patients diagnosed between 1973 and 1985." Cancer 72(1): 261-70.

Glidewell, O. J. and Holland, J. F. (1973). "Clinical trials of the acute leukemia group B in acute lymphocytic leukemia of childhood." Bibl Haematol 39: 1053-67.

Gozdasoglu, S., et al. (1999). "Fungal colonization and infection in children with acute leukemia and lymphoma during induction therapy." Med Pediatr Oncol 32(5): 344-8.

Gratwohl, A., et al. (1990). "Allogeneic bone marrow transplantation for leukemia in Europe: regional differences. Report from the Leukemia Working party of the European Group for Bone Marrow Transplantation." Bone Marrow Transplant 5(3): 159-65.

Gruber, F., et al. (2009). "Impact of tyrosine kinase inhibitors on patient outcomes in Philadelphia chromosome-positive acute lymphoblastic leukaemia." Br J Haematol 145(5): 581-97.

Hakim, H., et al. (2009). "Etiology and clinical course of febrile neutropenia in children with cancer." J Pediatr Hematol Oncol 31(9): 623-9.

Henze, G., et al. (1983). "[Results of preventive management of the central nervous system in 275 children with acute lymphoblastic leukemia]." Klin Padiatr 195(3): 168-75.

Henze, G., et al. (1981). "Treatment strategy for different risk groups in childhood acute lymphoblastic leukemia: A Report From the BFM Study Group." Haematol Blood Transfus 26: 87-93.

Herman, J. G., et al. (1996). "Hypermethylation-associated inactivation indicates a tumor suppressor role for p15INK4B." Cancer Res 56(4): 722-7.

Holland, P. and Holland, N. H. (1968). "Prevention and management of acute hyperuricemia in childhood leukemia." J Pediatr 72(3): 358-66.

Hovi, L., et al. (2007). "Prevention and monitoring of invasive fungal infections in pediatric patients with cancer and hematologic disorders." Pediatr Blood Cancer 48(1): 28-34.

Jeha, S. and Pui, C. H. (2009). "Risk-adapted treatment of pediatric acute lymphoblastic leukemia." Hematol Oncol Clin North Am 23(5): 973-90, v.

Johnson, F. L. (1990). "Role of bone marrow transplantation in childhood lymphoblastic leukemia." Hematol Oncol Clin North Am 4(5): 997-1008.

Jones, D. P., et al. (1995). "Tumor lysis syndrome: pathogenesis and management." Pediatr Nephrol 9(2): 206-12.

Jones, D. P., et al. (1990). "Renal dysfunction and hyperuricemia at presentation and relapse of acute lymphoblastic leukemia." Med Pediatr Oncol 18(4): 283-6.

Jones, G. R., et al. (1996). "Infection risk factors in febrile, neutropenic children and adolescents." Pediatr Hematol Oncol 13(3): 217-29.

Jones, L. K. and Saha, V. (2005). "Philadelphia positive acute lymphoblastic leukaemia of childhood." Br J Haematol 130(4): 489-500.

Katsibardi, K., et al. (2010). "Sequential monitoring of minimal residual disease in acute lymphoblastic leukemia: 7-year experience in a pediatric hematology/oncology unit." Leuk Lymphoma 51(5): 846-52.

Kawaguchi, H., et al. (2005). "In vitro drug resistance to imatinib and mutation of ABL gene in childhood Philadelphia chromosome-positive (Ph+) acute lymphoblastic leukemia." Leuk Lymphoma 46(2): 273-6.

Kedar, A., et al. (1995). "Clinical versus laboratory tumor lysis syndrome in children with acute leukemia." Pediatr Hematol Oncol 12(2): 129-34.

Kim, T., et al. (1972). "The role of central nervous system irradiation in children with acute lymphoblastic leukemia." Radiology 104(3): 635-41.

Kolb, E. A., et al. (2008). "Initial testing of dasatinib by the pediatric preclinical testing program." Pediatr Blood Cancer 50(6): 1198-206.

Koo, H. H. (2011). "Philadelphia chromosome-positive acute lymphoblastic leukemia in childhood." Korean J Pediatr 54(3): 106-10.

Kuhbock, J., et al. (1968). "[Hyperuricemia and kidney function in hemoblastoses]." Wildl Dis 49(10): 392-400.

Lee, A. C., et al. (2003). "Treatment of impending tumor lysis with single-dose rasburicase." Ann Pharmacother 37(11): 1614-7.

Liang, D. C., et al. (2010). "Long-term results of Taiwan Pediatric Oncology Group studies 1997 and 2002 for childhood acute lymphoblastic leukemia." Leukemia 24(2): 397-405.

Linger, R. M., et al. (2009). "Mer receptor tyrosine kinase is a novel therapeutic target in pediatric B-cell acute lymphoblastic leukemia." Blood 114(13): 2678-87.

Liu, Z., et al. (2009). "[Clinical characteristics and outcomes of 59 patients with acute lymphoblastic leukemia positive for BCR/ABL]." Nan Fang Yi Ke Da Xue Xue Bao 29(3): 512-5.

Ludwig, W. D., et al. (1990). "Possibilities and limitations of immunological marker analyses for the detection of minimal residual disease in childhood acute lymphoblastic leukemia." Onkologie 13(3): 166-74.

Makipernaa, A., et al. (1995). "Allogeneic bone marrow transplantation in children: single institution experience from 1974 to 1992." Acta Paediatr 84(6): 683-8.

Masera, G., et al. (1982). "Urate-oxidase prophylaxis of uric acid-induced renal damage in childhood leukemia." J Pediatr 100(1): 152-5.

McNutt, D. M., et al. (2006). "Rasburicase for the management of tumor lysis syndrome in neonates." Ann Pharmacother 40(7-8): 1445-50.

Milone, J. H. and Enrico, A. (2009). "Treatment of Philadelphia chromosome-positive acute lymphoblastic leukemia." Leuk Lymphoma 50 Suppl 2: 9-15.

Mitchell, C., et al. (2010). "Long-term follow-up of the United Kingdom medical research council protocols for childhood acute lymphoblastic leukaemia, 1980-2001." Leukemia 24(2): 406-18.

Moe, P. J. and Holen, A. (2000). "HIGH-DOSE METHOTREXATE IN CHILDHOOD ALL." Pediatric Hematology & Oncology 17(8): 615-622.

Moghrabi, A., et al. (2007). "Results of the Dana-Farber Cancer Institute ALL Consortium Protocol 95-01 for children with acute lymphoblastic leukemia." Blood 109(3): 896-904.

Mor, M., et al. (2011). "Invasive fungal infections in pediatric oncology." Pediatr Blood Cancer 56(7): 1092-7.

Moricke, A., et al. (2010). "Long-term results of five consecutive trials in childhood acute lymphoblastic leukemia performed by the ALL-BFM study group from 1981 to 2000." Leukemia 24(2): 265-84.

Moussalem, M., et al. (1995). "Allogeneic bone marrow transplantation for childhood acute lymphoblastic leukemia in second remission: factors predictive of survival, relapse and graft-versus-host disease." Bone Marrow Transplant 15(6): 943-7.

Neale, G. A., et al. (2004). "Comparative analysis of flow cytometry and polymerase chain reaction for the detection of minimal residual disease in childhood acute lymphoblastic leukemia." Leukemia 18(5): 934-8.

Neale, G. A., et al. (1994). "Molecular evidence for minimal residual bone marrow disease in children with 'isolated' extra-medullary relapse of T-cell acute lymphoblastic leukemia." Leukemia 8(5): 768-75.

Oriuchi, N., et al. (2005). "Current status of cancer therapy with radiolabeled monoclonal antibody." Ann Nucl Med 19(5): 355-65.

Ottmann, O. G. and Pfeifer, H. (2009). "Management of Philadelphia chromosome-positive acute lymphoblastic leukemia (Ph+ ALL)." Hematology Am Soc Hematol Educ Program: 371-81.

Patte, C., et al. (2001). "European experience in the treatment of hyperuricemia." Semin Hematol 38(4 Suppl 10): 9-12.

Peng, L. H., et al. (1981). "Fever in children with acute lymphoblastic leukemia." Cancer 47(3): 583-7.

Piccaluga, P. P., et al. (2007). "Tyrosine kinase inhibitors for the treatment of Philadelphia chromosome-positive adult acute lymphoblastic leukemia." Cancer 110(6): 1178-86.

Pinkel, D. (1994). "Role of bone marrow transplantation for acute lymphoid leukemia." J Pediatr 125(3): 506-7.

Porkka, K., et al. (2008). "Dasatinib crosses the blood-brain barrier and is an efficient therapy for central nervous system Philadelphia chromosome-positive leukemia." Blood 112(4): 1005-12.

Pui, C.-H., et al. (2001). "Recombinant Urate Oxidase for the Prophylaxis or Treatment of Hyperuricemia in Patients With Leukemia or Lymphoma." Journal of Clinical Oncology 19(3): 697-704.

Pui, C. H. (2001). "Urate oxidase in the prophylaxis or treatment of hyperuricemia: the United States experience." Semin Hematol 38(4 Suppl 10): 13-21.

Pui, C. H. (2010). "Recent research advances in childhood acute lymphoblastic leukemia." J Formos Med Assoc 109(11): 777-87.

Pui, C. H. and Campana, D. (2000). "New definition of remission in childhood acute lymphoblastic leukemia." Leukemia 14(5): 783-5.

Pui, C. H., et al. (2009). "Treating childhood acute lymphoblastic leukemia without cranial irradiation." N Engl J Med 360(26): 2730-41.

Pui, C. H., et al. (2010). "Long-term results of St Jude Total Therapy Studies 11, 12, 13A, 13B, and 14 for childhood acute lymphoblastic leukemia." Leukemia 24(2): 371-82.

Pui, C. H., et al. (1997). "Urate oxidase in prevention and treatment of hyperuricemia associated with lymphoid malignancies." Leukemia 11(11): 1813-6.

Pulsipher, M. A., et al. (2011). "High-risk pediatric acute lymphoblastic leukemia: to transplant or not to transplant?" Biol Blood Marrow Transplant 17(1 Suppl): S137-48.

Rackoff, W. R., et al. (1996). "Predicting the risk of bacteremia in childen with fever and neutropenia." J Clin Oncol 14(3): 919-24.

Reichert, J. M. and Valge-Archer, V. E. (2007). "Development trends for monoclonal antibody cancer therapeutics." Nat Rev Drug Discov 6(5): 349-56.

Renyi, I., et al. (2007). "Prevention and treatment of hyperuricemia with rasburicase in children with leukemia and non-Hodgkin's lymphoma." Pathol Oncol Res 13(1): 57-62.

Riehm, H., et al. (1977). "[The west-berlin therapy study of acute lymphoblastic leukemia in childhood--report after 6 years (author's transl)]." Klin Padiatr 189(8): 89-102.

Riehm, H., et al. (1987). "[Corticosteroid-dependent reduction of leukocyte count in blood as a prognostic factor in acute lymphoblastic leukemia in childhood (therapy study ALL-BFM 83)]." Klin Padiatr 199(3): 151-60.

Rieselbach, R. E., et al. (1964). "Uric Acid Excretion and Renal Function in the Acute Hyperuricemia of Leukemia. Pathogenesis and Therapy of Uric Acid Nephropathy." Am J Med 37: 872-83.

Rosner, F. and Grunwald, H. W. (1973). "Survival in acute lymphocytic leukemia." JAMA 224(10): 1426-7.

Rundles, R. W. (1966). "Effects of allopurinol on 6-mercaptopurine therapy in neoplastic diseases." Ann Rheum Dis 25(6 Suppl): 655-6.

Schotte, D., et al. (2011). "MicroRNA characterize genetic diversity and drug resistance in pediatric acute lymphoblastic leukemia." Haematologica 96(5): 703-11.

Schrappe, M., et al. (2010). "'Educational symposium on long-term results of large prospective clinical trials for childhood acute lymphoblastic leukemia (1985-2000)'." Leukemia 24(2): 253-4.

Schultz, K. R., et al. (2009). "Improved early event-free survival with imatinib in Philadelphia chromosome-positive acute lymphoblastic leukemia: a children's oncology group study." J Clin Oncol 27(31): 5175-81.

Simone, J. and Pinkel, D. (1973). "Rationale and results of combination chemotherapy and central nervous system irradiation in acute lymphocytic leukemia." Bibl Haematol 39: 1068-73.

Simone, J. V. (1973). "Editorial: Preventive central-nervous-system therapy in acute leukemia." N Engl J Med 289(23): 1248-9.

Simpson, L. D., et al. (1973). "Radiation dosimetry for large, irregularly-shaped fields in the treatment of acute lymphocytic leukemia." Radiology 109(1): 205-7.

Sood, A. R., et al. (2006). "Clarifying the Role of Rasburicase in Tumor Lysis Syndrome." Pharmacotherapy 27(1): 111-121.

Spiegler, B. J., et al. (2006). "Comparison of long-term neurocognitive outcomes in young children with acute lymphoblastic leukemia treated with cranial radiation or high-dose or very high-dose intravenous methotrexate." J Clin Oncol 24(24): 3858-64.

Stow, P., et al. (2010). "Clinical significance of low levels of minimal residual disease at the end of remission induction therapy in childhood acute lymphoblastic leukemia." Blood 115(23): 4657-63.

Sung, L., et al. (2004). "Prophylactic granulocyte colony-stimulating factor and granulocyte-macrophage colony-stimulating factor decrease febrile neutropenia after chemotherapy in children with cancer: a meta-analysis of randomized controlled trials." J Clin Oncol 22(16): 3350-6.

Topp, M. S., et al. (2011). "Targeted therapy with the T-cell-engaging antibody blinatumomab of chemotherapy-refractory minimal residual disease in B-lineage acute lymphoblastic leukemia patients results in high response rate and prolonged leukemia-free survival." J Clin Oncol 29(18): 2493-8.

Uderzo, C., et al. (1995). "Treatment of childhood acute lymphoblastic leukemia in second remission with allogeneic bone marrow transplantation and chemotherapy: ten-year experience of the Italian Bone Marrow Transplantation Group and the Italian Pediatric Hematology Oncology Association." J Clin Oncol 13(2): 352-8.

van Dongen, J. J., et al. (1999). "Standardized RT-PCR analysis of fusion gene transcripts from chromosome aberrations in acute leukemia for detection of minimal residual disease. Report of the BIOMED-1 Concerted Action: investigation of minimal residual disease in acute leukemia." Leukemia 13(12): 1901-28.

Wang, L. Y., et al. (2006). "Recombinant urate oxidase (rasburicase) for the prevention and treatment of tumor lysis syndrome in patients with hematologic malignancies." Acta Haematol 115(1-2): 35-8.

Watts, R. W. (1966). "Allopurinol in the therapy of neoplasia and blood diseases. Metabolic aspects." Ann Rheum Dis 25(6 Suppl): 657-9.

Wiley, J. M., et al. (1990). "Invasive fungal disease in pediatric acute leukemia patients with fever and neutropenia during induction chemotherapy: a multivariate analysis of risk factors." J Clin Oncol 8(2): 280-6.

Wingard, J. R., et al. (1990). "Allogeneic bone marrow transplantation for patients with high-risk acute lymphoblastic leukemia." J Clin Oncol 8(5): 820-30.

Wyngaarden, J. B. (1970). "Allopurinol and xanthine nephropathy." N Engl J Med 283(7): 371-2.

Yang, J. J., et al. (2009). "Genome-wide interrogation of germline genetic variation associated with treatment response in childhood acute lymphoblastic leukemia." JAMA 301(4): 393-403.

Young, J. L., Jr. and Miller, R. W. (1975). "Incidence of malignant tumors in U. S. children." Journal of Pediatrics 86(2): 254-8.

Yu, L., et al. (2011). "Microarray detection of multiple recurring submicroscopic chromosomal aberrations in pediatric T-cell acute lymphoblastic leukemia." Leukemia 25(6): 1042-6.

6

Cellular Therapy of ALL

Casey A. Moffa, Cyrus Khan and John Lister
Division of Hematology and Cellular Therapy, Western Pennsylvania Cancer Institute, West Penn Allegheny Health System, Pittsburgh, USA

1. Introduction

There are almost 6000 cases of acute lymphoblastic leukemia (ALL) diagnosed annually in the United States. Approximately two-thirds occur in children and adolescents making ALL the most common cancer in that age group.[1] The remaining third occurs in the adult population with the incidence increasing beyond age 50. The biology of the disease with advancing age confers a worse prognosis than with childhood ALL as the incidence of "very high risk" cytogenetic categories, such as Philadelphia chromosome–positive (Ph+) ALL, is much higher in the older population.[2] Treatment of childhood ALL has in general been relatively successful with five-year event-free survival rates ranging from 70 to 83% in developed countries, with an overall cure rate of approximately 80%. The experience with adult ALL has been far less successful with reported cure rates rarely exceeding 40% despite the use of hematopoietic stem cell transplantation (HSCT).[3] Historically there have been two separate approaches for treatment of adult patients, transplantation-based or attempts to optimize chemotherapy reserving transplantation only for patients who are Ph+.[4-8] Prior to the last decade, allogeneic transplantation in adult patients with ALL in first remission was reserved for patients who were Ph+ or those with advanced disease.[9] The recently published results from the landmark UKALL XII/ECOG E2993 trial compared these treatment options posing the question of whether the allogeneic graft versus leukemia (GVL) effect, could improve the outcome for all suitable adult patients.[10] The trial analysis, which will be discussed in detail later in the chapter, concluded that sibling donor allogeneic HSCT was superior to chemotherapy alone in standard risk first remission ALL patients with respect to overall survival.

Achieving a complete remission (CR) with induction chemotherapy is crucial for a favorable outcome in adult patients with ALL. Furthermore, relapse from complete remission is associated with dismal survival and overall only one-third of adult patients who achieve complete remission will survive 5 years. Thus prevention of relapse is vital for long-term survival. Strategy employed to maintain remission includes autologous and allogeneic HSCT. In the case of allogeneic HSCT, evidence is mounting that not only related donor but also matched unrelated donor and umbilical cord blood sources are equivalent options when overall survival is considered. Historically, it was felt that both autologous and allogeneic transplant could improve survival on the basis of phase two data.[11] More recently, this concept has been challenged by the findings of the UKALL XII/ECOG E2993 trial.[10] Phase two data demonstrated favorable leukemia free survival (LFS) with human leukocyte antigen (HLA)-matched sibling allogeneic HSCT in ALL in first or later CR. Considering that only one-third of patients have a matched sibling donor, other graft alternatives have to be considered including autologous transplant (auto), matched unrelated donor (MUD), umbilical cord blood (UCB) and haploidentical-related donors. Although transplant related mortality (TRM) is low with autologous transplant, typically less than 5%, the overall survival (OS) is disappointing due to an unacceptably high risk of relapse and because of these findings, enthusiasm for autologous HSCT has decreased over the past few years. In contrast, the appealing aspects of allogeneic transplantation, including the potential for an immune mediated GVL effect has been associated with decreased relapse rates and improved LFS.[11]

2. Graft versus leukemia

The GVL effect in recipients of allogeneic HSCT is an anecdotally described and statistically demonstrated phenomenon. The GVL effect is statistically evident by demonstration of a higher relapse rate after autologous or syngeneic HSCT compared to allogeneic HSCT. There is also a lower incidence of relapse in patients who experience graft versus host disease (GVHD), as well as increased relapse rates in recipients of T-cell-depleted marrow grafts. Both single institution and registry data provide evidence of an allogeneic GVL effect with relapse rates lower in patients who developed GVHD than in those who did not.[12, 13] The occurrence of acute, chronic or both forms of GVHD correlated with the best disease free survival (DFS).

Doney and colleagues described a study of 192 patients with ALL, mostly transplanted in second remission (CR2). They evaluated the probability of relapse among patients with or without GVHD.[12] Relapse was significantly higher in the group that had grade 0-I GVHD. In fact, in patients without significant GVHD, the actuarial risk of relapse approached 80% versus 40% in those who developed grade II or above. Subsequently, this observation was confirmed for both relapse and overall DFS by Appelbaum et al.[13] Passweg reported a study of 1132 patients with T-cell or B-cell ALL, which showed a decreased rate of relapse in patients with both acute and chronic GVHD.[14]

These data support the idea that T-cells in the graft mediate a potent GVL effect in patients with ALL. Augmenting the GVL effect may be possible by developing antigen-specific T-cell immunotherapy for patients with ALL.[13, 15-18]

3. Minimal residual disease

As mentioned previously, one of the most important prognostic factors in patients with ALL is the achievement of CR after induction chemotherapy, in addition to age and cytogenetic abnormalities at the time of diagnosis. These factors directly reflect the chemosensitivity of the disease. Consequently, a longer time to achieve CR during induction is an indicator of relative chemoresistance. Several studies have shown that patients who need more than one cycle of induction chemotherapy have a poor long-term prognosis and a shorter duration of remission.[19-21] Historically, clinical trials have defined success of induction chemotherapeutic regimens on the basis of morphology.

With the advent of ever more sensitive molecular and immunophenotypical methods, a single blast cell in 10,000 normal cells can now be reliably detected. Using these techniques a majority of patients with ALL will have markers identified that can be used to detect minimal residual disease (MRD) at different times throughout the treatment course. The presence of MRD as detected by these methods allows for the identification of groups at risk for relapse. MRD studies might be useful for identifying high-risk groups of patients who might benefit from early transplantation and also provide guidance to help determine the most suitable conditioning regimen.[22]

Bassan and colleagues reported results of the Northern Italy Leukemia Group (NILG) study 09/00 of 280 patients with ALL. Adequate probes for MRD detection were obtained in 223 patients (88%) with a single marker in 61% and two probes in 39%.[23] A sensitivity level of 10^{-4} or higher was found in 94% of these patients and data was available on 79% of patients who completed the first stage of treatment. The presence of MRD was the strongest predictor of LFS and bone marrow relapse in the multivariate model used. Detection of MRD was associated with hazard ratios of 5.88 for DFS and 5.33 for bone marrow relapse (p=0.001). The study used risk-adapted therapy based upon MRD detection.

Study	Year	No. Evaluable/ Studied (%)	Risk Subsets	MRD Study*	Survival/DFS of MRD Negative *v* Positive; Study Conclusions
Retrospective/descriptive MRD analysis					
MRC[109]	2010	161/NR	SR/HR BCP	RQ-PCR; < 10^{-4} at 1-9 months	DFS 74% *v* 30% at 5 years (*P* = .002) MRD at end of phase II induction best predictor of relapse (*P* = .0002) HSCT partially active in MRD-positive
PALG[110]	2008	116/132 (87.8%)	SR/HR BCP/TCP	IF; < 0.1% at end of induction	DFS 61% *v* 17% at 3 years (*P* = .0002) MRD best predictor of relapse (*P* < .001), higher value in SR and BCP
GRAALL[111]	2009	212/507 (41.8%)	SR/HR BCP/TCP	RQ-PCR; < 10^{-4} at end of induction/1st consolidation	DFS 82% at 3 years (84% after HSCT censoring) *v* relapse rate 56% (*P* < .001) MRD best predictor of relapse (*P* < .001) HSCT not needed in MRD negative, partially active in MRD positive
Prospective MRD analysis for therapy optimization†					
GMALL[24, 112]	2006, 2009	479/NR	SR/HR BCP/TCP	RQ-PCR; negative/<10^{-4} at end of induction I-II and 1st consolidation	SR: survival 67% *v* 38% at 5 years (*P* < .001) HR: survival 66% *v* 42% at 5 years (*P* = .003) MRD negative at days 11 and 24 (relapse risk 0%) *v* MRD positive until week 16 (relapse risk 94%) HSCT not needed in SR MRD negative and partially active in SR/HR MRD positive
NILG[23]	2009	223/253 (88.1%)	SR/HR BCP/TCP	RQ-PCR; < 10^{-4} at week 16, negative at week 22	DFS 72% *v* 14% at 5 years (*P* = .0000) MRD at weeks 10 to 22 best predictor of relapse (*P* < .0001) HSCT not needed in MRD negative and partially active in MRD positive
PETHEMA[113]	2009	156/202 (77.2%)	HR BCP/TCP	IF; < 0.1% at end of consolidation	DFS 54% at 4 years *v* 31% at 2 years (*P* = .043) MRD best predictor of relapse (*P* = .007) HSCT not needed in MRD negative and partially active in MRD positive

NOTE. Adapted from Bassan et al.[33]

Abbreviations: MRD, minimal residual disease; ALL, acute lymphoblastic leukemia; DFS, disease-free survival; MRC, Medical Research Council; NR, not reported; SR, standard risk; HR, high risk; BCP, B-cell precursor ALL; RQ-PCR, real-time quantitative polymerase chain reaction; HSCT, hematopoietic stem-cell transplantation; PALG, Polish Adult Leukemia Group; TCP, T-cell precursor ALL; IF, immunofluorescence study (flow cytometry); GRAALL, Group for Research on Adult ALL; GMALL, German Multicenter Study Group for Adult ALL; NILG, Northern Italy Leukemia Group; PETHEMA, Programa Espanol de Tratamiento en Hematologia; CR, complete response.

*Method and definition criteria for MRD negativity.

†GMALL: reporting MRD study results in 479 of 1,489 total study patients (CR 89%); includes pilot phase with two probes with sensitivity, 10^{-4}; MRD-oriented therapy (treatment stopped after 1 year in MRD negative, only pilot phase; intensification/HSCT in MRD positive); NILG: 280 study patients, 253 evaluated for MRD probe(s), 142 for risk-oriented (n = 30) or MRD-oriented (n = 112) therapy (maintenance in MRD negative; intensification/HSCT in MRD positive); PETHEMA: 253 study patients, 156 of 202 in CR reported MRD evaluable, 100 at end of consolidation (maintenance in MRD negative; HSCT in MRD positive).

Table 1. Clinical Significance of MRD Analysis in Adult ALL (selection of recent representative studies, mainly Ph- patients)

In an earlier study by the German study group GMALL, 196 patients with standard risk-ALL had their MRD status monitored prospectively.[24] At week 16 of therapy, subsets of patients could be identified with very different outcomes. Twenty three percent of patients who had MRD detectable until week 16 and beyond had a 3-year relapse rate of 94% whereas no relapses occurred in 10% of the patients who had a rapid decline to undetectable levels when measured at days 11 and 24. Other studies have also shown similar trends (Table 1).

Studies in MRD have also been performed in the pediatric population. A recent study used polymerase chain reaction (PCR) amplification of antigen-receptor genes to detect 1 leukemic cell per 100,000 normal mononuclear cells (0.001%).[25] Stow and colleagues examined 455 pediatric patients and compared 2 cohorts based on MRD levels at day 46 of therapy. Those patients with MRD $< 0.001\%$ had a 5 year risk of relapse of 5% compared with 13% for those with MRD levels of $< 0.01\%$ but $> 0.001\%$ ($p < 0.047$).

These studies show that a higher level of MRD either after consolidation chemotherapy or a rising level during treatment might predict for a higher relapse rate. Inversely, a low level of MRD might identify a group of patients who do not necessarily need transplantation, or perhaps can wait until there is clear evidence of rising levels of MRD before further therapy is initiated.[24, 26-28] In the future, MRD might be used to further refine the treatment options for patients with ALL, and may better define which patients should undergo transplantation.

4. Who should receive a HSCT?

Established predictors of poor long-term outcome in ALL patients undergoing aggressive chemotherapy have been used to determine which patients should proceed to transplantation in first remission. In the pediatric population, transplantation is reserved for the patients with the worst prognosis, whereas the adult patient is much more likely to benefit from allogeneic HSCT and the procedure is performed more frequently. Patients with high risk features are known to have a greater risk of relapse and have historically undergone HSCT in first remission (CR1) if they were deemed transplant candidates.[19, 29-31] High-risk features include: age greater than 35 years, leukocyte count > 30,000/μL for B-cell and > 100,000/μL in T-cell origin, non T-cell phenotype, lack of mediastinal adenopathy, poor performance status at diagnosis, t(9;22), t(4;11), t(1;19) or t(8;14). Patients who require more than four weeks of induction therapy to achieve remission or who have detectable molecular or immunophenotypical evidence of disease while in remission also have a poorer prognosis.[32]

The results of the UKALL XII/ ECOG E2993 trial demonstrated superior survival in standard risk patients who underwent allogeneic HSCT. Many centers have taken this as conclusive evidence that all patients with standard risk disease in CR 1 should undergo allogeneic HSCT, if they are suitable candidates and a suitable donor is available.[10] Whether allogeneic transplant should be performed in all ALL patients in CR 1 is debatable, given the excellent outcome observed with chemotherapy alone in subsets such as young males with standard risk T-ALL. The reduction of relapse risk with allogeneic HSCT is definitely superior to chemotherapy alone or autologous transplant.[5, 10, 33-37] Given the uncertainty, patient education and choice must be a priority for clinicians who treat such individuals.

Adolescents and young adults (AYA), ages 16-30, or subsets thereof appear to have less favorable outcome than younger pediatric patients. However, retrospective analyses comparing pediatric and adult therapy of ALL in AYA, have shown significantly better results with pediatric treatment protocols with survival rates at 5 years of 67% to 78% compared to 34% to 41% with adult protocols.[36, 38-42] The question of the applicability of pediatric style therapy is being formally tested in clinical trial to define the toxicity and feasibility of the pediatric approach to therapy in AYA. The CALGB is conducting study 10403 (http://www.clinicaltrials.gov ID:NCT00558519), which treats ALL patients 16 to 39 years of age on one arm of the Children's Oncology Group (COG) AALL0232 protocol. As the CALGB and COG protocols are running concurrently patient specific data from both trials will be used to compare the outcome of AYA treated in the pediatric and adult settings. Investigators at the Dana Farber Cancer Institute are conducting a phase 2 clinical trial that investigates the safety and efficacy of a pediatric regimen which includes pegylated L-asparaginase in patients age 18-50 (Study 06-254).[22] If the outcome appears to be improved by the application of the pediatric approach to therapy of ALL then subsequent trials might compare allogeneic transplant to pediatric chemotherapy regimens in a prospective fashion.

Although pediatric style treatment when retrospectively compared to adult therapy has created an interesting hypothesis, the UKALL XII/ECOG E2993 trial showed that in every age group up to 40 years, including those younger than 20, there was an OS advantage to having a donor. There is thus insufficient evidence at this point to conclude that allogeneic transplantation in CR1 should be abandoned in this age group, including those with high-risk disease.[22]

In patients with ALL greater than 50 years of age, treatment related mortality increases and the effectiveness of therapy decreases, as noted in previous studies and the UKALL XII/ECOG E2993 trial. The age at which the TRM exceeds the reduction in relapse risk may even be as low as age 35 to 40 years. A recent meta-analysis that included the UKALL XII/ECOG E2993 data also showed a survival advantage for standard risk patients and a non-significant survival advantage for high-risk patients.[43] This may be due in part to the fact that older patients have more high-risk features. These prospective trials have used full-intensity myeloablative conditioning regimens that include total body irradiation (TBI), whereas reduced intensity conditioning (RIC) might allow for the therapeutic benefit of a GVL effect with less transplant related toxicity. Reduced TRM with RIC regimens might permit allogeneic transplantation in older patients.[22] Conditioning regimens, including RIC regimens, are reviewed in more detail later in the chapter.

In patients with B-ALL that express CD20, the addition of the anti-CD20 monoclonal antibody rituximab to chemotherapy, might increase the survival rate by 20% to 30% to approximately 80%.[44, 45] In these patients, relapse tends to occur within the first year and a half after achieving remission. There are no validated prognostic factors that predict relapse. Thus the detection of MRD in CR1 might select patients for allogeneic HSCT since maintenance chemotherapy is associated with a high risk of relapse.[33]

Until more effective non-transplant therapy is developed for adult ALL, risk adapted selection of patients for allogeneic HSCT will likely increase. The co-morbid status, age of the patient and MRD status will most likely dictate the type of conditioning regimen selected for transplantation.[10] A summary of overall results of HSCT in adults with ALL can be found in table 2.

HSCT and Disease Stage	No.	DFS/OS*		Relapse*		TRM*		Decision	Recommendation
		No.	%	No.	%	No.	%		
Sibling donor									
CR1	1,100	50	21-71	24	10-50	27	12-42	HSCT *v* CHT	Comparable results; HSCT probably superior in HR
CR2	1,019	31	16-60	48	62-71	29	40-75		HSCT superior
Relapsed/refractory	216	18	8-33	75	60-77	47	46-47		
Matched unrelated donor									
CR1	318	39	32-51	10	6-19	47	32-54	Sibling *v* matched unrelated	Comparable results
> CR2	231	27	17-28	8†		75†			
Autologous									
CR1	1,369	42	15-65	51	27-68	5	0-8	Autologous *v* CHT	Comparable results
CR2	258	21	20-27	70	59-75	18		Autologous *v* allogeneic	Advantage for allogeneic
Non-myeloablative, all stages	132	23	0-50	47	30-56	42	10-72	RIC *v* TBI-based regimens	Advantage for TBI-based full intensity conditioning

NOTE. Adapted from Bassan et al.[33]

Abbreviations: HSCT, hematopoietic stem-cell transplantation; ALL, acute lymphoblastic leukemia; DFS, disease-free survival; OS, overall survival; TRM, transplantation-related mortality; CR1, first complete response; CHT, chemotherapy; HR, high risk; CR2, second complete response; RIC, reduced intensity conditioning; TBI, total body irradiation.

*Weighted mean and range of published studies.

†One study.

Table 2. Overall Results of HSCT in Adult ALL and Current Recommendations

5. Types of HSCT

Since 2000, there have been at least 10 trials that have compared the outcome of patients with ALL with high-risk features based upon related donor availability.[4, 7, 46, 47] Seven out of ten studies demonstrated statistically significant improvement in LFS with allografts. TRM varied considerably between 9% and 44% with the highest reported in the LALA-87 trial in sibling donor allogeneic HSCT compared to 2% to 24% in autologous transplant.[7] A meta-analysis was performed of all prospective trials, 1274 total patients, which confirmed a beneficial effect of allogeneic sibling HSCT.[48] Patients in the sibling donor group showed better survival, which was even more pronounced in the patients with high-risk features. The UKALL XII/ECOG E2993 trial reported its findings to prospectively determine what the optimal therapy should be for adult patients with newly diagnosed ALL. In individuals with standard risk ALL, defined as age < 30 years, Philadelphia chromosome negative and low white blood cell count at presentation, OS in allogeneic HSCT recipients was found to be superior to chemotherapy in CR1. The greatest benefit was apparent in patients < 30 years as higher TRM negated the benefit of a lower relapse rate in older patients.

HLA-matched unrelated donor transplantation is another HSCT option for patients with ALL. In high-risk ALL, matched unrelated donors have been used when matched siblings were not available, and there is preliminary evidence that a well-matched unrelated donor may be comparable to a sibling donor.[49] There have been no prospective randomized trials that investigate the use of this type of transplant compared to autologous transplant. In a large retrospective analysis from the Center for International Bone Marrow Transplant research (CIBMTR), outcome and toxicity of 712 patients < 50 years of age in CR1 or CR2 were compared based upon type of HSCT (517 MUD, 195 autologous).[50] TRM was significantly higher in the MUD treatment group as compared to those patients who underwent autologous transplant (p=0.004). The CIBMTR also performed a long-term update analysis that confirmed similar 5-year survival for patients in CR1 after MUD and autologous transplant (38% versus 39%), but superior 5-year survival after MUD transplantation in CR2 (30% versus 14%).[11] The rate of relapse was significantly different between the two types of transplant: 20% in CR1 and 25% in ≥ CR2 for MUD versus 58% in CR1 and 81% in ≥ CR2 in autologous transplant (P=<0.0001).

There have been two recent studies that compared the outcomes of MUD and sibling allogeneic transplantation.[8, 51] In these studies, HLA class I and II high resolution typing was used for most of the patients, which reflects more closely the current standard of donor selection. The first study found that disease free survival (DFS) for adults with high-risk ALL in CR1 is similar between siblings and MUD HSCT. The second study included 84 high-risk patients and showed a 3-year survival of 46% in patients who received a sibling allogeneic transplant versus 44% for those treated with MUD transplantation. There was no relevant difference noted in TRM rate (27% and 26%, respectively). These reports support comparable results whether the allogeneic donor is related or unrelated. Recent reports that present comparable outcomes after related and unrelated HSCT are not based on intention-to-treat analyses and need to be interpreted appropriately. Despite the widespread perception of a similar outcome, it is common practice for a discrepant approach in the policy of many transplant centers.[9]

Umbilical cord blood (UCB) transplantation is now a standard option for management of pediatric ALL. UCB grafts that are partially mismatched have been used without causing excessive GVHD or graft rejection. This may be a consequence of the naïve immune status of T-cells in the UCB unit. Collection of UCB from ethnic and racially underrepresented populations in the donor pool might increase the availability of allogeneic HSCT as a treatment option for these groups.[11] Since the collection of UCB is possible from every healthy live birth with no potential harm to the donor, this option is potentially unlimited as donation is uncomplicated. UCB samples are also prescreened for infection, HLA-typed and cryopreserved and are thus quickly available for transplantation. Three studies examined UCB transplantation in adults with different types of hematological malignancy and a meta-analysis was performed.[52] There were 316 total adults who received UCB transplant versus 996 patients who underwent mostly fully matched unrelated donor transplantation without in vitro T-cell depletion. The TRM and DFS were not statistically different between the two groups despite more HLA-disparity in the UCB transplant patients. This meta-analysis represents the most cogent data available for comparison of UCB and MUD transplantation. Logistical difficulty associated with designing and conducting a randomized comparison of UCB and MUD transplantation makes this comparison unlikely in the future.

Mismatched related donor and haploidentical HSCT is an experimental therapy whose usefulness is being explored in patients with very high-risk and late stage disease who do not have an HLA-matched sibling or alternative donor available.[22] The advantage of haploidentical HSCT is both real and theoretical. The most obvious advantage is the almost universal availability of a related donor who is at least haplotype identical to the patient in need of the transplant. Such donors are usually available quickly, and can serve as repeat donors in the event of engraftment failure or as donors of lymphocytes in order to convert mixed chimerism to full donor hematopoiesis or to treat disease relapse. A more potent graft versus tumor effect is also a theoretically attractive benefit from this type of transplant.[53]

6. Why Allogeneic HSCT?

6.1 UKALL XII/ECOG E2993

In 1993, the UK Medical Research Council (MRC) and the Eastern Cooperative Oncology Group (ECOG) of the United States collaboratively developed a large study to ask two fundamental questions regarding ALL.[10] Given that GVL was first described in adult ALL and given published data supporting allogeneic transplantation in first CR for Ph+ and other high risk patients; could the allogeneic effect improve the outcome for all suitable adult patients?[8, 54] The second question was, given the fact that protracted consolidation/maintenance therapy has been the mainstay of treatment for ALL, based on data mostly extrapolated from pediatric experience, could single autologous transplantation replace extended maintenance therapy? The UKALL XII/ECOG E2993 trial was designed so that all adult patients with a matched sibling donor would receive an allogeneic HSCT. The patients without a donor would be randomized to an autologous HSCT versus consolidation and maintenance chemotherapy. Maintenance therapy consisted of vincristine 1.4 mg/m^2 intravenously every 3 months, prednisone 60 mg/m^2 orally for 5 days every 3 months, 6-mercaptopurine 75 mg/m^2 orally each day, and methotrexate 20 mg/m^2 orally or intravenously once a week. Maintenance therapy was to continue for a total of 2.5 years from the start of intensification therapy.

Prior to randomization, all patients received intensification with high dose methotrexate. The primary outcome of the study was OS. Other measures of outcome to be assessed were event free survival (EFS) and non-relapse mortality defined as time to death censored at relapse.

A total of 1929 patients were recruited from 1993 to 2006, with 16 excluded, as pathology review did not substantiate the diagnosis of ALL. All patients age 15-59 with newly diagnosed ALL were included, including Ph+ patients. They received identical induction therapy, irrespective of risk assessment, including central nervous system (CNS) prophylaxis and treatment of CNS disease if present at diagnosis. In 2003, the upper age limit was increased to 64 and the upper age limit for allogeneic transplant was increased to 54. Patients that were Ph+ were also offered MUD transplantation.

High risk in this study was defined as patients older than 35 years, having a high WBC count at diagnosis ($\geq 30 \times 10^9$/L for B lineage and $\geq 100 \times 10^9$ /L for T lineage) and patients with t(9;22). All other patients were deemed standard risk. The median follow-up in this study was 4 years, 11 months. The OS of the 1913 patients at 5 years was 39% and was 43% for patients who were Ph- (Figure 1A and 1B) and there was no difference in survival between patients entered through MRC or ECOG (Figure 1C). Figure 1D demonstrates the overall survival benefit when all patients on study are included in this analysis with a 5-year survival of 53% (95% CI = 48% - 58%) for patients with a donor versus 45% (95% CI = 40% - 49%) for patients without a donor ($p = 0.1$). The high-risk patients had an OS of 41% versus 35% for donor versus no donor, respectively, which was not statistically significant; however, the OS was significantly improved in the standard risk patients, 62% versus 52% for donor versus no donor, respectively ($p = 0.02$) for survival at 5 years (Figure 1E and 1F). The relapse rate was significantly reduced in both risk groups who underwent allogeneic HSCT, confirming the potency of the graft versus leukemia effect in allogeneic transplantation.

There were 456 patients in the study that were randomized to the chemotherapy versus autologous transplantation arm of which 16 were Ph+. The patients who were randomized to receive chemotherapy had significantly improved 5 year EFS (41% versus 32%; $p = 0.02$) and OS (46% versus 37%; $p = 0.03$) (Figure 2A and 2B). The 5-year survival for chemotherapy versus autologous transplantation among the high-risk patients was 37% versus 31%, respectively and was 56% versus 46%, respectively for the standard risk patients (Figure 2C and 2D). Non-relapse mortality was 16% for the autologous versus 8% for the chemotherapy group (Figure 2E).

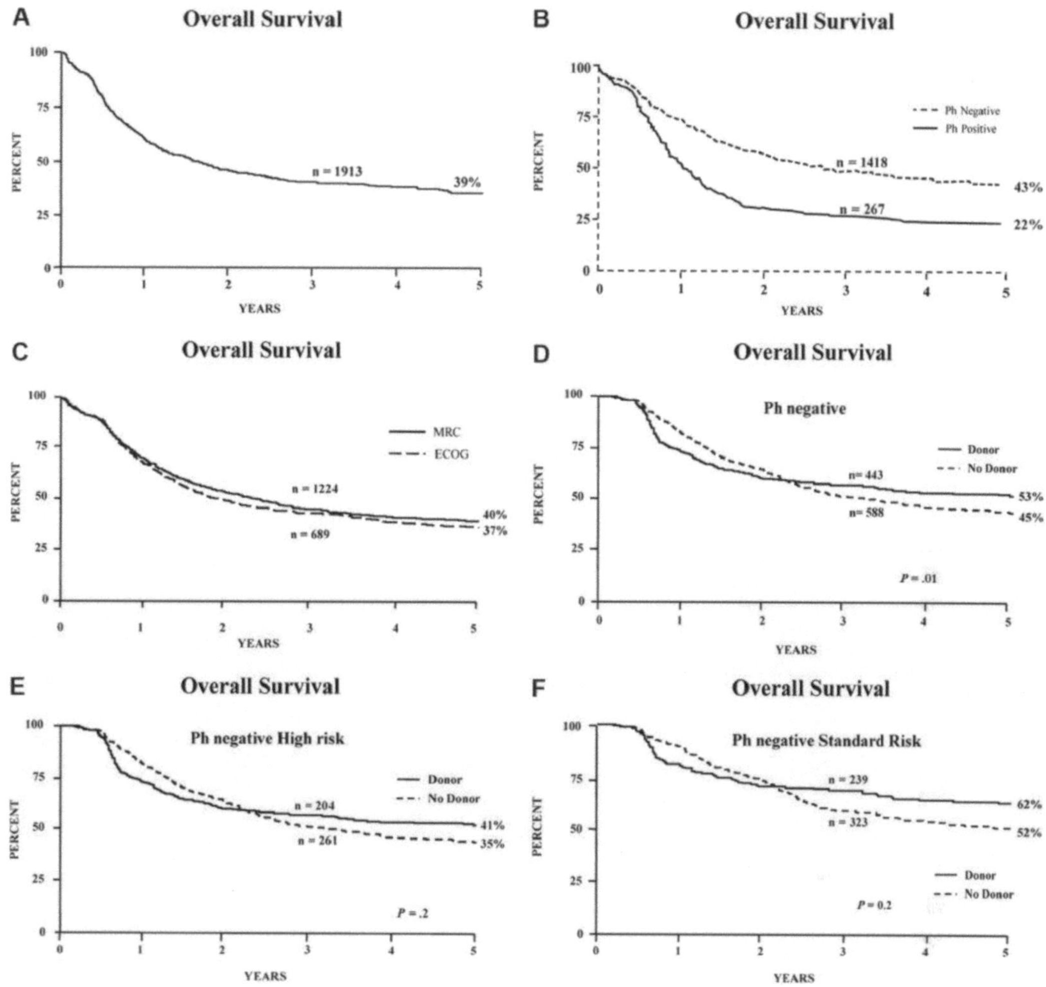

Note: Adapted from Goldstone, et al.[10]

Fig. 1. Survival of patients and donor versus no-donor analysis. Overall survival from diagnosis for (A) all patients entered on the study, including Ph-positive; (B) Ph-negative and Ph-positive patients; (C) patients entered via MRC or ECOG; (D) donor versus no-donor for all Ph-negative patients; (E) donor versus no-donor for Ph-negative patients with high risk; and (F) donor versus no-donor for Ph-negative patients with standard risk.

After reviewing the data and noting that patients randomized to chemotherapy had a better outcome than those undergoing autologous transplantation, an analysis was made that compared patients with a donor versus those without to investigate the effect of allogeneic transplantation versus chemotherapy alone. There was a superior OS noted for the patients with a donor, in the standard risk patients, with a 5-year survival of 62% for those with a donor versus 52% for those without. This same benefit could not be demonstrated for the high-risk patients. In high-risk patients, the donor versus no donor comparison showed a 5 year OS of 41% versus 35% which was not statistically significant. This finding questions the need for immediate allogeneic transplantation in high-risk patients, however for high-risk patients allogeneic transplantation remains the standard of care.

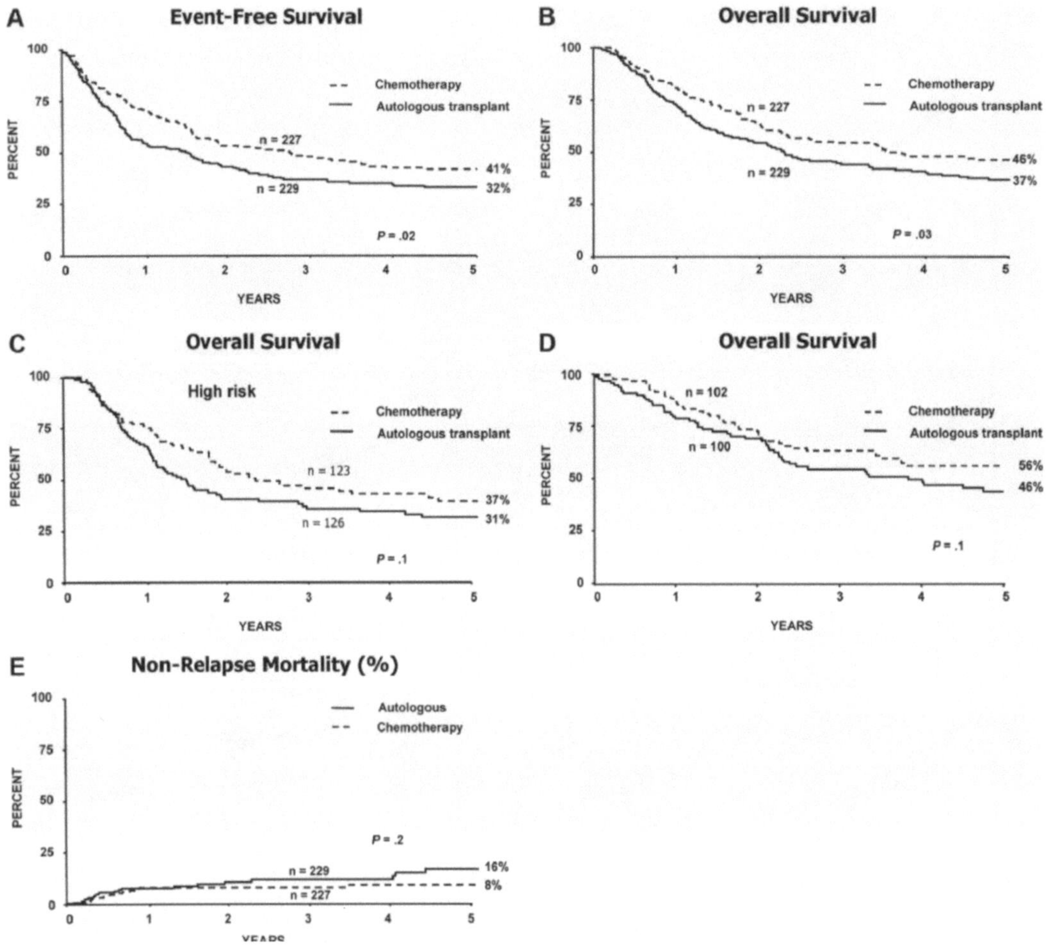

Note: Adapted from Goldstone, et al.10

Fig. 2. Randomized chemotherapy versus autologous transplantation, measured from time of randomization. (A) Event-free survival for all patients. (B) Overall survival for all (C) high-risk patients and (D) standard-risk patients. (E) Nonrelapse mortality for all patients undergoing chemotherapy or autologous transplantation.

One of the most noteworthy findings of the UKALL XII/ECOG E2993 trial was the potent anti-leukemic effect seen in adults who received allogeneic transplantation as demonstrated by a significantly reduced relapse rate. TRM in the high-risk patients was 36%, which is considered to be unacceptably high. In the low-risk group with a donor the TRM was 20%. However the high-risk group was older than the standard-risk group and would be expected to suffer more TRM. The TRM in the standard-risk group was 7% for no donor but rose to 14% in the high-risk group with no donor. The most benefit was seen in patients with standard risk disease where allogeneic transplant demonstrated a significant survival advantage over those who underwent conventional chemotherapy (Figure 3A, 3B and 3C). There have been small studies of autologous transplantation reported.[4-7, 55] Review of the data shows no clearly increased anti-leukemic benefit over conventional chemotherapy. The

UKALL XII/ECOG E2993 trial showed an inferior outcome for autologous transplantation as compared to chemotherapy and thus autologous HSCT cannot be recommended as the preferred modality. The study concluded that allogeneic transplantation is the treatment of choice for adults with standard risk disease in remission and provides the greatest chance for long-term survival.

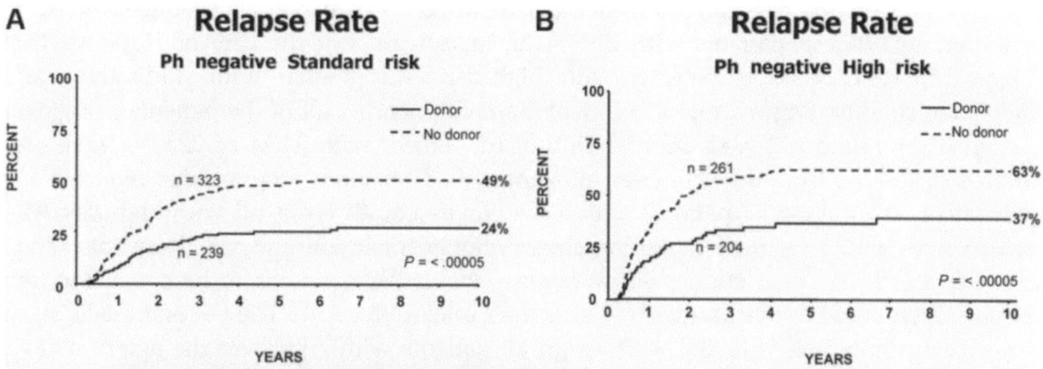

C **Non-Relapse Mortality (%)**

	3 months	6 months	1 year	2 years
High Risk				
Donor	1.5	7.3	26.0	35.8
No Donor	1.2	2.0	10.3	13.6
Standard Risk				
Donor	0.4	3.4	17.6	19.5
No Donor	0.3	1.2	5.3	6.9

Note: Adapted from Goldstone, et al.10

Fig. 3. Relapse on study and mortality not associated with relapse. Relapse rate for (A) Ph-negative patients at standard risk; (B) Ph-negative patients at high risk; and (C) nonrelapse mortality for high-risk and standard-risk patients. Note the underlying mortality at 1 and 2 years among the no-donor group.

7. Philadelphia positive ALL

ALL with t(9;22), also referred to as Philadelphia chromosome positive (Ph+), historically has a lower rate of CR and lower long-term OS than Ph negative disease. Ph+ ALL accounts for approximately one fourth of all adult ALL. Historically, clinical trials typically would assign this group to the very-high-risk treatment arms and most physicians treating outside of a clinical trial would recommend myeloablative HSCT. With the advent of tyrosine kinase inhibitors (TKI), there is now the question of whether HSCT is still necessary in this patient population.[49] There have been two large studies performed that support the overall benefit of a sibling transplant in unselected patients with Ph+ ALL in the pre-TKI era. The first study was the LALA-94 trial that prospectively studied 154 patients with Ph+ ALL and showed that among 103 patients eligible for HSCT, the presence of a sibling donor was independently predictive of remission duration.[47] The second trial, the previously mentioned UKALL XII/ECOG E2993 study, evaluated the outcome of 267 patients with Ph+ ALL and noted that those patients who had received a myeloablative sibling allogeneic or MUD transplantation had a better outcome than those who had received chemotherapy alone.[56]

There are no prospective randomized trials reported to date that use reduced intensity conditioning (RIC) in patients with Ph+ ALL. Investigators at the City of Hope Medical Center reported 24 adult patients with high-risk ALL treated with fludarabine and melphalan conditioning without T cell depletion with nearly half of the patients being over age 50. They found a 2-year OS and DFS of 62 percent with TRM of 22%.[57] There was another case series from the University of Minnesota Transplant program that reported a 3-year OS of 50% among 22 patients with a median age of 49 years, all with high-risk ALL treated with a RIC regimen of fludarabine, cyclophosphamide and low dose total body irradiation (TBI).[58] These studies show non-myeloablative regimens to be promising, but require careful prospective studies to define their role in Ph+ ALL. The UK National Cancer Research Institute, UKALL XIV, will assign all patients with ALL over the age of 40 to a non-myeloablative approach with fludarabine, melphalan and alemtuzumab in an attempt to decrease GVHD, which was seen in 86% of the City of Hope patients who did not undergo T cell depletion as part of their conditioning regimen.[49]

Prospective studies that randomize between allogeneic HSCT and continued chemotherapy introduce complexity in the analysis and interpretation of the trial data. Specifically the analysis might be biased by survivor treatment selection bias, also known as immortal time bias. Simply, patients with Ph+ ALL on a prospective study who undergo HSCT must have achieved, and remained in, a CR before transplant, resulting in a period of "immortal time." Patients dying of either disease or treatment-related causes within the immortal time window are never transplanted, resulting in an immortal time bias. This type of bias is present in studies of Ph+ ALL due to the lower rates of CR, short remission duration and toxicity of the initial treatment, as compared to Ph- patients.[49] The overall effect is to overestimate the effect of allogeneic HSCT as compared to chemotherapy when analyzed in an intent-to-treat fashion. The UKALL XII/ECOG E2993 trial is a good example of how the potential benefits of HSCT can be overestimated. Analysis by treatment received showed that those who received either a sibling or MUD HSCT had a much better 5-year OS (44% and 36%) than those who had received chemotherapy alone (19% at 5 years). All of these results, in addition to EFS and relapse free survival (RFS) were highly statistically significant. In contrast, when the analysis was repeated, adjusting for age, sex, presenting WBC and chemotherapy-treated patients who relapsed or died before median time to transplant were excluded; only RFS remained significantly superior in the transplanted group.[49]

Childhood ALL with t(9;22) remains an indication for HSCT. Due to the rarity of the disease, only 2% of cases, studies have been difficult to carry out. The Children's Oncology Group conducted a study using imatinib with intensive chemotherapy.59 The study evaluated 92 patients ages 1-21 who were divided into 5 cohorts who received progressively increased exposure to imatinib from 42 days to 280 continuous days (cohort 5, n=50) before maintenance therapy. Patients with an HLA identical sibling underwent HSCT with imatinib given for 6 months following their transplant. This allowed for comparison between the group that did not undergo transplantation and only received chemotherapy in combination, to the group that eventually went on to transplant. The concluding data was slightly confounded by the relatively high rate of off protocol use of MUD HSCT. Nevertheless, at 3 years, the outcomes were not significantly different for those treated with chemotherapy plus imatinib (n=25) compared to those treated with allogeneic HSCT (n=21). More than 85% of patients were alive and disease free at 3 years without allogeneic HSCT. This study was not powered to answer the question of whether imatinib plus chemotherapy could replace sibling allogeneic HSCT in Ph+ ALL, but the results encourage further investigation.

The UKALL XII/ECOG E2993 trial also reported in abstract form a large cohort of patients who were treated with imatinib and chemotherapy who did not undergo HSCT, in which the 3 year OS was 28%. By comparison, the 5 year OS of historical controls in the pre-TKI era was 19%.[60, 61]

A small series reported by Thomas et al added imatinib to hyper-CVAD induction chemotherapy and concluded superiority over historical controls treated with chemotherapy alone.[62] In older patients, for whom HSCT is not an option due to the presence of co-morbid conditions, the efficacy of imatinib alone can be studied more clearly. In a German study that included patients over 55 years of age (median 68 years), patients were randomized between co-administration of imatinib with induction chemotherapy or subsequent co-administration with consolidation chemotherapy.[61] The CR rates were 96% and 50%, respectively; however, there was no significant difference between the 2 cohorts in OS. Only 43% of the patients had undetectable *BCR-ABL* transcripts. Patients negative by reverse transcriptase polymerase chain retention assay (RT-PCR) for *BCR-ABL* had superior OS compared to those who remained positive.[2]

In other studies imatinib was given as monotherapy without subsequent HSCT, but the majority of those patients were older. These studies have shown similar impressive initial responses to that seen in the younger patients. CR rates of 90% to 100% have been documented, however relapse occurs quickly and long-term DFS remains low.[60, 61] A substantial number of patients treated with imatinib develop resistance which accounts for the high number of relapses. Second generation TKIs, such as dasatinib and nilotinib, have demonstrated promising efficacy in treatment of patients with imatinib resistance.[63-65] Long term survival however, remains elusive with monotherapy.

The CALGB has conducted a clinical trial (study 10001) to determine the activity and tolerability of imatinib used in initial treatment of Ph+ ALL. In that trial, imatinib is administered after sequential chemotherapy. Subsequently patients underwent autologous HSCT, allogeneic HSCT or consolidation chemotherapy with Etoposide and Cytarabine. All patients were given imatinib maintenance therapy beginning on day 30 post transplant or after consolidation chemotherapy and were continued on treatment for at least 1 year. Therapy was stopped before 1 year if the patient had 2 consecutive negative RT-PCR at least 3 months apart or until relapse. The final results of this study are not yet available and accrual closed April 2010 (https://www.clinicaltrials. gov ID:NCT00039377). Other trials compared alternating blocks of chemotherapy with single agent imatinib versus a concurrent treatment regimen. The simultaneous treatment schedule did induce greater reductions in the *BCR-ABL* transcripts than the alternating schedule ($p = 0.01$), however there was no significant improvement in overall survival.[66]

For patients with Ph+ ALL, myeloablative HSCT is still the treatment of choice if the patient is able to tolerate the procedure. There is a lack of prospective data showing TKIs alone or in combination with chemotherapy, have increased survival in ALL. Whether the incorporation of TKIs into the treatment of Ph+ ALL will increase the efficacy of allogeneic HSCT remains an open question. If TKI therapeutics were to be administered early in the treatment of Ph+ ALL, this strategy might facilitate allogeneic HSCT if CR is improved and extended. The use of TKI therapy after allogeneic HSCT might provide sufficient post-transplant leukemia suppression to allow a GVL effect to develop. In those patients with persistent MRD after transplant the GVL might be more potent with TKI suppression of MRD.

8. Conditioning regimens

Conditioning regimens previously employed in the treatment of ALL range from the fully myeloablative TBI containing regimens to the RIC regimens. Novel methods of radiation administration such as tomotherapy and radioimmunoconjugates are under clinical investigation.

8.1 Myeloablative conditioning regimens

Although many different regimens have been developed for ALL, the one most commonly used is cyclophosphamide (Cy) plus TBI.[32] TBI has remained the backbone of conditioning regimens for ALL since the decade beginning 1970. It is prudent to understand the details of TBI with respect to DFS and TRM and how the patient population under treatment influences these statistics.

8.2 Role of TBI

Initially, TBI was intended for eradication of disease or to reduce the tumor burden.[67-69] After TBI was established as a myeloablative agent in the setting of autologous and allogeneic transplantation, several groups also recognized its potential role as an immunosuppressive agent.[70] TBI can be employed as an immunosuppressant, facilitating engraftment of donor cells and allowing for an immunotherapeutic effect of donor cells against ALL. In this role, TBI is not used for its myeloablative properties.

Early myeloablative regimens employed TBI as single doses of 8-10 Gray (Gy).[67-69] These large dosages of radiation resulted in significant morbidity and mortality, particularly from interstitial pneumonitis.[71, 72] In order to decrease toxicity and improve tolerability, fractionation and dose rate reduction were employed.[72-76] Studies in both rodents and humans indicated that rates less than 10-12 cGy/min were associated with reduced morbidity.[73, 77, 78] Other studies showed that fractionated TBI given daily or even up to four times daily improved the therapeutic ratio, thus allowing for higher doses of radiation to be delivered safely.[68, 77, 79, 80] These data support reduced dose-rate, fractionated TBI as standard and myeloablative regimens containing TBI commonly employ a schedule delivering 12 Gy TBI administered twice daily in six fractions over three days (200 cGy per fraction), in combination with chemotherapy. These regimens provide both immunosuppressive and cytotoxic activity. Dose escalation to 15-16 Gy in hopes of further reducing relapse rates has not been shown to improve overall survival. Although relapse rates did decrease, there was an increase in non-relapse mortality, thus offsetting any benefit from the higher dose of TBI.[79, 81, 82]

8.3 Cy/TBI versus BuCy

Investigators substituted Busulfan (Bu) for TBI creating the regimen BuCy as some centers did not have TBI available.[83, 84] These studies showed that combined alkylating agents could replace Cy/TBI as conditioning for HSCT in the treatment of ALL.

There is conflicting data on the superiority of one regimen over another and various studies have tried to answer this question. A retrospective analysis from the CIBMTR concluded that the Cy/TBI regimen was superior to the non-TBI-containing regimen of BuCy, with a 3-year survival of 55% versus 40% for BuCy (P = 0.003). The study also found that the risk for relapse was similar between the groups.[85] A more recent meta-analysis of seven randomized controlled trials involving 730 patients compared Cy/TBI to BuCy in patients with acute leukemia and found that Cy/TBI was associated with a modest but non-significant reduction in all cause mortality (RR = 0.82, 95%CI: 0.64-1.05; p = 0.12) and relapse of leukemia (RR = 0.89, 95%CI: 0.72-1.10; p = 0.28). Treatment related mortality was significantly less with Cy/TBI compared to BuCy (RR-0.53, 95%CI: 0.31-0.90; p = 0.02) but the cumulative incidence of major complications was not significantly different between the two regimens.[86]

8.4 Other regimens

Several centers have employed high-dose fractionated TBI in combination with high-dose Ara-C in patients receiving allogeneic HSCT from sibling donors, and have not shown any significant improvement in DFS, except for a small series of pediatric patients in one study.[87, 88] Another study looked at combining Busulfan, Fludarabine and 400 cGy of TBI as a myeloablative regimen and showed low transplant-related mortality of 3% and projected DFS of 65%.[89] Significant interest has also been shown in evaluating the role of etoposide as part of conditioning regimens including a phase I/II study that evaluated substituting etoposide for Cyclophosphamide in combination with fractionated TBI (13.2Gy). This study found DFS to be 57% with a 32% relapse rate suggesting that this regimen had significant activity in patients with advanced ALL.[90] A subsequent randomized controlled trial also confirmed these findings.[91] The UKALL XII/ECOG E2993 trial utilized Etoposide/TBI as their conditioning regimen for patients with ALL in CR1. Another study that compared Cy/TBI to Etoposide/TBI (60mg/kg) in 502 patients with ALL found that relapse rates, treatment failure and mortality were lower with etoposide/TBI, regardless of TBI dose (*P*=0.001).[92] However, in patients receiving Cy/TBI, OS was significantly improved with TBI doses less than 13 Gy (p = 0.0005).

We conclude that both the chemotherapeutic agents used, as well as the dose of radiation therapy, interact in altering the outcome of patients with ALL undergoing HSCT. There is still no conclusive evidence of one regimen's superiority over another but most centers are still inclined to include TBI as part of any regimen used for myeloablative conditioning in patients with ALL.

8.5 Role of reduced intensity conditioning

As mentioned previously, the UKALL XII/ECOG E2993 trial showed that allogeneic HSCT confers the greatest durable benefit for standard risk adult patients and is more effective than either chemotherapy or autologous HSCT.[10] However, the same trial also showed that in patients over 45 years of age and others with high-risk ALL, a high non-relapse mortality (NRM) of 36% would offset any potential survival advantage of a reduced relapse rate conferred by myeloablative transplant. Thus, myeloablative regimens are often limited to patients who are less than 50 years of age and have an excellent performance status. RIC regimens have been developed over the last decade to allow engraftment with reduced regimen related toxicity. Once donor engraftment is achieved and immune reconstitution has started a GVL effect might be operative. Hence the benefit of allogeneic transplantation might be retained and with decreased regimen related toxicity this type of transplant could be offered to older patients with greater safety.

Investigation of RIC in ALL has somewhat lagged behind studies of other hematological malignancies such as AML, despite evidence of a GVL effect.[93] Gyurkocza and collaborators reported 247 patients with AML with a median age of 60 who underwent allogeneic HSCT from both related as well as unrelated donors.[94] The estimated OS at 5 years was 33% and the estimated 5-year relapse/progression rate and non-relapse mortality were 42% and 26%, respectively.

There have been several reports published with regards to using RIC in adult patients with ALL. One series of 24 patients, primarily with high risk ALL, who received Fludarabine and Melphalan conditioning, followed by matched related (33%) or unrelated (67%) HSCT.[57] Only 10 patients in the series were in CR1 and there was a median follow-up of 28.5 months for living patients. Both OS and DFS at 2 years was 62%, relapse incidence was 21% and non-relapse mortality was 22% at two years.

The European Group for Blood and Marrow Transplantation (EBMT) reported the outcome of 97 adult patients with ALL who received RIC allogeneic HSCT.[95] Only 29% of patients were in CR1 and the 2-year OS for this sub-group was 52%. Inclusive of all patients, the 2-year OS was 31% with a non-relapse mortality of 18%. Marks et al reported 93 adult patients with Philadelphia negative ALL receiving RIC allogeneic HSCT compared to 1428 patients receiving full-intensity allografts using sibling and unrelated donors in first or second CR.[96] Surprisingly, the RIC cohort had a similar OS to the full intensity cohort at 3 years (38% versus 43%, $p = 0.39$) despite a substantially older median age (45 versus 28, $p < 0.01$).

A retrospective study reported by the EBMT compared the outcome of 576 adult ALL patients aged 45 and over in CR who received RIC (n=127) or full intensity conditioning (n=449) followed by allogeneic HSCT from an HLA-identical sibling.[97] With a median follow-up of 16 months, the non-relapse mortality was significantly higher in the cohort of patients receiving the full intensity conditioning while rates of relapse were significantly higher in the RIC cohort. In a multivariate analysis, the type of conditioning regimen was not significantly associated with leukemia-free survival.

Ram et al evaluated the utility of RIC in patients with high-risk ALL.[98] Fifty-one patients, median age 56 years, underwent allogeneic HSCT from a sibling or MUD after fludarabine and 2 Gy TBI. Twenty-five patients were Ph+ ALL. Eighteen of these patients received post-grafting imatinib. With a median follow-up of 43 months, the 3-year overall survival was 34%. The 3-year relapse/progression and non-relapse mortality rates were 40% and 28%, respectively. Three-year OS for patients with Ph- ALL in CR1 and beyond was 52% and 8%, respectively. For patients with Ph+ ALL in CR1 who received post-grafting imatinib, the 3-year OS was 62%; for the subgroup without evidence of MRD at transplantation, the overall survival was 73%.

Data from the pediatric population also suggests that RIC might be a viable option. Verneris et al reported on 38 pediatric patients median age of 12 years who received a RIC allogeneic HSCT.[99] Only 13% of the patients were in CR1. A third of the patients received

MUD transplantation. At 3 years, the probability of TRM was 40%, relapse 37%, and DFS was 30%.

These results show consistently that OS is not decreased with RIC when compared to fully myeloablative regimens. The improved tolerability of RIC regimens, when compared to myeloablative regimens, makes RIC an option for older patients. RIC may also extend the option of an allogeneic HSCT to patients who would not otherwise be transplant candidates because of co-morbid conditions.

8.6 Novel conditioning regimens

Studies performed on patients with other hematological malignancies have suggested that with higher doses of TBI the rates of relapse are lower.[32] These findings suggest that methods that can selectively deliver radiation to sites of leukemia without increasing toxicity might be of benefit. Two such radiation delivery methods are currently being explored, one is helical tomotherapy and the other is utilization of tumor-reactive monoclonal antibody (MAB) conjugated with locally acting radionucleotides such as Iodine-131 or yttrium-90.

8.7 Radioimmunotherapy

A phase I trial of iodine-131 MAB plus Cy and TBI for advanced leukemia looked primarily at the biodistribution and toxicity of escalating doses of targeted radiation therapy combined with 120 mg/kg Cy and 12 Gy TBI followed by matched related or autologous HSCT.[100] A total of 44 patients were included in this study, 10 had ALL, 5 of which had ALL in relapse or refractory disease. Five of the patients were in CR2 or third CR. The study demonstrated that by utilizing iodine-131 anti-CD45 MAB, appreciable supplemental doses of radiation could be delivered to the marrow (approximately 24 Gy) and spleen when combined with conventional fractionated TBI.

Bethge et al reported a phase II study evaluating the utility of yttrium-90 as the radionucleotide.[101] Forty patients with advanced non-Hodgkin lymphoma were enrolled in this study combining radioimmunotherapy (RIT) using yttrium-90-ibritumomab-tiuxetan with RIC employing fludarabine and 2 Gy TBI followed by allogeneic HSCT from related (n = 13) or unrelated (n = 27) donors. Median age in the study was 55 years. All patients were high-risk with refractory disease or relapse after preceding autologous HSCT. No additional toxicity attributable to RIT was observed. Engraftment was rapid and sustained and estimated NRM was 45% at 2 years. Estimated 2-year OS was reported to be 51%.

These early results point the way to strategy that effectively increases the intensity of the conditioning regimen without increased toxicity. Further study is needed to assess the efficacy and safety of RIT in adult patients with ALL. Other radioconjugated MAB are needed to target ALL as the majority do not express CD20.

8.8 Helical tomotherapy

Helical tomotherapy is a newer method of delivering radiation therapy. With its ability to focus and intensify local radiation treatment, there is potential to augment the radiation to the marrow containing bones without increasing toxicity to other organs. This technology employs a megavoltage linear accelerator mounted on a computed tomography gantry that allows the beam source to continually rotate around the patient. Simultaneously, the couch, or patient placement device, moves perpendicularly to the beam source. The beam moves in a spiral or helical pattern relative to the patient. The beam can be modulated with a multileaf collimator. During treatment planning, these qualities allow large volumes to be delineated and treated, while neighboring volumes are spared.[102]

Because conventional TBI can be associated with significant toxicity, there remains an interest in exploring helical tomotherapy as a means of delivering TBI because of its ability to deliver minimal radiation to sensitive organs such as the lungs and kidneys. Interstitial pneumonitis is an important toxicity seen with TBI and has been observed to occur in approximately 50% of patients receiving a single fraction of 8-10 Gy, with 50% of cases proving fatal.[71] Even when low-dose-rate, fractionated TBI is employed with concurrent chemotherapy, the rate of interstitial pneumonitis may approach 25%.[103] Important acute toxicity associated with TBI includes nausea, vomiting, parotitis, dry mouth and mucositis. These can be a source of significant morbidity for patients. TBI may also result in significant end-organ damage. Cataract formation is seen in 30-40% of patients, and gonadal failure, thyroid dysfunction, kidney dysfunction and decreased bone mineral density have all been documented.[102] Survivors are also at known risk for chronic oral and dental complications especially xerostomia which greatly affects quality of life. Other long term complications may also include the development of secondary neoplasms with a 3 to 7% increase in risk at 15 years following transplant.[104, 105] Thus, hypothetically, delivering TBI via helical tomotherapy might minimize these complications while allowing dose escalation of radiotherapy to the target tissues.

Zhuang et al reported a dosimetric comparison of TBI delivered via helical tomotherapy compared with the more traditional extended source to surface distance (SSD) approach.[106] Results from this study showed that the average dose delivered to the target volume was improved with tomotherapy while a lesser dose was delivered to the lungs, which were excluded from the target volume. Another similar study evaluated the use of tomotherapy to treat the marrow cavity (target region skeletal bone) as well as the major lymph node chains, spleen and sanctuary sites.[107] A 1.7 to 7.5-fold reduction in median organ dose was demonstrated and a dose-volume histogram analysis predicted that dose escalation up to 20 Gy was feasible and potentially safe with this technique.

Penagaricano et al reported the utility of TBI with helical tomotherapy in patients with AML.[108] Four patients with AML received TBI by tomotherapy as part of their conditioning regimen prior to allogeneic transplantation. They each received 12 Gy in six equal fractions at two fractions per day, over 3 days. TBI planning was set up so that the lungs and kidneys would receive minimal radiation. Analysis showed that although the delivered clinical target volume doses ranged from 11.9 to 12.3 Gy, the delivered lung doses ranged from 6.5 to 7.4 Gy and the delivered kidney doses ranged from 7.2 to 8.6 Gy. Overall toxicity was limited to grade I asymptomatic radiation dermatitis and grade I headache.

These studies have demonstrated the feasibility of helical tomotherapy to deliver TBI. Tomotherapy delivers an elegant and dosimetrically superior solution to the conventional technique of TBI. With tomotherapy, there is no need for blocks or compensators, low dose rates, extended source to skin distances, beam spoilers or uncomfortable patient positioning. Further investigation in this area might allow delivery of higher doses of radiation to sites of disease while limiting exposure to critical structures and thus reducing toxicity and long-term complications.

9. Conclusion

Allogeneic HSCT remains integral to the treatment of adult patients with ALL. Preliminary evidence supports the use of alternative donors in HSCT for ALL. As in other forms of hematological malignancy the use of fully matched unrelated donors shows similar outcome to matched related donor HSCT in patients with ALL. The use of UCB as the donor source appears feasible in children and also in adults. Whether the use of less well matched donors, such as haploidentical siblings, or unrelated multiple UCB units has utility in the treatment of ALL needs further study of efficacy but is certainly feasible.

The UKALL XII/ECOG E2993 trial confirmed the presence of GVL in allogeneic HSCT for ALL. It also showed that the benefit of allogeneic HSCT was operative in standard-risk ALL. Surprisingly, the benefit of allogeneic HSCT was not clearly demonstrated in patients with high-risk ALL, but was certainly not inferior to other therapy. Autologous HSCT proved inferior to allogeneic HSCT and chemotherapy only treatment. Despite these findings the trial has been the focus of much debate and alternative analyses have been presented that question the magnitude of the benefit from allogeneic HSCT. Nevertheless we conclude that allogeneic HSCT should be included as a therapeutic option for all patients with ALL eligible for HSCT.

The applicability of pediatric style chemotherapeutic regimens to adult patients is currently under investigation. If these regimens can be safely administered to adult patients and yield improved results particularly in the AYA population, then the benefit from GVL might be reduced negating the need for allogeneic HSCT in first remission.

Ph+ ALL presents a unique therapeutic opportunity with TKIs such as imatinib, nilotinib and dasatinib. The combination of TKIs and chemotherapy has been demonstrated to be feasible and they may also be effectively administered after both autologous and allogeneic HSCT. The utility of allogeneic transplantation will need to be tested again in Ph+ ALL, if recently conducted studies show superiority of TKIs in combination with chemotherapy over historical data.

Moreover, the expanded use of MRD monitoring and a better understanding of its utility might further refine selection of patients who would benefit from allogeneic HSCT.

Innovative approaches to conditioning regimens including RIC, radioimmunoconjugates and helical tomotherapy offer the possibility of reduced toxicity and thus wider applicability of HSCT. The more elderly patient with ALL might then become a candidate for allogeneic HSCT with consequent improvement in survival. In younger patients the ability to escalate the intensity of the conditioning regimen might improve disease control without adding to toxicity.

The treatment of adult ALL has improved but remains inferior to the results seen in the pediatric population. Further research into the biological diversity of ALL may help explain this difference and allow therapy to be tailored to individual circumstance. Ultimately only well designed and conducted clinical trials will allow us to address these questions and refine therapy. Given the relative rarity of this disease, international collaboration remains the most efficient way of obtaining timely answers to questions surrounding the treatment of adult ALL.

10. References

[1] Pui CH, Evans WE. Acute lymphoblastic leukemia. N Engl J Med. 1998; 339(9): 605-15.

[2] Fielding A. The treatment of adults with acute lymphoblastic leukemia. Hematology Am Soc Hematol Educ Program. 2008: 381-9.

[3] Pui C-H, Evans WE. Treatment of acute lymphoblastic leukemia. N Engl J Med. 2006; 354(2): 166-78.

[4] Thomas X, Boiron J-M, Huguet F, Dombret H, Bradstock K, Vey N, et al. Outcome of treatment in adults with acute lymphoblastic leukemia: analysis of the LALA-94 trial. J Clin Oncol. 2004; 22(20): 4075-86.

[5] Hunault M, Harousseau J-L, Delain M, Truchan-Graczyk M, Cahn J-Y, Witz F, et al. Better outcome of adult acute lymphoblastic leukemia after early genoidentical allogeneic bone marrow transplantation (BMT) than after late high-dose therapy and autologous BMT: a GOELAMS trial. Blood. 2004; 104(10): 3028-37.

[6] Fiere D, Lepage E, Sebban C, Boucheix C, Gisselbrecht C, Vernant JP, et al. Adult acute lymphoblastic leukemia: a multicentric randomized trial testing bone marrow transplantation as postremission therapy. The French Group on Therapy for Adult Acute Lymphoblastic Leukemia. J Clin Oncol. 1993; 11(10): 1990-2001.

[7] Thiebaut A, Vernant JP, Degos L, Huguet FR, Reiffers J, Sebban C, et al. Adult acute lymphocytic leukemia study testing chemotherapy and autologous and allogeneic transplantation. A follow-up report of the French protocol LALA 87. Hematol Oncol Clin North Am. 2000; 14(6): 1353-66.

[8] Kiehl MG, Kraut L, Schwerdtfeger R, Hertenstein B, Remberger M, Kroeger N, et al. Outcome of allogeneic hematopoietic stem-cell transplantation in adult patients with acute lymphoblastic leukemia: no difference in related compared with unrelated transplant in first complete remission. J Clin Oncol. 2004; 22(14): 2816-25.

[9] Rowe JM. Interpreting data on transplant selection and outcome in adult acute lymphoblastic leukemia (ALL). Biol Blood Marrow Transplant. 2011; 17(1 Suppl): S76-83.

[10] Goldstone AH, Richards SM, Lazarus HM, Tallman MS, Buck G, Fielding AK, et al. In adults with standard-risk acute lymphoblastic leukemia, the greatest benefit is achieved from a matched sibling allogeneic transplantation in first complete remission, and an autologous transplantation is less effective than conventional consolidation/maintenance chemotherapy in all patients: final results of the International ALL Trial (MRC UKALL XII/ECOG E2993). Blood. 2008; 111(4): 1827-33.

[11] Bachanova V, Weisdorf D. Unrelated donor allogeneic transplantation for adult acute lymphoblastic leukemia: a review. Bone Marrow Transplant. 2008; 41(5): 455-64.

[12] Doney K, Fisher LD, Appelbaum FR, Buckner CD, Storb R, Singer J, et al. Treatment of adult acute lymphoblastic leukemia with allogeneic bone marrow transplantation. Multivariate analysis of factors affecting acute graft-versus-host disease, relapse, and relapse-free survival. Bone Marrow Transplant. 1991; 7(6): 453-9.

[13] Appelbaum FR. Graft versus leukemia (GVL) in the therapy of acute lymphoblastic leukemia (ALL). Leukemia. 1997; 11 Suppl 4: S15-7.

[14] Passweg JR, Tiberghien P, Cahn JY, Vowels MR, Camitta BM, Gale RP, et al. Graft-versus-leukemia effects in T lineage and B lineage acute lymphoblastic leukemia. Bone Marrow Transplant. 1998; 21(2): 153-8.

[15] Mutis T, Verdijk R, Schrama E, Esendam B, Brand A, Goulmy E. Feasibility of immunotherapy of relapsed leukemia with ex vivo-generated cytotoxic T lymphocytes specific for hematopoietic system-restricted minor histocompatibility antigens. Blood. 1999; 93(7): 2336-41.

[16] Warren EH, Greenberg PD, Riddell SR. Cytotoxic T-lymphocyte-defined human minor histocompatibility antigens with a restricted tissue distribution. Blood. 1998; 91(6): 2197-207.

[17] Jensen MC, Clarke P, Tan G, Wright C, Chung-Chang W, Clark TN, et al. Human T lymphocyte genetic modification with naked DNA. Mol Ther. 2000; 1(1): 49-55.

[18] Cooper LJ, Topp MS, Serrano LM, Gonzalez S, Chang WC, Naranjo A, et al. T-cell clones can be rendered specific for CD19: toward the selective augmentation of the graft-versus-B-lineage leukemia effect. Blood. 2003; 101(4): 1637-44.

[19] Rowe JM, Buck G, Burnett AK, Chopra R, Wiernik PH, Richards SM, et al. Induction therapy for adults with acute lymphoblastic leukemia: results of more than 1500 patients from the international ALL trial: MRC UKALL XII/ECOG E2993. Blood. 2005; 106(12): 3760-7.

[20] Larson RA, Dodge RK, Burns CP, Lee EJ, Stone RM, Schulman P, et al. A five-drug remission induction regimen with intensive consolidation for adults with acute lymphoblastic leukemia: cancer and leukemia group B study 8811. Blood. 1995; 85(8): 2025-37.

[21] Hoelzer D, Thiel E, Loffler H, Buchner T, Ganser A, Heil G, et al. Prognostic factors in a multicenter study for treatment of acute lymphoblastic leukemia in adults. Blood. 1988; 71(1): 123-31.

[22] Sellar RS, Goldstone AH. Transplants for the old but not for the young?--The enigma of adult ALL. Biol Blood Marrow Transplant. 2011; 17(1 Suppl): S71-5.

[23] Bassan R, Spinelli O, Oldani E, Intermesoli T, Tosi M, Peruta B, et al. Improved risk classification for risk-specific therapy based on the molecular study of minimal residual disease (MRD) in adult acute lymphoblastic leukemia (ALL). Blood. 2009; 113(18): 4153-62.

[24] Bruggemann M, Raff T, Flohr T, Gokbuget N, Nakao M, Droese J, et al. Clinical significance of minimal residual disease quantification in adult patients with standard-risk acute lymphoblastic leukemia. Blood. 2006; 107(3): 1116-23.

[25] Stow P, Key L, Chen X, Pan Q, Neale GA, Coustan-Smith E, et al. Clinical significance of low levels of minimal residual disease at the end of remission induction therapy in childhood acute lymphoblastic leukemia. Blood. 2010; 115(23): 4657-63.

[26] Cave H, van der Werff ten Bosch J, Suciu S, Guidal C, Waterkeyn C, Otten J, et al. Clinical significance of minimal residual disease in childhood acute lymphoblastic leukemia. European Organization for Research and Treatment of Cancer--Childhood Leukemia Cooperative Group. N Engl J Med. 1998; 339(9): 591-8.

[27] Yamada M, Wasserman R, Lange B, Reichard BA, Womer RB, Rovera G. Minimal residual disease in childhood B-lineage lymphoblastic leukemia. Persistence of leukemic cells during the first 18 months of treatment. N Engl J Med. 1990; 323(7): 448-55.

[28] Mortuza FY, Papaioannou M, Moreira IM, Coyle LA, Gameiro P, Gandini D, et al. Minimal residual disease tests provide an independent predictor of clinical outcome in adult acute lymphoblastic leukemia. J Clin Oncol. 2002; 20(4): 1094-104.

[29] Hoelzer D, Ludwig WD, Thiel E, Gassmann W, Loffler H, Fonatsch C, et al. Improved outcome in adult B-cell acute lymphoblastic leukemia. Blood. 1996; 87(2): 495-508.

[30] Laport GF, Larson RA. Treatment of adult acute lymphoblastic leukemia. Semin Oncol. 1997; 24(1): 70-82.

[31] Hoelzer D, Gokbuget N. New approaches to acute lymphoblastic leukemia in adults: where do we go? Semin Oncol. 2000; 27(5): 540-59.

[32] Stein A, Forman SJ. Allogeneic transplantation for ALL in adults. Bone Marrow Transplant. 2008; 41(5): 439-46.

[33] Bassan R, Hoelzer D. Modern therapy of acute lymphoblastic leukemia. J Clin Oncol. 2011; 29(5): 532-43.

[34] Takeuchi J, Kyo T, Naito K, Sao H, Takahashi M, Miyawaki S, et al. Induction therapy by frequent administration of doxorubicin with four other drugs, followed by intensive consolidation and maintenance therapy for adult acute lymphoblastic leukemia: the JALSG-ALL93 study. Leukemia. 2002; 16(7): 1259-66.

[35] Ribera J-M, Oriol A, Bethencourt C, Parody R, Hernandez-Rivas J-M, Moreno M-J, et al. Comparison of intensive chemotherapy, allogeneic or autologous stem cell transplantation as post-remission treatment for adult patients with high-risk acute lymphoblastic leukemia. Results of the PETHEMA ALL-93 trial. Haematologica. 2005; 90(10): 1346-56.

[36] Cornelissen JJ, van der Holt B, Verhoef GE, van't Veer MB, van Oers MH, Schouten HC, et al. Myeloablative allogeneic versus autologous stem cell transplantation in adult patients with acute lymphoblastic leukemia in first remission: a prospective sibling donor versus no-donor comparison. Blood. 2009; 113(6): 1375-82.

[37] Labar B, Suciu S, Zittoun R, Muus P, Marie JP, Fillet G, et al. Allogeneic stem cell transplantation in acute lymphoblastic leukemia and non-Hodgkin's lymphoma for patients <or=50 years old in first complete remission: results of the EORTC ALL-3 trial. Haematologica. 2004; 89(7): 809-17.

[38] Huguet F, Leguay T, Raffoux E, Thomas X, Beldjord K, Delabesse E, et al. Pediatric-inspired therapy in adults with Philadelphia chromosome-negative acute lymphoblastic leukemia: the GRAALL-2003 study. J Clin Oncol. 2009; 27(6): 911-8.

[39] Barry E, DeAngelo DJ, Neuberg D, Stevenson K, Loh ML, Asselin BL, et al. Favorable outcome for adolescents with acute lymphoblastic leukemia treated on Dana-Farber Cancer Institute Acute Lymphoblastic Leukemia Consortium Protocols. J Clin Oncol. 2007; 25(7): 813-9.

[40] Ribera J-M, Oriol A, Sanz M-A, Tormo M, Fernandez-Abellan P, del Potro E, et al. Comparison of the results of the treatment of adolescents and young adults with standard-risk acute lymphoblastic leukemia with the Programa Espanol de Tratamiento en Hematologia pediatric-based protocol ALL-96. J Clin Oncol. 2008; 26(11): 1843-9.

[41] Stock W, La M, Sanford B, Bloomfield CD, Vardiman JW, Gaynon P, et al. What determines the outcomes for adolescents and young adults with acute lymphoblastic leukemia treated on cooperative group protocols? A comparison of Children's Cancer Group and Cancer and Leukemia Group B studies. Blood. 2008; 112(5): 1646-54.

[42] Storring JM, Minden MD, Kao S, Gupta V, Schuh AC, Schimmer AD, et al. Treatment of adults with BCR-ABL negative acute lymphoblastic leukaemia with a modified paediatric regimen. Br J Haematol. 2009; 146(1): 76-85.

[43] Ram R, Gafter-Gvili A, Vidal L, Paul M, Ben-Bassat I, Shpilberg O, et al. Management of adult patients with acute lymphoblastic leukemia in first complete remission: systematic review and meta-analysis. Cancer. 2010; 116(14): 3447-57.

[44] Thomas DA, Kantarjian H, Cortes J. Long term outcome after Hyper-CVAD and Rituximab chemoimmunotherapy for Burkitt (BL) or Burkitt-like (BLL) leukemia/lymphoma and mature B-Cell acute lymphocytic leukemia (B-ALL). Blood (ASH Annual Meeting Abstracts). 2007; 110:831A (abstract 2825).
[45] Hoelzer D, Hiddemann W, Baumann A. High survival rate in adult Burkitt's lymphoma/leukemia and diffuse large B-cell lymphoma with mediastinal involvement. Blood (ASH Annual Meeting Abstracts). 2007; 110:159a (abstract 518).
[46] Hahn T, Wall D, Camitta B, Davies S, Dillon H, Gaynon P, et al. The role of cytotoxic therapy with hematopoietic stem cell transplantation in the therapy of acute lymphoblastic leukemia in adults: an evidence-based review. Biol Blood Marrow Transplant. 2006; 12(1): 1-30.
[47] Dombret H, Gabert J, Boiron JM, Rigal-Huguet F, Blaise D, Thomas X, et al. Outcome of treatment in adults with Philadelphia chromosome-positive acute lymphoblastic leukemia--results of the prospective multicenter LALA-94 trial. Blood. 2002; 100(7): 2357-66.
[48] Yanada M, Matsuo K, Suzuki T, Naoe T. Allogeneic hematopoietic stem cell transplantation as part of postremission therapy improves survival for adult patients with high-risk acute lymphoblastic leukemia: a metaanalysis. Cancer. 2006; 106(12): 2657-63.
[49] Fielding AK. Philadelphia-positive acute lymphoblastic leukemia--is bone marrow transplant still necessary? Biol Blood Marrow Transplant. 2011; 17(1 Suppl): S84-8.
[50] Weisdorf D, Bishop M, Dharan B, Bolwell B, Cahn JY, Cairo M, et al. Autologous versus allogeneic unrelated donor transplantation for acute lymphoblastic leukemia: comparative toxicity and outcomes. Biol Blood Marrow Transplant. 2002; 8(4): 213-20.
[51] Dahlke J, Kroger N, Zabelina T, Ayuk F, Fehse N, Wolschke C, et al. Comparable results in patients with acute lymphoblastic leukemia after related and unrelated stem cell transplantation. Bone Marrow Transplant. 2006; 37(2): 155-63.
[52] Hwang WY, Samuel M, Tan D, Koh LP, Lim W, Linn YC. A meta-analysis of unrelated donor umbilical cord blood transplantation versus unrelated donor bone marrow transplantation in adult and pediatric patients. Biol Blood Marrow Transplant. 2007; 13(4): 444-53.
[53] Ballen KK, Spitzer TR. The great debate: haploidentical or cord blood transplant. Bone Marrow Transplant. 2011; 46(3): 323-9.
[54] Weiden PL, Flournoy N, Thomas ED, Prentice R, Fefer A, Buckner CD, et al. Antileukemic effect of graft-versus-host disease in human recipients of allogeneic-marrow grafts. N Engl J Med. 1979; 300(19): 1068-73.
[55] Mato AR, Luger SM. Autologous stem cell transplant in ALL: who should we be transplanting in first remission? Bone Marrow Transplant. 2006; 37(11): 989-95.
[56] Fielding AK, Rowe JM, Richards SM, Buck G, Moorman AV, Durrant IJ, et al. Prospective outcome data on 267 unselected adult patients with Philadelphia chromosome-positive acute lymphoblastic leukemia confirms superiority of allogeneic transplantation over chemotherapy in the pre-imatinib era: results from the International ALL Trial MRC UKALLXII/ECOG2993. Blood. 2009; 113(19): 4489-96.

[57] Stein AS, Palmer JM, O'Donnell MR, Kogut NM, Spielberger RT, Slovak ML, et al. Reduced-intensity conditioning followed by peripheral blood stem cell transplantation for adult patients with high-risk acute lymphoblastic leukemia. Biol Blood Marrow Transplant. 2009; 15(11): 1407-14.

[58] Bachanova V, Verneris MR, DeFor T, Brunstein CG, Weisdorf DJ. Prolonged survival in adults with acute lymphoblastic leukemia after reduced-intensity conditioning with cord blood or sibling donor transplantation. Blood. 2009; 113(13): 2902-5.

[59] Schultz KR, Bowman WP, Aledo A, Slayton WB, Sather H, Devidas M, et al. Improved early event-free survival with imatinib in Philadelphia chromosome-positive acute lymphoblastic leukemia: a children's oncology group study. J Clin Oncol. 2009; 27(31): 5175-81.

[60] Vignetti M, Fazi P, Cimino G, Martinelli G, Di Raimondo F, Ferrara F, et al. Imatinib plus steroids induces complete remissions and prolonged survival in elderly Philadelphia chromosome-positive patients with acute lymphoblastic leukemia without additional chemotherapy: results of the Gruppo Italiano Malattie Ematologiche dell'Adulto (GIMEMA) LAL0201-B protocol. Blood. 2007; 109(9): 3676-8.

[61] Ottmann OG, Wassmann B, Pfeifer H, Giagounidis A, Stelljes M, Duhrsen U, et al. Imatinib compared with chemotherapy as front-line treatment of elderly patients with Philadelphia chromosome-positive acute lymphoblastic leukemia (Ph+ALL). Cancer. 2007; 109(11): 2068-76.

[62] Thomas DA, Faderl S, Cortes J, O'Brien S, Giles FJ, Kornblau SM, et al. Treatment of Philadelphia chromosome-positive acute lymphocytic leukemia with hyper-CVAD and imatinib mesylate. Blood. 2004; 103(12): 4396-407.

[63] Kantarjian H, Giles F, Wunderle L, Bhalla K, O'Brien S, Wassmann B, et al. Nilotinib in imatinib-resistant CML and Philadelphia chromosome-positive ALL. N Engl J Med. 2006; 354(24): 2542-51.

[64] Ottmann O, Dombret H, Martinelli G, Simonsson B, Guilhot F, Larson RA, et al. Dasatinib induces rapid hematologic and cytogenetic responses in adult patients with Philadelphia chromosome positive acute lymphoblastic leukemia with resistance or intolerance to imatinib: interim results of a phase 2 study. Blood. 2007; 110(7): 2309-15.

[65] Talpaz M, Shah NP, Kantarjian H, Donato N, Nicoll J, Paquette R, et al. Dasatinib in imatinib-resistant Philadelphia chromosome-positive leukemias. N Engl J Med. 2006; 354(24): 2531-41.

[66] Wassmann B, Pfeifer H, Goekbuget N, Beelen DW, Beck J, Stelljes M, et al. Alternating versus concurrent schedules of imatinib and chemotherapy as front-line therapy for Philadelphia-positive acute lymphoblastic leukemia (Ph+ ALL). Blood. 2006; 108(5): 1469-77.

[67] Thomas E, Storb R, Clift RA, Fefer A, Johnson FL, Neiman PE, et al. Bone-marrow transplantation (first of two parts). N Engl J Med. 1975; 292(16): 832-43.

[68] Altschuler C, Resbeut M, Blaise D, Maraninchi D, Stoppa AM, Lagrange JL, et al. Fractionated total body irradiation and bone marrow transplantation in acute lymphoblastic leukemia. Int J Radiat Oncol Biol Phys. 1990; 19(5): 1151-4.

[69] Gale RP, Butturini A, Bortin MM. What does total body irradiation do in bone marrow transplants for leukemia? Int J Radiat Oncol Biol Phys. 1991; 20(3): 631-4.

[70] Gough MJ, Crittenden MR. Combination approaches to immunotherapy: the radiotherapy example. Immunotherapy. 2009; 1(6): 1025-37.

[71] Keane TJ, Van Dyk J, Rider WD. Idiopathic interstitial pneumonia following bone marrow transplantation: the relationship with total body irradiation. Int J Radiat Oncol Biol Phys. 1981; 7(10): 1365-70.

[72] Kim TH, Rybka WB, Lehnert S, Podgorsak EB, Freeman CR. Interstitial pneumonitis following total body irradiation for bone marrow transplantation using two different dose rates. Int J Radiat Oncol Biol Phys. 1985; 11(7): 1285-91.

[73] Barrett AJ. Bone marrow transplantation. Cancer Treat Rev. 1987; 14(3-4): 203-13.

[74] Barrett A, Depledge MH, Powles RL. Interstitial pneumonitis following bone marrow transplantation after low dose rate total body irradiation. Int J Radiat Oncol Biol Phys. 1983; 9(7): 1029-33.

[75] Cosset JM, Girinsky T, Malaise E, Chaillet MP, Dutreix J. Clinical basis for TBI fractionation. Radiother Oncol. 1990; 18 Suppl 1: 60-7.

[76] Shank B, Chu FC, Dinsmore R, Kapoor N, Kirkpatrick D, Teitelbaum H, et al. Hyperfractionated total body irradiation for bone marrow transplantation. Results in seventy leukemia patients with allogeneic transplants. Int J Radiat Oncol Biol Phys. 1983; 9(11): 1607-11.

[77] Thomas ED, Clift RA, Hersman J, Sanders JE, Stewart P, Buckner CD, et al. Marrow transplantation for acute nonlymphoblastic leukemic in first remission using fractionated or single-dose irradiation. Int J Radiat Oncol Biol Phys. 1982; 8(5): 817-21.

[78] Katz R, Sharma SC, Homayoonfar M. Irradiation equivalence. Health Phys. 1972; 23(5): 740-1.

[79] Clift RA, Buckner CD, Appelbaum FR, Bearman SI, Petersen FB, Fisher LD, et al. Allogeneic marrow transplantation in patients with acute myeloid leukemia in first remission: a randomized trial of two irradiation regimens. Blood. 1990; 76(9): 1867-71.

[80] Clift RA, Buckner CD, Appelbaum FR, Sullivan KM, Storb R, Thomas ED. Long-term follow-Up of a randomized trial of two irradiation regimens for patients receiving allogeneic marrow transplants during first remission of acute myeloid leukemia. Blood. 1998; 92(4): 1455-6.

[81] Clift RA, Buckner CD, Appelbaum FR, Bryant E, Bearman SI, Petersen FB, et al. Allogeneic marrow transplantation in patients with chronic myeloid leukemia in the chronic phase: a randomized trial of two irradiation regimens. Blood. 1991; 77(8): 1660-5.

[82] Bieri S, Helg C, Chapuis B, Miralbell R. Total body irradiation before allogeneic bone marrow transplantation: is more dose better? Int J Radiat Oncol Biol Phys. 2001; 49(4): 1071-7.

[83] Santos GW, Tutschka PJ, Brookmeyer R, Saral R, Beschorner WE, Bias WB, et al. Marrow transplantation for acute nonlymphocytic leukemia after treatment with busulfan and cyclophosphamide. N Engl J Med. 1983; 309(22): 1347-53.

[84] Tutschka PJ, Copelan EA, Klein JP. Bone marrow transplantation for leukemia following a new busulfan and cyclophosphamide regimen. Blood. 1987; 70(5): 1382-8.

[85] Davies SM, Ramsay NK, Klein JP, Weisdorf DJ, Bolwell B, Cahn JY, et al. Comparison of preparative regimens in transplants for children with acute lymphoblastic leukemia. J Clin Oncol. 2000; 18(2): 340-7.
[86] Gupta T, Kannan S, Dantkale V, Laskar S. Cyclophosphamide plus total body irradiation compared with busulfan plus cyclophosphamide as a conditioning regimen prior to hematopoietic stem cell transplantation in patients with leukemia: a systematic review and meta-analysis. Hematol Oncol Stem Cell Ther. 2011; 4(1): 17-29.
[87] Coccia PF, Strandjord SE, Warkentin PI, Cheung NK, Gordon EM, Novak LJ, et al. High-dose cytosine arabinoside and fractionated total-body irradiation: an improved preparative regimen for bone marrow transplantation of children with acute lymphoblastic leukemia in remission. Blood. 1988; 71(4): 888-93.
[88] Champlin R, Jacobs A, Gale RP, Ho W, Selch M, Lenarsky C, et al. High-dose cytarabine in consolidation chemotherapy or with bone marrow transplantation for patients with acute leukemia: preliminary results. Semin Oncol. 1985; 12(2 Suppl 3): 190-5.
[89] Russell JA, Savoie ML, Balogh A, Turner AR, Larratt L, Chaudhry MA, et al. Allogeneic transplantation for adult acute leukemia in first and second remission with a novel regimen incorporating daily intravenous busulfan, fludarabine, 400 CGY total-body irradiation, and thymoglobulin. Biol Blood Marrow Transplant. 2007; 13(7): 814-21.
[90] Blume KG, Forman SJ, O'Donnell MR, Doroshow JH, Krance RA, Nademanee AP, et al. Total body irradiation and high-dose etoposide: a new preparatory regimen for bone marrow transplantation in patients with advanced hematologic malignancies. Blood. 1987; 69(4): 1015-20.
[91] Blume KG, Kopecky KJ, Henslee-Downey JP, Forman SJ, Stiff PJ, LeMaistre CF, et al. A prospective randomized comparison of total body irradiation-etoposide versus busulfan-cyclophosphamide as preparatory regimens for bone marrow transplantation in patients with leukemia who were not in first remission: a Southwest Oncology Group study. Blood. 1993; 81(8): 2187-93.
[92] Marks DI, Forman SJ, Blume KG, Perez WS, Weisdorf DJ, Keating A, et al. A comparison of cyclophosphamide and total body irradiation with etoposide and total body irradiation as conditioning regimens for patients undergoing sibling allografting for acute lymphoblastic leukemia in first or second complete remission. Biol Blood Marrow Transplant. 2006; 12(4): 438-53.
[93] Sullivan KM, Weiden PL, Storb R, Witherspoon RP, Fefer A, Fisher L, et al. Influence of acute and chronic graft-versus-host disease on relapse and survival after bone marrow transplantation from HLA-identical siblings as treatment of acute and chronic leukemia. Blood. 1989; 73(6): 1720-8.
[94] Gyurkocza B, Storb R, Storer BE, Chauncey TR, Lange T, Shizuru JA, et al. Nonmyeloablative allogeneic hematopoietic cell transplantation in patients with acute myeloid leukemia. J Clin Oncol. 2010; 28(17): 2859-67.
[95] Mohty M, Labopin M, Tabrizzi R, Theorin N, Fauser AA, Rambaldi A, et al. Reduced intensity conditioning allogeneic stem cell transplantation for adult patients with acute lymphoblastic leukemia: a retrospective study from the European Group for Blood and Marrow Transplantation. Haematologica. 2008; 93(2): 303-6.

[96] Marks DI, Wang T, Perez WS, Antin JH, Copelan E, Gale RP, et al. The outcome of full-intensity and reduced-intensity conditioning matched sibling or unrelated donor transplantation in adults with Philadelphia chromosome-negative acute lymphoblastic leukemia in first and second complete remission. Blood. 2010; 116(3): 366-74.

[97] Mohty M, Labopin M, Volin L, Gratwohl A, Socie G, Esteve J, et al. Reduced-intensity versus conventional myeloablative conditioning allogeneic stem cell transplantation for patients with acute lymphoblastic leukemia: a retrospective study from the European Group for Blood and Marrow Transplantation. Blood. 2010; 116(22): 4439-43.

[98] Ram R, Storb R, Sandmaier BM, Maloney DG, Woolfrey AE, Flowers ME, et al. Nonmyeloablative conditioning with allogeneic hematopoietic cell transplantation for the treatment of high risk acute lymphoblastic leukemia. Haematologica. 2011; 96:xxx (epub ahead of print).

[99] Verneris MR, Eapen M, Duerst R, Carpenter PA, Burke MJ, Afanasyev BV, et al. Reduced-intensity conditioning regimens for allogeneic transplantation in children with acute lymphoblastic leukemia. Biol Blood Marrow Transplant. 2010; 16(9): 1237-44.

[100] Matthews DC, Appelbaum FR, Eary JF, Fisher DR, Durack LD, Hui TE, et al. Phase I study of (131)I-anti-CD45 antibody plus cyclophosphamide and total body irradiation for advanced acute leukemia and myelodysplastic syndrome. Blood. 1999; 94(4): 1237-47.

[101] Bethge WA, Lange T, Meisner C, von Harsdorf S, Bornhaeuser M, Federmann B, et al. Radioimmunotherapy with yttrium-90-ibritumomab tiuxetan as part of a reduced-intensity conditioning regimen for allogeneic hematopoietic cell transplantation in patients with advanced non-Hodgkin lymphoma: results of a phase 2 study. Blood. 2010; 116(10): 1795-802.

[102] Hill-Kayser CE, Plastaras JP, Tochner Z, Glatstein E. TBI during BM and SCT: review of the past, discussion of the present and consideration of future directions. Bone Marrow Transplant. 2011; 46(4): 475-84.

[103] Pecego R, Hill R, Appelbaum FR, Amos D, Buckner CD, Fefer A, et al. Interstitial pneumonitis following autologous bone marrow transplantation. Transplantation. 1986; 42(5): 515-7.

[104] Rizzo JD, Curtis RE, Socie G, Sobocinski KA, Gilbert E, Landgren O, et al. Solid cancers after allogeneic hematopoietic cell transplantation. Blood. 2009; 113(5): 1175-83.

[105] Curtis RE, Rowlings PA, Deeg HJ, Shriner DA, Socie G, Travis LB, et al. Solid cancers after bone marrow transplantation. N Engl J Med. 1997; 336(13): 897-904.

[106] Zhuang AH, Liu A, Schultheiss TE, Wong JY. Dosimetric study and verification of total body irradiation using helical tomotherapy and its comparison to extended SSD technique. Med Dosim. 2010; 35(4): 243-9.

[107] Wong JY, Liu A, Schultheiss T, Popplewell L, Stein A, Rosenthal J, et al. Targeted total marrow irradiation using three-dimensional image-guided tomographic intensity-modulated radiation therapy: an alternative to standard total body irradiation. Biol Blood Marrow Transplant. 2006; 12(3): 306-15.

[108] Penagaricano JA, Chao M, Van Rhee F, Moros EG, Corry PM, Ratanatharathorn V. Clinical feasibility of TBI with helical tomotherapy. Bone Marrow Transplant. 2011; 46(7): 929-35.

[109] Patel B, Rai L, Buck G, Richards SM, Mortuza Y, Mitchell W, et al. Minimal residual disease is a significant predictor of treatment failure in non T-lineage adult acute lymphoblastic leukaemia: final results of the international trial UKALL XII/ECOG2993. Br J Haematol. 2010; 148(1): 80-9.

[110] Holowiecki J, Krawczyk-Kulis M, Giebel S, Jagoda K, Stella-Holowiecka B, Piatkowska-Jakubas B, et al. Status of minimal residual disease after induction predicts outcome in both standard and high-risk Ph-negative adult acute lymphoblastic leukaemia. The Polish Adult Leukemia Group ALL 4-2002 MRD Study. Br J Haematol. 2008; 142(2): 227-37.

[111] Beldjord K, Lheritier V, Boulland M-L. Post-induction minimal residual disease (MRD) defines a large subset of adults with favorable Ph-negative acute lymphoblastic leukemia (ALL), who do not benefit from allogeneic stem cell transplantation (SCT) in first complete remission: A GRALL study. Blood (ASH Annual Meeting Abstracts). 2009; 114:239 (abstract 577).

[112] Goekbuget N, Bruggemann M, Arnold R. New definition of treatment response in adult lymphoblastic leukemia (ALL): use of molecular markers for minimal residual disease (MRD). Blood (ASH Annual Meeting Abstracts). 2009; 114:42 (abstract 90).

[113] Ribera JM, Oriol A, Morgades M. Treatment of high-risk (HR) Philadelphia chromosome negative (Ph-) adult acute lymphoblastic leukemia (ALL) according to baseline risk factors and minimal residual disease (MRD): Results of the PETHEMA ALL-AR-03 trial including the use of propensity score (PS) method to reduce assignment bias. Blood (ASH Annual Meeting Abstracts). 2009; 114:136 (abstract 322).

Part 5

Resistance to Therapy

7

Multidrug Resistance Mechanism of Acute Lymphoblastic Leukemia

Zhaoliang Su, Haitao Zhu, Yanfang Liu,
Hongyan Yuan, Jingping Yin and Huaxi Xu
*Department of Immunology, Jiangsu University,
P. R. China*

1. Introduction

Multidrug resistance is recognized as the key factor of many anticancer drugs invalidity. Anticancer treatments such as chemotherapy or radiation must hit their cellular targets and then cause cellular alteration or damage. However, in most cases the damage inflicted by the anticancer agent triggers apoptosis [1]. Acute lymphoblastic leukemia (ALL) is the most frequently occurring cancer in children. Chemotherapy to childhood ALL has markedly improved during the past years [2]. The remission rate of chemotherapy patients is more than 95%, and the long term free survival rate about 75-80%. However, 25–30% of the patients will experience a relapsing, that leads to die of teenagers. Which may be explained by unfavourable pharmacokinetics, by leukemic stem cells regrowth and by cellular drug resistance [2, 3].

Since the early 1970s, multidrug resistance (MDR) has been known to exist in cancer cells and is thought to be attributable to a membrane-bound, energy-dependent pump protein (P-glycoprotein [P-gp]) capable of excluding various related and unrelated chemotherapeutic drugs. In this chapter, we would discussed the multidrug resistance mechanism of cancer cell.

2. Prognostic factors

Prognosis of patients with ALL depends on several interrelated factors including sex, age, race, leukocyte burden, immunophenotype, and chromosomal abnormalities, central nervous system (CNS) involvement and response to therapy [4-7]. It is important to recognize prognostic factors depending on the efficacy of therapy; more effective regimens decreasing the importance of prognostic variables. And identification of prognostic factors has become an essential element in the design and analysis of current therapeutic protocols in ALL. The biologic explanation of the prognostic significance of these features is unclear, but is often assumed to be related to cellular drug resistance [8, 9].

Age is an important but complex risk factor in ALL [10-12]. Children aged 2 to 10 years have the best prognosis. Adults and infants younger than 12 months of age have the worst prognosis. The poor prognosis in infants is most likely related to a higher incidence of undifferentiated and hybrid leukemias [8, 13, 14]. For adults, increasing age is associated with lower remission rates and shorter remissions. To analyze results of any therapeutic trial, it is important to consider the age limits and distribution, since these factors have a major effect on outcome.

The initial leukocyte burden is the most important conventional predictor of clinical outcome. There is a linear relationship between the initial leukocyte counts and outcome in children with ALL. Children with high leukocyte count tend to have a worse prognosis. Although there is no sharp dividing line, patients with an initial leukocyte count more than 50000 cells/mm^3 blood are universally recognized as having a particularly poor prognosis; however, the worst survival experience was exhibited by those with initial leukocyte from 100000 - 200000 cells/mm^3 blood.

Immunophenotype is one of the prognostic factors in ALL. B-ALL cases had the worst prognosis; although this has improved, while patients with B cell precursor ALL have the most favourable prognosis. Among the patient with B cell precursor ALL, those with the early pre-B cell phenotype have a more favourable prognosis compared with patients with pre-B cell phenotype, who have a relatively poor prognosis [15, 16]. T cell ALL is usually associated with male, sex, high leukocyte count, mediastinal mass, and CNS infiltration, and formerly had a poor outcome [17-21].

Chromosomal abnormalities can be identified at least 80% to 90% acute childhood leukemia [22]. The karyotypes of leukemic cells not only have diagnostic and prognostic importance but may also indicate the sites of molecular lesions involved in leukemic transformation and proliferation. Childhood ALL can be classified by the number of chromosomes/leukemic cell. Although several ploidy groups have been recognized, only two have clinical relevance. Hyperdiploidy (>50 chromosomes/cell) is associated with a better prognosis than that indicated by more traditional measures [23]. The biologic basis for the association between ploidy and prognosis is not yet clear but may stem from the tendency of hyperdiploid blasts to accumulate increased amounts of methotrexate and its polyglutamates as well as the marked propensity of these cells for apoptosis. Hypodiploidy (<45 chromosomes) is associated with an exceptionally poor prognosis. Phenotype-specific reciprocal translocations are the most common cytogenetic hallmarks of the childhood leukemias [24-28]. The majority of rearrangements are well characterized both clinically and molecularly and are thought to have a causative role in leukemogenesis. Chromosomal rearrangements can contribute to leukemia by moving proto-oncogenes into the vicinity of normally active enhancer or promoter sequences. the prototype of this mechanism is t(8;14)(q24;q32.3) in B-cell ALL, which brings the MYC proto-oncogene on chromosome 8 under the control of immunoglobulin-gene regulatory sequences on chromosome 14. Through a series of complex molecular changes, including coincident mutations, MYC is dysregulated, leading to inappropriately increased expression of the MYC product, a nuclear regulatory protein (transcription factor) that interacts with the other cellular protein (MAX) to influence the expression of other genes involved in cellular proliferation [29, 30]. A similar mechanism operates in T-cell ALL.

The BCR-ABL gene in ALL, which results from the classic t(9;22)(q34;q11) translocation that forms the Philadelphia chromosome, is perhaps the best known fusion gene in the childhood leukemias. In adult-type chronic myelogenous leukemia (CML) , the Philadelphia chromosome gives rise to a 210kd BCR-ABL product, whereas in most cases of childhood ALL with this rearrangement, the breakpoint within the BCR region is more centromeric, yielding a smaller (185 kd) chimeric protein [31]. Both proteins are tyrosine kinases, but the 185 kd form has more potent transforming activity. Regardless of the type of BCR-ABL protein, blast cells with the Philadelphia chromosome show extraordinary resistance to chemotherapy.

Approximately one fourth of patients with pre-B-cell ALL have a t(1;19)(q23;p13) translocation, which fuses the E2A gene on chromosome 19 with the PBX1 gene on chromosome 1.19. Paradoxically, the chimeric transcription factor induces both proliferation and apoptosis of lymphoid cells in transgenic mice [32, 33].

Structural chromosomal abnormalities affecting the q23 region of chromosome 11 are common in the acute childhood leukemias. Approximately 5% all children with ALL and 70% infants have 11q23 rearrangements, primarily the t(4;11)(q21;q23) translocation. This rearrangement, which creates the MLL-AF4 fusion gene, is associated with hyperleukocytosis and a poor prognosis. In fact, the extremely poor outcome of treatment in infants with ALL appears to be limited to those with the t(4;11) translocation or other 11q23 abnormalities.

3. Drug resistance

As mentioned previously, the prognostic significance of these factors may partly be caused by cellular drug resistance. Cellular drug resistance is generally recognized as an important determinant of the clinical outcome after chemotherapy. Even if optimal tumor cell exposure is achieved, a number of cellular factors may be responsible for drug resistance. The mechanisms would be described as following:

3.1 Drug transporters mediate resistance

Classical resistance is associated with transmembrane protein-mediated efflux of cytotoxic compounds leading to a decreased cellular drug accumulation and toxicity. Most of them belong to ATP-binding cassette (ABC) transporters superfamily including P-glycoprotein, multidrug resistance-associated protein (MRP) family, breast cancer resistance protein (BCRP), lung resistance protein (LRP) *et al.*

3.1.1 P-glycoprotein (P-gp)

P-gp expression occurs in about 30% acute myeloid leukemia (AML) patients at diagnosis and >50% at relapse and correlates with a reduced complete remission rate and shorter duration of survival of the patients. P-gp expression is also observed in CML blast crisis, chronic lymphocytic leukemia (CLL), multiple myeloma, non-Hodgkin's lymphoma and in ALL [34].P-gp is a member of the ABC (MDR/TAP) subfamily. In humans, P-gp is encoded by two MDR genes, including MDR1 and MDR3,which are located on the long arm of chromosome 7 (7q21) [35]. Human P-gp is a 170 kDa polypeptide, consisting of 1280 amino acids. The protein appears to have arisen by a gene duplication, fusing two related half molecules, each consisting of one nucleotide-binding domain and one transmembrane domain. The multidrug-resistant phenotype is associated with MDR1. However, under certain conditions, human MDR3 may transport selected MDR1 substrates, albeit inefficiently [36-41].

P-gp primary sequence displays 3 putative glycosylation sites in a region that appears to lie in the first extracellular loop of the protein; however, it seems unlikely that glycosylation affects the function of P-gp because of tunicamycin treatment, which blocks N-linked glycosylation, does not alter drug sensitivity in human multidrug resistant cells. P-gp has been shown to be phosphorylated on several sites through several kinases, including protein kinase C and the cAMP-dependent protein kinase A. Phosphorylation of P-gp appears was also associated with drug resistance. Indeed, treatment with the phorbolester TPA, which stimulates P-gp phosphorylation, results in increasing drug resistance and decreasing drug accmnulation in some multidrug-resistant cell lines. By contrast, protein kinase inhibitors, such as staurosporine, decreased phosphorylation and impaired anticancer drug transport [42, 43].

P-gp has a wide variety of substrates. All its substrates are large hydrophobic and amphipathic molecules, although they have no structural dissimilarity. These molecules are able to intercalate into the membrane and enter the cytosol by passive diffusion. It is no longer believed that P-gp is a classical pump, which binds substrates from the extracellular fluid and then transports these over the membrane. Hydrophobic compounds that are substrates for P-gp do not fully penetrate into the cytoplasm of cells that express P-gp [44]. Interaction of substrate with P-gp has been shown to take place within the membrane[21]. This mechanism of transport is also postulated for a prokaryotic homologue of P-gp with a similar broad substrate specificity in Lactococcus lactis. However, the exact mechanism by which this protein removes hydrophobic drugs from the cell is still unclear. It may translocate drugs actively from the cytosolic inner lipid leaflet of the plasma membrane to the outer lipid leaflet. Then these drugs are able to leave the plasma membrane by diffusion.

Besides anti-cancer drugs, P-gp also mediates the transport of various structurally unrelated compounds including toxic peptides, such as gramicidin D, valinomycin and N-acetyl-leucyl-leu -cyl-norleucinal (ALLN), digoxin, opiates, fluorescent dyes. Endogenous compounds, such as some steroid hormones, have also been demonstrated to be substrates for P-gp. In addition, the pump may serve as an ATP channel and is involved in volume-regulated chloride channel activity. A great number of studies have been conducted during the last few years to analyze the relation of P-gp expression and hematological malignancies, then to determine its clinical relevance. Various methods for determining P-gp gene expression have been used, such as northern blot, dot blot, RNase protection assay, hybridation and RT-PCR. In addition, western blot, immunohistochemistry and flow cytometry (FCM) were also used to analyze P-gp protein level. Furthermore, P-gp activity has also been evaluated by FCM.

Mutational analysis of P-gp has indicated that some point mutations may result in altering drug transport activity. Indeed a change Gly185Val led to reduce vinblastine transport, whereas colchicine transport was improved. However, two different groups showed that a mutation of the major phosphorylation sites within P-gp doesn't affect its transport function.

3.1.2 MRP

The human MRP1 gene is mapped to chromosome16p13.1[45-47]. It encodes a membrane-bound glycoprotein consisting of 1531 amino acids. This protein has a similar topologic structure to that of P-gp. However, in addition to the two half transporters connected by a linker region L1 as in P-gp, MRP1 protein contains an extra N-terminal segment, TMD 0, which connects TMD1 with a L0 linker region. The L0 linker region is essential for drug transport, whereas TMD0 is not required for transport. Although MRP1 also requires two ATPs as the energy source to transport chemotherapeutic drugs, the mechanism in the cycle of transportation is somewhat different from that of P-gp. In P-gp, the functions of the two NBDs are "equal", and the two

ATP-binding sites operate randomly but alternately. In MRP1, the function of NBD1 and NMD2 is nonequivalent. NBD1 has higher affinity than NBD2 for ATP. Therefore, when the substrate binds to TMDs of MRP1, the conformational change of MRP1 protein first induces ATP binding at NBD1. It then further alters the conformation of the protein and enhances ATP binding at NBD2. When both NBD1 and NBD2 are occupied by the two ATPs simultaneously, the bound substrate is transported out of the cell. After substrate extrusion, the ATP bound at NBD2 is hydrolyzed first. The release of ADP and inorganic phosphate from NBD2 partially brings the MRP1 protein back to its original conformation, and facilitates the dissociation of ATP bound at NBD1. Subsequent release of ADP and inorganic phosphate from NBD1 returns the MRP1 protein to its original conformation.

MRP1 is expressed almost ubiquitously in many different organs and cell types. Unlike P-gp, which is invariably located in the apical membranes of epithelial cells, MRP1 is located basolaterally and tends to pump drugs into the body, rather than excrete them into the bile, urine or gut. Cells overexpressing MRP1 protein are resistant to a variety of anticancer drugs, e.g. doxorubicin, epirubicin, vinblastine, vincristine, andetoposide. However, MRP1 cannot transport the unmodified anticancer drugs without the presence of glutathione (GSH). This implies that MRP1 may cotransport the anticancer drugs with GSH, or GSH may bind to the MRP1 protein to enhance the transport of these hydrophobic anticancer drugs across biological membrane.

3.1.3 BCRP

The initial demonstration that BCRP transfection directly confers MDR supports evidence that BCRP might be able to function by homodimerization [48-50]. The exogenous BCRP proteins migrated as 70 kDa bands in SDS–PAGE under reducing conditions, but as a 140 kDa complex in the absence of reducing agents. The 140 kDa BCRP complex dissociated into 70 kDa polypeptides with the addition of 2-mercaptoethanol. The 140 kDa BCRP complex was immunoprecipitated with anti-Myc antibody from lysates of cells co-transfected with Myc- and HA-tagged BCRP constructs. The 140 kDa complex reacted with anti-HA and anti-BCRP antibodies. After the addition of reducing agents, a 70 kDa BCRP band was seen, reactive with both anti-HA and anti-Mycantibodies. Furthermore, a dominant-negative mutant of BCRP was found to inhibit BCRP function partially when cotransfected with BCRP. These results elegantly demonstrate that BCRP forms a homodimer bridged by disulfide bonds. A molecular mass shift from a 72 kDa band under denaturing conditions to a 180 kDa band after treatment with crosslinking agents was also noted using polyclonal antibodies directed against peptide epitopes of BCRP.

The BCRP promoter is TATA-less, contains a CAAT box. Unlike ABCG1 promoter, the BCRP promoter does not contain a sterol response element, strengthening the argument that BCRP is not involved with lipid transport. The reporter analysis indicated that a 312 bp sequence directly upstream from the transcriptional start site conferred basal promoter activity, with positive and negative cis-regulatory elements identified in the region between 1285 and 1362 relative to the transcriptional start site. Strong resistance to mitoxantrone characterizes most drug-selected cell lines that overexpress BCRP, even if the selecting agent is not mitoxantrone.

3.1.4 LRP

LRP also known as the major vault protein (MVP), is not an ABC transporter but it is frequently expressed at high levels in drug-resistant cell lines and tumor samples [51, 52].

LRP/MVP is the most abundant component of the vault complex. Vaults are ribonucleoprotein (RNP) particles that are present in the cytoplasm of most eukaryotic cells and might be involved in intracellular transport processes. However, the physiological role of vaults is poorly understood.Vaults might confer drug resistance by transporting drugs away from their intracellular targets and/or by the sequestration of drugs. Several studies showed that LRP/MVP expression was an independent adverse prognostic factor for response to chemotherapy. With regard to clinical drug resistance, LRP/MVP expression in AML, multiple myeloma and diffuse large B cell lymphoma was associated with poor response to chemotherapy. LRP/MVP is an indicator of poor response to chemotherapy with platin or alkylating agents.

3.2 Resistance related to cell death mechanisms and apoptosis

Many investigators have considered apoptosis as the essential response of cancer cells to chemotherapeutic agents. Many data supported the association of functional apoptotic pathways in cancer cells with chemotherapy sensitivity. The discovery of the bcl proteins family altered the threshold of recognition of cell damage as a cell death signal, which suggests novel mechanisms of MDR [46, 49, 53-56]. The anti-apoptotic protein bcl-x_L and bcl-2 were strong associated with drug resistance.

Bcl-2 gene, discovered by Tsujimoto and Croce, is widely expressed in human tumor. Bcl-2 gene is translocated in many follicular B cell lymphomas from its normal 18q21 position to 14q32 where its location adjacent to enhancers in the immunoglobulin H gene leads to high level expression. Alternative splicing yields two proteins, bcl-2a and bcl-2b, differing only at their C terminus. Bcl-2 inhibited cell death and altered the normal cell death versus cell division ratio, which may allow tumor cells to accumulate the mutations, then cause the cells to become invasive and metastatic. Most publications about bcl-2 showed that transfection of immature pre-B cells with bcl-2 expression vectors protected against cell death due to IL-3 deprivation, thus indicating a role in antagonizing apoptosis.Transfection and antisense experiments confirmed an important role for bcl-2 in resistance to apoptosis induced by chemotherapeutic drugs. It is clear that bcl-2 is just one component of a large and complex family of proteins which determine particular cells die in response to particular physiological or pharmacological environments (e.g. growth factor deprivation, drug exposure). Apotosis may be particularly important in determining organ shape and size during development.

More recent research indicates a key role of bcl-x_L in apoptosis regulation in follicular lymphoma. Transfection with bcl-x_L cDNA has been shown to protect several cell types *in vitro* against apoptosis induced by a wide range of chemotherapeutic drugs. Transfection human bcl-x_L cDNA into the murine IL-3-dependent prolymphocytic cell line FL5.12, then increased resistance to the anticancer drugs bleomycin, cisplatin, etoposide and vincristine.

3.3 Telomerase involved in resistance

Telomerase is responsible for the renewal of the chromosomal ends, the so-called telomeres [57]. By preventing them from **shortening** with each cell cycle, telomerase is able to inhibit cellular senescence and apoptosis. Telomerase activity, which is detectable in the majority of cancer cells, allows them to maintain their proliferative capacity. The thus obtained immortality of those cells again is a key to their malignancy.

3.4 DNA mismatch repair deficiency led to resistance

DNA mismatch repair deficiency results in a high risk of malignant tumorigenesis [58-61]. A defect in this system may cause accumulation of mutations in several proto-oncogenes or tumor-suppresser genes, which results in the transformation to cancer. DNA mismatch repair deficiency was thought to be an early event in multi-step carcinogenesis. It could be speculated that an abnormality in the DNA mismatch repair system increases the risk of multidrug resistance.

DNA damage caused by cisplatin is recognized by DNA damage recognition proteins, such as high mobility group proteins (HMG1 and HMG2) and mismatch repair complexes (hMSH2 or hMutSα), which transducer DNA damage signals to various downstream effectors.Cell death or cell survival after DNA damage depends on the relative intensity of the signals generated and the crosstalk between the effectors involved. Among these effectors, the p53 tumor suppressor gene plays a central role in determining the final fate of the cell. DNA damage recognition proteins activate the mitogen-activated protein kinase signal transduction pathway, which activates the function of p53 and causes cell cycle arrest at the G2/M checkpoint for DNA repair [60, 62-65]. If the DNA damage is too excessive to repair, apoptosis occurs through the bax and caspase system. In addition, DNA damage may also result in apoptosis through the p53-related gene, p73. The other mechanisms involved in the resistance include enhanced DNA repair capacity and increased antiapoptotic activity.

3.5 Leukemia stem cell contribute to resistance

Current investigations in the field of cancer multidrug resistance research intensively focus upon the "cancer stem cell (CSC) [66-68]". The CSC theory appears to be well established and now widely accepted. The CSC, similar to a normal stem cell, is capable of self-renewal and the production of differentiated progeny. In addition, the human CSC has a capacity to form secondary tumors. Such features of CSCs reflect the activity of cancer initiation, therapy-resistance, all of which are critical in cancer therapy. Stem cells are primarily characterized by the properties of unlimited self-renewal, which maintains and expands the undifferentiated cell pool over the lifetime of the host, and multi-lineage differentiation, which produces progeny of diverse mature phenotypes to generate and regenerate tissues. These stem cell attributes are tightly regulated in normal development, yet their alteration may lead to many human diseases ncluding cancer. In fact, because stem cells and some cancer cells share self-renewal and differentiation capacities, it was suggested that tumors were derived from mutated stem cells, "called cancer stem cells" [69-72]. Although this hypothesis was postulated in early reports, definite proof of their existence came from recent studies in leukemia, where among the complete tumor cell population only a small subset of cells could initiate, regenerate and maintain the leukemia after transplantation into immunocompromised mice. Using similar functional approaches, a variety of cancer stem cells have been identified in an increasing number of epithelial tumors, including breast, prostate, pancreatic, and head and neck carcinomas, all of which were distinguished by the expression of the cell-surface glycoprotein CD44. Another cell surface marker, the CD133 glycoprotein, defined the tumor-initiating cells of brain and colon carcinomas.The concept of cancer stem cells is not only changing our current understanding of cancer biology, but may also have profound consequences on cancer diagnostics and therapeutics.

Cancer stem cells have been identified in leukemias. Many researchers now suspect that all cancers are composed of a mixture of stem cells and proliferative cells. These cancer stem cells make up as few as 1% of the total tumor cells, making them difficult to detect and study. Therefore, the existence of cancer stem cells provides a tumor reservoir that is the source of disease recurrence and metastasis. ABCB1 and ABCG2 genes are expressed in most tumor stem cells [41, 73]. Thus, the major barrier to therapy is the quiescent tumor stem cell with constitutive MDR. In fact, dose-limiting toxicities of many antineoplastic agents occur precisely at drug concentrations that damage normal tissue stem cells. If the proposed relationships between normal and neoplastic stem cells prove correct, the inescapable conclusion is that systemic cytotoxic therapies are doomed to failure because regimens that spare resting normal stem cells will also likely spare resting tumor stem cells. Similarly, inhibition of drug transporters may also cause toxicity of the patient's normal stem cells, particularly those of the bone marrow. Successful therapy awaits the discernment of biological and immunologic differences between the tumor and normal stem cells so that approaches can be developed to eliminate thetumor stem cells without excessive toxicity to normal stem cells, which can be measured *in vitro*.

General decreased transport of drug into the cell, defective intracellular metabolism of the drug to its active compound, increased drug inactivation, enhanced cellular repair mechanisms, altered target molecules, altered cell death regulators could increased MDR. Because many drugs are used in the treatment of leukemia and many factors may be responsible for resistance to each drug, it is unlikely that one single mechanism is responsible for clinical resistance to the complete treatment. And the resistant mechanism to some drugs were listed as following (Table 1).

4. Drug resistance assay

There are many different assays to asses the chemosensitivity of leukemia cells. Clonogenic assays have long been considered to be the golden standard for chemosensitivity testing *in-vitro* [74-76]. However, there were a number of drawbacks. Firstly, the number of patient samples of which the leukemic cells will be clonogenic is limited, especially in ALL samples *in vitro*. Secondly, the drug effect is measured on a small proportion of cells, *i.e.* those cells that can be induced to proliferation *in vitro*, and not on cells that are non dividing or resting. Practical disadvantages are that these assays are very time consuming and laborious. Therefore, these drawbacks make clonogenic assays less suitable for its use in ALL patients.

Recently, non clonogenic assays, an increasing number of authors has been studying cellular drug resistance in childhood leukemia. Examples of these assays are the colorimetric tetrazolium based assays such as the MTT, INT [77-79], DiSC [80], and the fluorometric microculture cytotoxicity assay (FMCA)[81]. The DiSC assay relies on the intactness of the cell membrane in living cells as opposed to dead cells after several days of incubation with drugs. Relatively low numbers of cells are needed to test a range of drugs in different concentrations. A main advantage of this assay is that it can discriminate between malignant and non-malignant cells, in contrast to the MTT assay and FMCA. However, the DiSC assay has the disadvantages of being subjective, laborious, and time consuming, which makes it less suited for large-scale patient studies.

Since drug resistance has a major impact on the success of chemotherapy, it is of clinical importance to identify possibilities to modulate or circumvent each type of drug resistance, which contribute to decreasing the unnecessary toxicity of drugs and increasing the efficacy of treatment by a more rational design of effective chemotherapies.

Type of Drug	Possible Mechanisms
Glucocorticoids (GC)	Affinity of receptor Function of receptor Nuclear translocation of the GCR complex DNA binding of the GC R complex GCR polymorphism (?)
L-Asparaginase	Asparagine synthetase
Methotrexate (MTX)	Membrane transport MTX polyglutamylation and folylpolyglutamate synthetase (FPGS) / folylpolyglutamate hydrolase Active efflux Intracellular normal folate pools Dihydrofolate reductase, Thymidylate synthase (TS) Methylenetetrahydrofolate reductase(MTHFR) (?)
Thiopurines	Nucleoside concentration, ecto-5′ nucleotidase Cyto-5′ nucleotidase and phosphatases Phosphoribosyl pyyrophosphate (PRPP) and PRPP Amidotransferase Hypoxanthine-guanine phosphoribosyl transferase Thiopurine methyltransferase (TPMT)
Cytosine arabinoside (ara-C)	Ara CTP formation Ara C transport Ara-C and Ara-CTP deamination DNA incorporation
Anthracylines, Vinca-alkaloids and Epipodophyllotoxins	MDR-1/P-glycoprotein Multidrug resistance related protein (MRP) Lung resistance protein (LRP) Topoisomerase II BCRP (breast cancer resistance protein)
Alkylating agents	Glutathione Glutathione and glutathione S-transferases DNA repair

Table 1. Drug resistance mechanisms in ALL

5. References

[1] Ross DD. Novel mechanisms of drug resistance in leukemia. Leukemia 2000 Mar; 14(3): 467-473.

[2] Norgaard JM, Hokland P. Biology of multiple drug resistance in acute leukemia. International journal of hematology 2000 Oct; 72(3): 290-297.

[3] Pieters R, Klumper E, Kaspers GJ, Veerman AJ. Everything you always wanted to know about cellular drug resistance in childhood acute lymphoblastic leukemia. Critical reviews in oncology/hematology 1997 Jan; 25(1): 11-26.

[4] Matsuzaki A, Ishii E, Okamura J, Eguchi H, Yoshida N, Yanai F, Inoue T, Miyake K, Ishihara T, Tsuboi C, et al. Treatment of high-risk acute lymphoblastic leukemia in children using the AL851 and ALHR88 protocols: a report from the Kyushu-Yamaguchi Children's Cancer Study Group in Japan. Medical and pediatric oncology 1996 Jan; 26(1): 10-19.

[5] Rask C, Albertioni F, Bentzen SM, Schroeder H, Peterson C. Clinical and pharmacokinetic risk factors for high-dose methotrexate-induced toxicity in children with acute lymphoblastic leukemia--a logistic regression analysis. Acta oncologica (Stockholm, Sweden) 1998; 37(3): 277-284.

[6] Steinherz PG, Gaynon P, Miller DR, Reaman G, Bleyer A, Finklestein J, Evans RG, Meyers P, Steinherz LJ, Sather H, et al. Improved disease-free survival of children with acute lymphoblastic leukemia at high risk for early relapse with the New York regimen--a new intensive therapy protocol: a report from the Childrens Cancer Study Group. J Clin Oncol 1986 May; 4(5): 744-752.

[7] Waber DP, Shapiro BL, Carpentieri SC, Gelber RD, Zou G, Dufresne A, Romero I, Tarbell NJ, Silverman LB, Sallan SE. Excellent therapeutic efficacy and minimal late neurotoxicity in children treated with 18 grays of cranial radiation therapy for high-risk acute lymphoblastic leukemia: a 7-year follow-up study of the Dana-Farber Cancer Institute Consortium Protocol 87-01. Cancer 2001 Jul 1; 92(1): 15-22.

[8] Hammond D, Sather H, Nesbit M, Miller D, Coccia P, Bleyer A, Lukens J, Siegel S. Analysis of prognostic factors in acute lymphoblastic leukemia. Medical and pediatric oncology 1986; 14(3): 124-134.

[9] Hiyoshi Y, Fujimoto T, Kuriya N, Otani Y, Mibu K, Yanai M, Sasaki K, Shingaki Y, Yokoyama T, Kadoya S. Prognostic factors in children with acute lymphoblastic leukemia. Part I: Univariate analysis. Children's Cancer and Leukemia Study Group. Japanese journal of clinical oncology 1985 Mar; 15(1): 3-12.

[10] Improvement in treatment for children with acute lymphoblastic leukaemia. The Medical Research Council UKALL trials, 1972-84. Report to the Council by the Working Party on Leukaemia in Childhood. Lancet 1986 Feb 22; 1(8478): 408-411.

[11] Hoelzer D, Gale RP. Acute lymphoblastic leukemia in adults: recent progress, future directions. Seminars in hematology 1987 Jan; 24(1): 27-39.

[12] Sather HN. Age at diagnosis in childhood acute lymphoblastic leukemia. Medical and pediatric oncology 1986; 14(3): 166-172.

[13] Crist W, Boyett J, Pullen J, van Eys J, Vietti T. Clinical and biologic features predict poor prognosis in acute lymphoid leukemias in children and adolescents: a Pediatric Oncology Group review. Medical and pediatric oncology 1986; 14(3): 135-139.

[14] Crist W, Pullen J, Boyett J, Falletta J, van Eys J, Borowitz M, Jackson J, Dowell B, Frankel L, Quddus F, et al. Clinical and biologic features predict a poor prognosis in acute lymphoid leukemias in infants: a Pediatric Oncology Group Study. Blood 1986 Jan; 67(1): 135-140.

[15] Catts VS, Farnsworth ML, Haber M, Norris MD, Lutze-Mann LH, Lock RB. High level resistance to glucocorticoids, associated with a dysfunctional glucocorticoid receptor, in childhood acute lymphoblastic leukemia cells selected for methotrexate resistance. Leukemia 2001 Jun; 15(6): 929-935.

[16] Gaynon PS, Lustig RH. The use of glucocorticoids in acute lymphoblastic leukemia of childhood. Molecular, cellular, and clinical considerations. J Pediatr Hematol Oncol 1995 Feb; 17(1): 1-12.

[17] Banker DS, Pahwa RN, Miller DR, Hilgartner MW, Good RA, Pahwa SG. Immunoregulatory properties of childhood leukemias. Journal of clinical immunology 1982 Jul; 2(3): 230-236.

[18] Favara BE, Mierau GW, McCarthy RC, Waldstein G, McGavran L. The leukemias of childhood. Perspectives in pediatric pathology 1987; 9: 75-132.

[19] Klujber V, Koos R, Schuler D, Bocsi J. [Immunophenotyping of childhood leukemias--results of the first 100 bone marrow tests]. Orvosi hetilap 1996 May 26; 137(21): 1139-1142.

[20] Morisot S, Wayne AS, Bohana-Kashtan O, Kaplan IM, Gocke CD, Hildreth R, Stetler-Stevenson M, Walker RL, Davis S, Meltzer PS, Wheelan SJ, Brown P, Jones RJ, Shultz LD, Civin CI. High frequencies of leukemia stem cells in poor-outcome childhood precursor-B acute lymphoblastic leukemias. Leukemia Nov; 24(11): 1859-1866.

[21] Thone I, Kabisch H, Muller J, Winkler K, Landbeck G. [Immunological classification of acute lymphoblastic leukemias (ALL) in childhood. Origin and clinical significance of phenotypic variability]. Monatsschr Kinderheilkd 1982 Dec; 130(12): 883-890.

[22] Pui CH, Crist WM, Look AT. Biology and clinical significance of cytogenetic abnormalities in childhood acute lymphoblastic leukemia. Blood 1990 Oct 15; 76(8): 1449-1463.

[23] Trueworthy R, Shuster J, Look T, Crist W, Borowitz M, Carroll A, Frankel L, Harris M, Wagner H, Haggard M, et al. Ploidy of lymphoblasts is the strongest predictor of treatment outcome in B-progenitor cell acute lymphoblastic leukemia of childhood: a Pediatric Oncology Group study. J Clin Oncol 1992 Apr; 10(4): 606-613.

[24] Faderl S, O'Brien S, Pui CH, Stock W, Wetzler M, Hoelzer D, Kantarjian HM. Adult acute lymphoblastic leukemia: concepts and strategies. Cancer Mar 1; 116(5): 1165-1176.

[25] Graux C, Cools J, Michaux L, Vandenberghe P, Hagemeijer A. Cytogenetics and molecular genetics of T-cell acute lymphoblastic leukemia: from thymocyte to lymphoblast. Leukemia 2006 Sep; 20(9): 1496-1510.

[26] Harrison CJ, Foroni L. Cytogenetics and molecular genetics of acute lymphoblastic leukemia. Reviews in clinical and experimental hematology 2002 Jun; 6(2): 91-113; discussion 200-112.

[27] Hayne CC, Winer E, Williams T, Chaves F, Khorsand J, Mark HF. Acute lymphoblastic leukemia with 4;11 translocation analyzed by a multi-modal strategy of conventional cytogenetics, FISH, morphology, flow cytometry and molecular genetics, and review of the literature. Experimental and molecular pathology 2006 Aug; 81(1): 62-71.

[28] Mrozek K, Harper DP, Aplan PD. Cytogenetics and molecular genetics of acute lymphoblastic leukemia. Hematology/oncology clinics of North America 2009 Oct; 23(5): 991-1010, v.

[29] Landrigan PJ. Childhood leukemias. The New England journal of medicine 1995 Nov 9; 333(19): 1286.

[30] Pui CH. Childhood leukemias. The New England journal of medicine 1995 Jun 15; 332(24): 1618-1630.

[31] Bash RO, Crist WM, Shuster JJ, Link MP, Amylon M, Pullen J, Carroll AJ, Buchanan GR, Smith RG, Baer R. Clinical features and outcome of T-cell acute lymphoblastic leukemia in childhood with respect to alterations at the TAL1 locus: a Pediatric Oncology Group study. Blood 1993 Apr 15; 81(8): 2110-2117.

[32] Adhya S. Harrison Echols (1933-1993). Cell 1993 Jun 4; 73(5): 833-834.

[33] Dedera DA, Waller EK, LeBrun DP, Sen-Majumdar A, Stevens ME, Barsh GS, Cleary ML. Chimeric homeobox gene E2A-PBX1 induces proliferation, apoptosis, and malignant lymphomas in transgenic mice. Cell 1993 Sep 10; 74(5): 833-843. 34van den Heuvel-Eibrink MM, Sonneveld P, Pieters R. The prognostic significance of membrane transport-associated multidrug resistance (MDR) proteins in leukemia. International journal of clinical pharmacology and therapeutics 2000 Mar; 38(3): 94-110.

[34] Chin JE, Soffir R, Noonan KE, Choi K, Roninson IB. Structure and expression of the human MDR (P-glycoprotein) gene family. Molecular and cellular biology 1989 Sep; 9(9): 3808-3820.

[35] Abd El-Ghaffar HA, Aladle DA, Farahat SE, Abd El-Hady N. P-glycoprotein (P-170) expression in acute leukemias. Hematology (Amsterdam, Netherlands) 2006 Feb; 11(1): 35-41.

[36] Buda G, Orciuolo E, Maggini V, Galimberti S, Barale R, Rossi AM, Petrini M. MDR1 pump: more than a drug transporter comment on "Regulatory polymorphisms of multidrug resistance 1 (MDR1) gene are associated with the development of childhood acute lymphoblastic leukaemia" by Hattori et al. [Leuk. Res. (in press)]. Leukemia research 2008 Feb; 32(2): 359-360.

[37] Fazlina N, Maha A, Zarina AL, Hamidah A, Zulkifli SZ, Cheong SK, Ainoon O, Jamal R, Hamidah NH. Assessment of P-gp and MRP1 activities using MultiDrugQuant Assay Kit: a preliminary study of correlation between protein expressions and its functional activities in newly diagnosed acute leukaemia patients. The Malaysian journal of pathology 2008 Dec; 30(2): 87-93.

[38] Hartman A, van Schaik RH, van der Heiden IP, Broekhuis MJ, Meier M, den Boer ML, Pieters R. Polymorphisms in genes involved in vincristine pharmacokinetics or pharmacodynamics are not related to impaired motor performance in children with leukemia. Leukemia research Feb; 34(2): 154-159.

[39] Rao DN, Anuradha C, Vishnupriya S, Sailaja K, Surekha D, Raghunadharao D, Rajappa S. Association of an MDR1 gene (C3435T) polymorphism with acute leukemia in India. Asian Pac J Cancer Prev; 11(4): 1063-1066.

[40] Svirnovski AI, Shman TV, Serhiyenka TF, Savitski VP, Smolnikova VV, Fedasenka UU. ABCB1 and ABCG2 proteins, their functional activity and gene expression in concert with drug sensitivity of leukemia cells. Hematology (Amsterdam, Netherlands) 2009 Aug; 14(4): 204-212.

[41] Gayet L, Dayan G, Barakat S, Labialle S, Michaud M, Cogne S, Mazane A, Coleman AW, Rigal D, Baggetto LG. Control of P-glycoprotein activity by membrane cholesterol amounts and their relation to multidrug resistance in human CEM leukemia cells. Biochemistry 2005 Mar 22; 44(11): 4499-4509.

[42] Olson DP, Taylor BJ, La M, Sather H, Reaman GH, Ivy SP. The prognostic significance of P-glycoprotein, multidrug resistance-related protein 1 and lung resistance protein in pediatric acute lymphoblastic leukemia: a retrospective study of 295 newly diagnosed patients by the Children's Oncology Group. Leukemia & lymphoma 2005 May; 46(5): 681-691.

[43] Kanerva J, Tiirikainen M, Makipernaa A, Riikonen P, Mottonen M, Salmi TT, Krusius T, Saarinen-Pihkala UM. Multiple drug resistance mediated by P-glycoprotein is not a major factor in a slow response to therapy in childhood ALL. Pediatric hematology and oncology 1998 Jan-Feb; 15(1): 11-21.

[44] Gurbuxani S, Singh Arya L, Raina V, Sazawal S, Khattar A, Magrath I, Marie J, Bhargava M. Significance of MDR1, MRP1, GSTpi and GSTmu mRNA expression in acute lymphoblastic leukemia in Indian patients. Cancer letters 2001 Jun 10; 167(1): 73-83.

[45] Kourti M, Vavatsi N, Gombakis N, Sidi V, Tzimagiorgis G, Papageorgiou T, Koliouskas D, Athanassiadou F. Expression of multidrug resistance 1 (MDR1), multidrug resistance-related protein 1 (MRP1), lung resistance protein (LRP), and breast cancer resistance protein (BCRP) genes and clinical outcome in childhood acute lymphoblastic leukemia. International journal of hematology 2007 Aug; 86(2): 166-173.

[46] Sauerbrey A, Voigt A, Wittig S, Hafer R, Zintl F. Messenger RNA analysis of the multidrug resistance related protein (MRP1) and the lung resistance protein (LRP) in de novo and relapsed childhood acute lymphoblastic leukemia. Leukemia & lymphoma 2002 Apr; 43(4): 875-879.

[47] Sauerbrey A, Sell W, Steinbach D, Voigt A, Zintl F. Expression of the BCRP gene (ABCG2/MXR/ABCP) in childhood acute lymphoblastic leukaemia. British journal of haematology 2002 Jul; 118(1): 147-150.

[48] Stam RW, van den Heuvel-Eibrink MM, den Boer ML, Ebus ME, Janka-Schaub GE, Allen JD, Pieters R. Multidrug resistance genes in infant acute lymphoblastic leukemia: Ara-C is not a substrate for the breast cancer resistance protein. Leukemia 2004 Jan; 18(1): 78-83.

[49] Su Y, Lee SH, Sinko PJ. Inhibition of efflux transporter ABCG2/BCRP does not restore mitoxantrone sensitivity in irinotecan-selected human leukemia CPT-K5 cells: evidence for multifactorial multidrug resistance. Eur J Pharm Sci 2006 Oct 1; 29(2): 102-110.

[50] Ogretmen B, Barredo JC, Safa AR. Increased expression of lung resistance-related protein and multidrug resistance-associated protein messenger RNA in childhood acute lymphoblastic leukemia. J Pediatr Hematol Oncol 2000 Jan-Feb; 22(1): 45-49.

[51] Kakihara T, Tanaka A, Watanabe A, Yamamoto K, Kanto K, Kataoka S, Ogawa A, Asami K, Uchiyama M. Expression of multidrug resistance-related genes does not contribute to risk factors in newly diagnosed childhood acute lymphoblastic leukemia. Pediatr Int 1999 Dec; 41(6): 641-647.

[52] Ramakers-van Woerden NL, Beverloo HB, Veerman AJ, Camitta BM, Loonen AH, van Wering ER, Slater RM, Harbott J, den Boer ML, Ludwig WD, Haas OA, Janka-Schaub GE, Pieters R. In vitro drug-resistance profile in infant acute lymphoblastic

leukemia in relation to age, MLL rearrangements and immunophenotype. Leukemia 2004 Mar; 18(3): 521-529.
[53] High LM, Szymanska B, Wilczynska-Kalak U, Barber N, O'Brien R, Khaw SL, Vikstrom IB, Roberts AW, Lock RB. The Bcl-2 homology domain 3 mimetic ABT-737 targets the apoptotic machinery in acute lymphoblastic leukemia resulting in synergistic in vitro and in vivo interactions with established drugs. Molecular pharmacology Mar; 77(3): 483-494.
[54] Srinivas G, Kusumakumary P, Nair MK, Panicker KR, Pillai MR. Bcl-2 protein and apoptosis in pediatric acute lymphoblastic leukemia. International journal of molecular medicine 1998 Apr; 1(4): 755-759.
[55] Coustan-Smith E, Kitanaka A, Pui CH, McNinch L, Evans WE, Raimondi SC, Behm FG, Arico M, Campana D. Clinical relevance of BCL-2 overexpression in childhood acute lymphoblastic leukemia. Blood 1996 Feb 1; 87(3): 1140-1146.
[56] Rabi T, Banerjee S. Novel semisynthetic triterpenoid AMR-Me inhibits telomerase activity in human leukemic CEM cells and exhibits in vivo antitumor activity against Dalton's lymphoma ascites tumor. Cancer letters 2009 Jun 18; 278(2): 156-163.
[57] Best A, Matheson E, Minto L, Hall AG, Irving JA. Mismatch repair and the downstream target genes, PAX5 and Ikaros, in childhood acute lymphoblastic leukemia. Leukemia research Aug; 34(8): 1098-1102.
[58] Leone G, Pagano L, Ben-Yehuda D, Voso MT. Therapy-related leukemia and myelodysplasia: susceptibility and incidence. Haematologica 2007 Oct; 92(10): 1389-1398.
[59] Mathonnet G, Krajinovic M, Labuda D, Sinnett D. Role of DNA mismatch repair genetic polymorphisms in the risk of childhood acute lymphoblastic leukaemia. British journal of haematology 2003 Oct; 123(1): 45-48.
[60] Thoms KM, Baesecke J, Emmert B, Hermann J, Roedling T, Laspe P, Leibeling D, Truemper L, Emmert S. Functional DNA repair system analysis in haematopoietic progenitor cells using host cell reactivation. Scandinavian journal of clinical and laboratory investigation 2007; 67(6): 580-588.
[61] Infante-Rivard C. Diagnostic x rays, DNA repair genes and childhood acute lymphoblastic leukemia. Health physics 2003 Jul; 85(1): 60-64.
[62] Matheson EC, Hall AG. Assessment of mismatch repair function in leukaemic cell lines and blasts from children with acute lymphoblastic leukaemia. Carcinogenesis 2003 Jan; 24(1): 31-38.
[63] Molenaar JJ, Gerard B, Chambon-Pautas C, Cave H, Duval M, Vilmer E, Grandchamp B. Microsatellite instability and frameshift mutations in BAX and transforming growth factor-beta RII genes are very uncommon in acute lymphoblastic leukemia in vivo but not in cell lines. Blood 1998 Jul 1; 92(1): 230-233.
[64] Zhu YM, Das-Gupta EP, Russell NH. Microsatellite instability and p53 mutations are associated with abnormal expression of the MSH2 gene in adult acute leukemia. Blood 1999 Jul 15; 94(2): 733-740.
[65] Holleman A, den Boer ML, Kazemier KM, Janka-Schaub GE, Pieters R. Resistance to different classes of drugs is associated with impaired apoptosis in childhood acute lymphoblastic leukemia. Blood 2003 Dec 15; 102(13): 4541-4546.

[66] Jansson J, Hsu YC, Kuzin, II, Campbell A, Mullen CA. Acute lymphoblastic leukemia cells that survive combination chemotherapy in vivo remain sensitive to allogeneic immune effects. Leukemia research Nov 11.

[67] Yamazaki H, Xu CW, Naito M, Nishida H, Okamoto T, Ghani FI, Iwata S, Inukai T, Sugita K, Morimoto C. Regulation of cancer stem cell properties by CD9 in human B-acute lymphoblastic leukemia. Biochemical and biophysical research communications May 27; 409(1): 14-21.

[68] Copelan EA, McGuire EA. The biology and treatment of acute lymphoblastic leukemia in adults. Blood 1995 Mar 1; 85(5): 1151-1168.

[69] Gale RP, Butturini A. Controversies in therapy of acute lymphoblastic leukemia. Leukemia 1992; 6 Suppl 2: 144-147.

[70] Hofmann WK, Komor M, Wassmann B, Jones LC, Gschaidmeier H, Hoelzer D, Koeffler HP, Ottmann OG. Presence of the BCR-ABL mutation Glu255Lys prior to STI571 (imatinib) treatment in patients with Ph+ acute lymphoblastic leukemia. Blood 2003 Jul 15; 102(2): 659-661.

[71] Zwaan CM, Kaspers GJ, Pieters R, Ramakers-Van Woerden NL, den Boer ML, Wunsche R, Rottier MM, Hahlen K, van Wering ER, Janka-Schaub GE, Creutzig U, Veerman AJ. Cellular drug resistance profiles in childhood acute myeloid leukemia: differences between FAB types and comparison with acute lymphoblastic leukemia. Blood 2000 Oct 15; 96(8): 2879-2886.

[72] Erdilyi DJ, Kamory E, Csokay B, Andrikovics H, Tordai A, Kiss C, Filni-Semsei A, Janszky I, Zalka A, Fekete G, Falus A, Kovacs GT, Szalai C. Synergistic interaction of ABCB1 and ABCG2 polymorphisms predicts the prevalence of toxic encephalopathy during anticancer chemotherapy. The pharmacogenomics journal 2008 Oct; 8(5): 321-327.

[73] Kirkwood JM, Marsh JC. In vivo drug sensitivity assay of clonogenic human melanoma cells and correlation with treatment outcome. Cancer research 1983 Jul; 43(7): 3434-3440.

[74] Lieber MM, Kovach JS. Soft agar clonogenic assay for primary human renal carcinoma: in vitro chemotherapeutic drug sensitivity testing. Investigative urology 1981 Sep; 19(2): 111-114.

[75] Salmon SE. Human tumor clonogenic assays: growth conditions and applications. Cancer genetics and cytogenetics 1986 Jan 1; 19(1-2): 21-28.

[76] Karakas Z, Agaoglu L, Erdem S, Anak S, Hacibektasoglu A, Gedikoglu G. MTT assay for drug resistance in childhood acute leukemia and effect of cyclosporin and interferon. A preliminary report. Advances in experimental medicine and biology 1999; 457: 453-459.

[77] Sargent J, Elgie A, Taylor CG, Wilson J, Alton P, Hill JG. The identification of drug resistance in ovarian cancer and breast cancer: application of the MTT assay. Contributions to gynecology and obstetrics 1994; 19: 64-75.

[78] Stute N, Kohler T, Lehmann L, Wetzstein W, Ehninger G. Drug resistance testing of acute myeloid leukemia in adults using the MTT assay. Advances in experimental medicine and biology 1999; 457: 445-452.

[79] Li QY, Wang Y, Yin ZF, Wu MC. [Application of the improved MTT assay in predicting the intrinsic drug resistance of liver cancer]. Zhonghua yi xue za zhi 2007 Jan 30; 87(5): 333-335.

[80] Poulain S, Lepelley P, Cambier N, Cosson A, Fenaux P, Wattel E. Assessment of P-glycoprotein expression by immunocytochemistry and flow cytometry using two different monoclonal antibodies coupled with functional efflux analysis in 34 patients with acute myeloid leukemia. Advances in experimental medicine and biology 1999; 457: 57-63.

Part 6

Pathophysiology and Novel Targets

8

Novel Therapeutic Targets in ALL Therapy

Roman Crazzolara
Department of Pediatrics, Medical University of Innsbruck
Austria

1. Introduction

ALL is a malignant disorder of the blood system characterized by uncontrolled proliferation of bone marrow-derived B- and T-lymphocyte progenitors that are arrested in an early stage of development (Pui et al, 2008). This arrest is caused by aberrant gene fusions or inappropriate expression of oncogenes. The lymphoblasts replace the normal marrow elements, resulting in a substantial decrease in the production of normal blood cells. Consequently, anemia, thrombocytopenia, and neutropenia occur to varying degrees. Moreover, the expanding lymphoblasts can escape the bone marrow niche, and manifest as heptospenomegaly, enlargement of lymph nodes, thymus, and gonads, and infiltration of the meninges (Pui et al, 2008).

ALL has a peak incidence between the ages of 2 to 5 years, representing 25% of the malignant disorders in childhood (Pui et al, 2006). Currently, ALL is treated by administration of cyclic induction chemotherapy, which is intended to kill the majority of leukemic cells, followed by a consolidation chemotherapy, which should destroy any remaining leukemic cells (Freycon et al, 2008; Pui et al, 2008). For high risk patients, myeloablative regimens followed by allogeneic hematopoietic stem-cell transplantation are indicated to achieve more extensive eradication of leukemia and to induce graft versus leukemia effects against the disease. The implementation of risk-adapted strategies, which tailor the intensity of therapy to the risk of relapse, has resulted in a cure rate of more than 80% in children being long-term survivors (Pui et al, 2006). In contrast to the successes obtained with paediatric patients, treatment outcomes for adult patients remain poor with less than 40% being long-term survivors (Vitale et al, 2006). Due to relative nonspecific action and narrow therapeutic indices of antileukemic medications, serious short and long-term complications arise as a result of the intensification of many current therapies (Barr et al, 2008).

The identification of genetic and epigenetic changes that are associated with leukemogenesis and altered drug response provides insights into the molecular basis of ALL. The translation to the clinic might serve as a model for optimizing the treatment and generate innovative therapeutic agents. Finally, these could be implemented in more effective, and potentially less toxic, individually tailored treatment protocols, based on the underlying molecular abnormalities of a patient's leukemia. This review will concentrate on novel agents that show promising anti-leukemic activity in pre-clinical studies or clinical trials.

2. CXCR4 inhibitors

Several studies have been reported on the involvement of chemokines and adhesion molecules in the process of mobilization of ALL cells. Among the most studied molecules are the chemokine receptor CXCR4 and the chemokine stromal cell-derived factor-1 (SDF-1, CXCL12); in particular CXCR4, was found to be highly expressed in bone-marrow derived ALL cells enabling these cells to migrate across a gradient of CXCL12 concentrations (Crazzolara et al, 2001). Elevated levels of CXCL12 are not only found in the bone marrow environment, but also at extramedullary sites associated with ALL induced organ infiltration (Muller et al, 2001). Subsequently CXCL12 can act as survival and proliferation factor for CXCR4 positive cells and protect them from spontaneous and chemotherapy-induced apoptosis (Burger et al, 2000). In several studies, CXCL12 is also reported in the process of homing of CXCR4 positive cells in NOD/SCID xenograft mouse models (Nagasawa et al, 1996). Of note is the direct correlation between high CXCR4 expression on lymphoblasts and the extent of extramedullary infiltration in patients with ALL (Crazzolara et al, 2001).

Direct evidence for the involvement of CXCR4 and CXCL12 in the release of ALL cells in the blood is demonstrated from the finding that treatment of mice with small compounds that target CXCR4 and its ligand can disrupt the interaction between ALL cells and the stromal microenvironment. The polyphemusin II-derived inhibitors T140, TC140012, T134, and the bicyclam AMD3100 effectively inhibit CXCR4, and CXCL12-driven migration into bone marrow layers *in vitro,* thus enhancing the cytotoxic and anti-proliferative effects of the currently used agents vincristine and dexamethasone (Juarez et al, 2003). Disruption of the interaction of CXCR4 and its ligand *in vivo* mobilizes leukemic cells into the peripheral blood, potentially rendering them more susceptible to cytotoxic effects (Juarez et al, 2006). The importance of CXCR4 in the context of therapy is further supported by the observation, that CXCR4 expression is dynamically up regulated by chemotherapy exposure in ALL cells. Up regulation of surface CXCR4 may therefore be considered as a mechanism of chemo resistance in acute leukaemias that is potentially reversible with CXCR4-targeted therapy.

Concerns have been raised regarding potential side effects from CXCR4 inhibition, since CXCR4 knockout mice display severe defects in hematopoesis, vascular and cardiac development (Nagasawa et al, 1996). However, these defects are related to CXCR4 functions in early development, and short-term exposure to AMD3100 for stem cell mobilization does not result in any significant toxicity (Broxmeyer et al, 2005). Activity of different CXCR4 antagonists in animal models for solid tumors (Smith et al, 2004) generalizes the potential anti-neoplastic activity and suggests further clinical development of these agents in ALL. It is anticipated, that a phase I pediatric study has recently started to study the addition of the selective CXCR4 antagonist plerixafor to enhance the conditioning regimen cytotoxicity (NCT01068301, www.clinicaltrials.gov). Though the primary goal is to determine the maximum tolerated dose (MTD), additional trials are necessary to study the use of plerixafor as a complimentary agent with conditioning as well as other chemotherapeutic regimens for patients with relapsed or refractory hematologic malignancies.

3. CD22 immunoconjugates

The approval of antibody-targeted agents for cancer treatment has provoked increased interest in the development of new and improved antibody-mediated therapies. This emerging approach centers on targeting cell clusters of differentiation on ALL cells with a monoclonal antibody (mAb), conjugated to a cytotoxic agent. After internalization of the antibody-drug complex, vital survival pathways for malignant cells can be blocked or dyregulated. Among these, CD22 antibody-targeted agents have more extensively been explored with significant preclinical success in models of acute leukemia (Dijoseph et al, 2004).

CMC-544 (inotuzumab ozogamicin) is a conjugate of a recombinant humanized antibody directed against the CD22 antigen and calicheamicin. After internalization into the target cell, calicheamicin binds to DNA in the minor groove in a sequence specific manner, causing double-strand DNA breaks followed by apoptotic death. *In vitro*, CMC-544 binds to CD22 with subnanomolar affinity and potently inhibits growth of ALL cell lines (Dijoseph et al, 2007). When administered to xenograft models, CMC-544 prevents engraftment, but also induces dose-dependent tumor regression in mice presenting with leukemia. Whereas the level of CD22 expression is significantly reduced after incubation with CMC-544, the CD20 level can be increased (Takeshita et al, 2009). Therefore, sequential administration of rituximab increases the cytotoxic effect and supports the rationale for a combination with other antibodies.

Currently, a phase I study is recruiting patients for the aminstration of CMC-544 with or without rituximab in relapsed or primary refractory ALL patients (NCT01134575, www.clinicaltrials.gov). Preliminary results indicate liver function abnormalities in 25% of patients, including periportal fibrosis and venoocclusive disease after allo SCT, among the most relevant side effects (Jabbour et al, 2011). Overall, complete response plus complete bone marrow response is achieved in more than 50% of the patients.

Additional phase I studies are soon expected to open, including a single use of CMC-544 in refractory ALL patients (NCT01363297, www.clinicaltrials.gov) and a 2 dose level study in combination with cyclophosphamide, vincristine, dexamethasone, methotrexate, cytarabine in elderly ALL patients (NCT01371630, www.clinicaltrials.gov).

4. BCL-2 Antisense therapy

In several clinical studies alterations in the apoptotic threshold were proven to be predictive of poor response to treatment and adverse clinical outcome in patients with a variety of hematologic malignancies, including acute leukemia. Specifically, the up regulation of the BCL-2 family of proteins has been demonstrated to suppress caspase- and non-caspase-mediated apoptosis mediated by several agents, including γ-irradiation and chemotherapy (Reed et al, 1995). As such, over expression of BCL-2 has been associated with an increased risk of relapse in childhood ALL (Hogarth et al, 1999), suggesting the use of factors that override the BCL-2 pathway might restore chemo sensitivity in chemo resistant leukemic cells.

Since the discovery of BCL-2, a single antisense oligodeoxynucleotide - Genasense (G3139, oblimersen; Genta Inc.) - has been explored. *In vitro* studies have shown that when administered alone or in combination with chemotherapy, G3139 inhibits BCL2 expression, resulting in increased tumor cell apoptosis (Webb et al, 1997). Subsequently, its ability to effectively reduce BCL-2 protein levels has clearly been demonstrated in a mouse model transplanted with leukemia. This effect is correlated with enhanced induction of apoptosis, when cells are cultured with the anti-leukemic agents imatinib, daunorubicin, cytarabine and etoposide. Mice treated with G3139 have prolonged survival with some showing complete tumor regression. Of particular interest is the efficacy of G3139 in STI571 resistant

BCR-ABL transformed cells, suggesting its use in clinically acquired STI571 resistance (Tauchi et al, 2003). The very low toxicity observed in a phase I study of relapsed acute leukemia, demonstrates that G3139 can safely be administered with fludarabine and cytarabine salvage chemotherapy (FLAG) without dose limiting toxicity. Common side effects of this combination include fever, nausea; emesis, electrolyte imbalance, and fluid retention that are not dose limiting. Pharmacokinetics indicates steady-state concentrations within 24 hours and is associated with significant down-regulation of BCL-2 mRNA levels in 75% of patients (Marcucci et al, 2003). Despite an encouraging result of 45% overall survival is achieved, the specific role of G3139 cannot be discriminated from the antileukemic activity of FLAG. Based upon the results obtained so far, validation of the G3139 efficacy, still needs to be completed with phase II/III trials.

5. Proteasome inhibitors

Malignant cells can harbour altered expression of proteasome subunits and their distribution between nucleus and cytoplasm can differ from normal cells. Subsequently, the ubiquitin-proteasome pathway is involved in malignant cellular hemostasis since it regulates the degradation of damaged, oxidized, or misfolded proteins and regulatory proteins that govern cell cycle, transcription factor activation, apoptosis, and cell trafficking. Key proteins degraded by this pathway include cyclins A, B and E, p21, p27, p53, cJun, cFos, IkB, Bcl2, BclX, and MAPK (Laney et al, 1999; Maki et al, 1996). Targeting proteasome subunits by proteasome inhibitors offers the possibility to sensitize surviving tumor cells to the effect of chemotherapy and to induce apoptosis in tumor cells.

Bortezomib (Velcade, PS-341; Millenium Pharmaceuticals) is the first proteasome inhibitor to be tested in humans and is currently approved for the treatment of relapsed multiple myeloma and mantle cell lymphoma. It is a potent and selective, reversible inhibitor of the 26S proteosome, a key regulatory multi-subunit protease, that controls cell cycle and apoptosis (Adams et al, 1998). As in a broad range of tumor cells, bortezomib has demonstrated significant activity in ALL cells, inducing apoptosis *in vitro* and *in vivo*. Additional studies have indicated that it may also potentiate the cytotoxic effects of chemotherapy. In particular, it enhances the *in vitro* cytotoxicity of dexamethasone, vincristine, asparaginase, cytarabine, doxorubicin, phenyl butyrate, trichostatin and HA14.1 (Horton et al, 2006; Sutheesophon et al, 2006).

A recent phase I clinical study in adults with refractory or relapsed acute leukemias indicates the dose of 1.25 mg/m^2 to be safely administered on a twice weekly schedule for a 4 week period (Cortes et al, 2004). This is similar to the currently recommended dose of 1.3 mg/m^2, given in multiple myeloma. Dose limiting toxicity includes orthostatic hypotension, nausea, diarrhoea and fluid retention. Evidence of biological activity is demonstrated by significant proteasome inhibition. It is anticipated, that few patients have achieved transient reduction of bone marrow blasts, with eventual recurrence of the initial blasts, usually during the time off therapy.

Unfortunately, experience in childhood is limited to a phase I trial of bortezomib in pediatric patients with solid tumors, showing minimal toxicity. Since it has non-overlapping toxicities with myelosuppressive agents used to treat ALL and promising *in vitro* activity, further investigation of bortezomib in this setting is warranted, particularly in studies with multimodal chemotherapy.

6. Inhibitors of γ-secretase

The detection of NOTCH1 gain-of-function mutations in more than 50% of T-cell ALL patients has attracted much interest in the understanding of its role in the molecular pathogenesis of this leukemic subtype. Although expression of an activated NOTCH1 allele has been shown to cause T-cell leukemia in mice, the molecular mechanism for cellular transformation is largely unknown. However, the identification of c-myc as a direct and critical NOTCH1 target gene (Weng et al, 2004) has urged the screening and development of NOTCH1 pathway therapeutics.

The NOTCH1 inhibitor MK-0752 (Merck & Co.) has been developed for the treatment of Alzheimer's disease, since it cleaves amyloid precursor protein and prevents the formation of amyloid ß-peptides (Evin et al, 2006). Its activity in leukemia is demonstrated by the conservation of the NOTCH1 receptor within the transmembrane domain, preventing the release of the NOTCH intracellular domain, and thereby suppressing the transcription of target genes. This results in the arrest of cells in $G_{0/1}$, reduces viability, and increases apoptosis (DeAngelo et al, 2006). In a phase I trial of adult and pediatric patients with T-cell malignancies MK-0752 has been shown to be well-tolerated with diarrhoea being the dose-limiting toxicity. Measurements of γ-secretase inhibition have shown a 24-69% decrease in plasma $Abeta_{40}$ peptide levels compared to predose levels (DeAngelo et al, 2006). Only one patient with a NOTCH1 activating mutation has achieved a significant reduction of a mediastinal mass at the end of the treatment, but has subsequently progressed.

Currently, an additional phase I study is examining the safety of a newer NOTCH1 inhibitor with improved biological availability (PF-03084014, Pfizer; NCT01068301, www.clinicaltrials.gov) in adult patients with relapsed T-ALL.

7. Heat-shock-protein antagonists

Heat shock protein 90 (Hsp90) is currently receiving considerable attention as a potential anticancer drug target. It is a molecular chaperone that regulates structural folding and active configuration of a variety of signal transduction and cell cycle regulatory proteins, including tyrosine and serine kinases such as c-src and Akt (Isaacs et al, 2003; Hawkins et al, 2005). Inhibition of Hsp90 disrupts the folding of these proteins, thus increasing their susceptibility to ubiquitination and proteosomal degradation. Although the exact mechanism by which Hsp90 inhibitors kill tumor cells remain to be defined, the ability to abrogate the AKT and BCR-ABL pathways makes these compounds particularly attractive for ALL therapy.

17-allylamino-17-demethoxygeldanamycin (17-AAG) is a toxic derivative of geldanamycin and is undergoing clinical examination as it has significant Hsp90-dependent antitumor activity and a favorable toxicity profile (Goetz et al, 2005). Following exposure to 17-AAG results in a rapid decrease of AKT phosphorylation and total AKT protein levels in pediatric ALL patients. This effect can be relevant when 17-AAG is combined with drugs that induce AKT activation, such as arsenic trioxide (Pelicano et al, 2006). Sequential administration causes rapid decline of phosphorylated AKT, increasing the number of cells accumulating in $G_{0/1}$ phase as well as the rate of cleaved caspase-3.

Beyond the effect of 17-AAG on AKT function, BCR-ABL has also been shown to be a client protein for Hsp90 (Gorre et al, 2002). Treatment with 17-AAG results in significant down-

regulation of intracellular levels of BCR-ABL, followed by a decrease in cell survival and the induction of apoptosis. Of interest is the effect on imatinib mesylate-resistant cells, in which sensitivity to imatinib can be restored.
Based on this selective toxicity, 17-AAG has been examined in phase I and II clinical trials in patients with acute myeloid and chronic lymphatic leukemia. These studies have shown that 17-AAG is reasonably well tolerated, with transient elevation of serum transaminases, nausea, vomiting, and diarrhoea being dose-limiting when this agent is administered as a 60-minute infusion on a weekly schedule. Further studies are required to determine tolerability and effectiveness in leukemic patients.

8. Resveratrol

Recently, several natural or dietary substances have been shown to have antineoplastic activity. Much attention has been paid to the polyphenolic phytoalexin resveratrol (3,5,4'-trihydroxy-trans-stilbene), since it inhibits events associated with tumor initiation, promotion and progress (Jang et al, 1997). Potentially, it inhibits free-radical formation and reduces oxidative and mutagenic stress (Aggarwal et al, 2004). Subsequently, resveratrol suppresses the growth of transformed cells and induces apoptosis through interaction with kinase pathways and activation of the caspase cascade (Bernhard et al, 2000).
In leukemic cells resveratrol arrests cells in the S-phase of the cell cycle. A mechanism, by which the replication machinery is arrested, is demonstrated by the inhibition of the ribonucleotide reductase in murine lymphoblastic leukemic cells. Additionally, both the NOTCH and the PI3K/AKT pathway are inhibited at higher concentrations of resveratrol. This is modulated by the activation of signalling systems, such as p53, p21waf-1 and Bax (Cecchinato et al, 2007). Also, resveratrol has been shown to induce mitochondrial depolarization and subsequent activation of downstream caspases associated with the intrinsic apoptotic pathway (Dorrie et al, 2001; Fontecave et al, 1998). Independence of Fas- and TNFα signalling in resveratrol-induced apoptosis might be a desirable property of a potential new therapeutic agent, since tumor cells develop strategies to escape Fas-mediated apoptosis (Bernhard et al, 2000).
Preliminary results of a phase II study of the synthetic resveratrol derivative SRT501 (GlaxoSmithKline) in multiple myeloma patients reveal, that administration of this formulation is limited by the development of the acute renal failure (NCT00920556, www.clinicaltrials.gov). Whereas this complication might be restricted to the underlying disease, tolerability and efficacy of resveratrol in leukemic patients still remain to be clarified in further clinical investigations.

9. Fms-like tyrosine kinase-3 inhibitors

The fms-like tyrosine kinase-3 (FLT3) is a member of the class III receptor tyrosine kinase family and is largely expressed along with CD34 and CD117 in immature hematopoetic progenitor cells. Knock-out mice are associated with deficiencies in B-cell lymphopoesis and reconstitution of both T cells and myeloid cells after BMT, indicating a crucial role of FLT3 in the development of multipotent hematopoetic and lymphoid cells.
Similarly, FLT3 has been implicated in the pathogenesis of leukemia (Carow et al, 1996). In addition to the near-universal FLT3 expression in adult precursor B-ALL, gene expression analysis have shown, that the highest levels of FLT3 expression occur in infant and

childhood ALL with rearrangement of the MLL gene and in ALL patients with hyperdiploidy (Armstrong et al, 2002, 2004); . *In vitro* studies have shown that coexpression of FLT3 ligand and activating mutations on the FLT3 gene can constitutively activate downstream targets. These include signal transducers and activators of transcription (STAT), MAPK, and AKT pathways that regulate proliferation, differentiation, and survival (Mizuki et al, 2000). Considering the worse prognosis of MLL patients and understanding the molecular mechanism of FLT3, has prompted the development of specific FLT3 inhibitors.

Small-molecular FLT3 inhibitors have initially been developed for AML, in which FLT3 mutations represent the most common somatic genetic alteration. FLT3 inhibitors induce significant cytotoxic responses, and several of these agents have been tested in adult trials of AML (Fiedler et al, 2005; Smith et al, 2004). FLT3 inhibitors are well tolerated; toxicities include mild nausea, emesis and generalized weakness with the highest doses administered. In MLL-rearranged ALL, treatment with the FLT3 inhibitor PKC-412 (Midostaurin, Novartis Pharmaceuticals) has proved to be cytotoxic to Ba/F3 cells dependent upon activating mutations of FLT3 (Armstrong et al, 2003). Similarly, ALL with high hyperdiploidy and t (4;11), has shown pronounced apoptotic responses to treatment with CEP-701 (Lesaurtinib, Cephalon) (Brown et al, 2005). Synergistic effects have not been noted, when FLT3 inhibitors are used simultaneously or immediately following exposure to cytarabine, daunorubicin, mitoxantrone or etoposide. These effects might be of interest, if used to overcome rapid development of resistance to FLT3 inhibitors (Levis et al, 2004). Of note, pretreatment with CEP-701 in combination with cytarabine may act antagonistically, due to its cell-cycle inhibitory effect in AML.

In MLL-rearranged ALL with wild type FLT3, FLT3 ligand induces quiescence and chemoresistance that can be overcome by FLT3 inhibition (Furuichi et al, 2007). It is possible that ligation of FLT3 in these ALL cases contributes to the poor response to chemotherapy by activating quiescence and self-renewal functions. It is therefore worth examining the ability of FLT3 inhibitors to reverse this response and increase chemosensitivity in this particularly difficult to treat group of patients. More specific FLT3 targeting has recently been developed by the application of anti-FLT3 antibodies (Piloto et al, 2006). IMC-NC7 consistently inhibits FLT3 phosphorylation, whereas IMC-EB10 stimulates its activation. Both treatments prolong survival and/or reduced engraftment of leukemic cells in a NOD/SCID mouse model, mainly through the recruitment of the host's immune system against targeted cells, independently of receptor activation.

A phase I/II clinical trial is currently recruiting patients that will evaluate the safety, tolerability, clinical response, pharmacokinetics and pharmacodynamics of PKC-412 in children who have relapsed or refractory acute leukemias, including MLL-rearranged ALL (NCT00866281, www.clinicaltrials.gov).

10. Farnesyl transferase inhibitors

Inhibitors of farnesyl transferase (FTI) have originally been developed to prevent attachment of intracellular Ras to the inner leaflet of the plasma membrane and, therefore, transduction of proliferative and survival signals (Gelb et al, 1997). Subsequent studies, however, have suggested that the cytotoxic actions of FTIs might also involve oncoproteins other than Ras, such as RhoB and members of phosphoinositide 3/OH kinase (PI3K)/AKT-2 pathway (Lebowitz et al, 1998), suggesting that the mechanism of action of FTIs is significantly more complex than initially presumed.

Results of *in vitro* exposure of several leukemic cells provide evidence for the efficacy of FTIs in suppressing tumor cell proliferation. Particularly, the nonpeptidomimetic enzyme-specific inhibitor R115777 (Tipifarnib, Johnson & Johnson) has been shown to decrease proliferation and sensitize apoptosis to chemotherapy-induced cell death. A phase I trial of R115777 in adults with poor-risk acute leukemia provides first evidence for *in vivo* efficacy. 29% of the 34 evaluable patients have shown a clinical response, including 2 patients with complete remission (Karp et al, 2001). Dose limiting toxicities on various schedules include central neurotoxicity and reversible nausea, renal insufficiency, polydipsia, paresthesia and myelosuppression.

Of note is the novel, orally active FTI SCH66336 (Lonafarnib, Schering-Plough), which competes with the enzyme for the CAAX portion of Ras and induces apoptosis in acute myeloid leukemia. It might be particularly attractive for a combination therapy with STI571, since it has been shown to inhibit the proliferation of STI571-resistant BCR-ABL-positive cell lines and synergize for the induction of apoptosis (Borthakur et al, 2006; Hoover et al, 2002).

11. DNA methylase inhibitors

Aberrant DNA methylation of multiple promoter CpG islands is frequently observed in patients with ALL both at initial presentation and at the time of relapse. Indeed these methylation marks are stable in over 70% of patients with ALL at the time of relapse. Importantly, methylation of specific molecular pathways has been associated with an extremely poor prognosis in patients with ALL. This has been demonstrated in the aberrant methylation of the promotor region within tumor suppressor genes such as the fragile histidine triad (FHIT) of members of the cell cycle pathway such as p73, the cyclin dependent kinase inhibitors p57KIP2 and p15 (Bueso-Ramos et al, 2005). Pharmacologic modification of aberrant methylation can therefore be an attractive approach to regulate leukemic cell proliferation.

Recently, the pyrimidine nucleoside analog 5-Aza-2'-deoxycytidine (decitabine/Daco-gene, SuperGen) has received much interest as a strong hypomethylating agent with clinical activity in myelodysplastic syndrome, and acute and chronic myelogeous leukemia (Richel et al, 1991). *In vitro* exposure of decitabine results in hypomethylation and reactivation of putative tumor suppressor genes. As a result, low concentrations of decitabine stimulate cellular differentiation, whereas high concentrations directly interfere with DNA synthesis and mediate cytotoxicity in acute leukemias (Pinto et al, 1984). Combination therapy with cytarabine achieves complete remission in the majority of patients in a clinical trial of ALL (Richel et al, 1991). Analysis of cell membrane markers shows a loss of the early differentiation antigens CD34 and CD33 in leukemic bone marrow cells, which is suggestive of leukemic cell differentiation. Addition of HDACIs might synergize in controlling gene transcription as has successfully been shown in a clinical trial for t(8;14) AML (Klisovic et al, 2003).

Temozolomide (Temodal, Schering-Plough) is a second-generation oral alkylating agent with DNA methylating properties. Although the exact mechanism for methylation is not fully elucidated, it results in an active mismatch-repair pathway with consequent DNA strand breakage and apoptosis (D'Atri et al, 1998). Temozolomide is well tolerated when it is administered as a single agent (Seiter el al, 2002). Because of the chance to deplete O^6-

alkylguanine DNA alkyltransferase levels, a potential mechanism of drug resistance, temozolomide should be administered in an extended low-dose schedule, as has been suggested in a clinical trial of malignant gliomas (Khan et al, 2002).

12. Histone deacetylase inhibitors

Epigenetic changes to promoter regions have been identified in recent years as important factors in the pathogenesis of acute leukemia. They include DNA modifications that regulate chromatin structure and change gene expression without altering the nucleotide sequence. A promising new therapeutic strategy is aimed at removal of acetyl groups from histone proteins as well as other non-histone protein targets with histone deacetylation inhibitors (HDACIs), which results in chromatin remodeling that permits re-expression of silenced tumor suppressor genes in cancer cells (Brown et al, 2002). This in turn, can potentially result in cellular differentiation, inhibition of proliferation and/or apoptosis.

Several classes of HDACIs are currently under development for treatment of leukemia, including the short-chain fatty acids sodium phenylbutyrate and valproic acid, the hydroxamic acids suberoylanilide hydroxamic acid (SAHA, Vorinostat, Merck & Co.), FK-228 (Depsipeptide, Gloucester Pharmaceuticals) and LBH589 (Panobinostat, Novartis Pharmaceuticals), and the benzamides MS-275 and C1-994.

In vitro studies have demonstrated that HDACIs trigger maturation, when administered at low concentrations, whereas at higher concentrations, apoptosis is induced. The factors that determine whether HDACIs engage apoptosis versus differentiation remain the subject of investigation, but they may involve the induction of death receptors such as Fas- and tumor-necrosis-factor-related apoptosis-inducing ligand (TRAIL) (Bernhard et al, 2001; Inoue et al, 2004), the production of reactive oxygen species, which leads to mitochondrial disruption (Bernhard et al, 2001), independently of activation of caspase-8 or -3, followed by internucleosomal DNA fragmentation. Specifically in Philadelphia chromosome-positive (Ph+) ALL, HDACIs reduce viability and increase expression of the apoptosis associated proteins FANCG, FOXO3A, GADD45A, GADD45B and GADD45G (Scuto et al, 2008). If HDACIs are used at lower concentrations, they induce either $G_{0/1}$ or G_2-M arrest. These events are accompanied by induction of p53 and $p21^{WAF1}$, and down-regulation of cell cycle-promoting proteins, including cyclin D1 and D2.

In vivo FK-228 effectively inhibits HDAC in patients with chronic lymphatic leukemia (CLL) and acute myeloid leukemia (AML) (Byrd et al, 2005), but its use in the current schedule of administration is limited by progressive constitutional symptoms. Dose-limiting toxicities include anorexia, dehydration, diarrhoea, and fatigue. Several patients have evidence of anti-tumor activity following treatment, but no partial or complete response is noted. Both, SAHA and LBH589, have been reported to be tolerable for short- and long-term application in phase I clinical trials of adult refractory hematological malignancies (Garcia-Manero et al, 2008). Based on the safety and efficacy demonstrated in phase I/II trials, a single HDACI compound, SAHA, has been approved for the treatment of cutaneous T-cell lymphoma, after demonstrating activity in heavily pre-treated patients.

Regarding childhood ALL data, a recent phase I study of vorinostat has just been published. Drug disposition and tolerance in children is similar to that observed in adult patients, whereas the maximum tolerated dose (MTD) seems to be lower due to liver dysfunction. Furthermore, a phase II study is reported as currently recruiting participants (NCT00882206, www.clinicaltrials.gov). Specifically, this trial is investigating the use of decitabine and vorinostat together with combination chemotherapy in treating patients with relapsed/refractory ALL or lymphoblastic lymphoma.

13. Mammalian target of rapamycin inhibitors

The mammalian target of rapamycin (mTOR) is a critical effector in cell-signalling pathways, such as the PI3K/AKT transduction pathway, that are up regulated in malignant transformed cells (Dann et al, 2006). After activation of G-protein coupled receptors by various growth factors, mTOR mediates the phosphorylation of the 70 kDa S6 ribosomal protein kinase and the initiation factor 4E-binding protein 1 (Vignot et al, 2005). Subsequently, activated cyclin D1, CDK4, and Rb initiate the $G_{0/1}$ to S phase progression. Accordingly, targeting the mTOR signalling pathway has extensively been analyzed for suppression of leukemic cell proliferation.

Inhibitors of mTOR include rapamycin (Sirolimus, Wyeth Pharmaceuticals) and the second generation analogs RAD001 (Everolimus, Novartis Pharmaceuticals), and CCI-779 (Temsirolimus, Wyeth Pharmaceuticals). Rapamycin was initially developed as immunosuppressive agent and was the first inhibitor to be used in a clinical setting for leukemic therapy. Rapamycin induces apoptosis in precursor B ALL lines *in vitro* and has *in vivo* activity in transgenic mice with pre-B leukemia/lymphoma (Brown et al, 2003). CCI-779 inhibits the growth of adult human ALL on bone marrow layers and reduces the number of blasts in the peripheral-blood and the degree of organ infiltration in human ALL engrafted NOD/SCID mice (Teachey et al, 2006). RAD001 reduces tumor mass *in vivo,* conferring prolonged survival of NOD/SCID mice engrafted with childhood ALL (Crazzolara et al, 2009). Mechanistic insight demonstrates the induction of autophagy in the absence of apoptosis, which is particular interesting in ALL, since resistance to current chemotherapies, such as dexamethasone, has been linked to certain defects in the apoptotic machinery.

Phase I trials in patients with various cancers show that mTOR inhibitors when used as monotherapy are well tolerated in humans, with little nephrotoxicity and neurotoxicity (Calne et al, 1989). They may further cause hyperlipidemia, mild myelosuppression, hypertension, skin rashes and mucositis. However, the toxicities of combining mTOR inhibitors with conventional cytotoxic agents have not been fully explored in both preclinical and clinical studies. Based on the preclinical work, a number of clinical trials evaluating the efficacy of mTOR inhibitors in ALL as single agents and in combination with other agents have been performed are still on-going (NCT01162551, www.clinicaltrials.gov). Two phase I/II trials of MTIs in patients with relapsed or refractory malignances, including one patient each with ALL, have shown that both patients have tolerated therapy, but neither have had an objective response. A recent interim result of an on-going phase 1 trial of sirolimus in children reveals that 3 of 7 patients relapsed/refractory ALL have stable disease.

14. Cyclin dependent kinase inhibitors

Loss of p16 (INK4A) in hematopoietic stem cells is associated with enhanced self-renewal capacity and might facilitate progression of damaged stem cells into pre-cancerous cells that give rise to leukemia (Bhojwani et al, 2006). Based on higher frequency of p16 (INK4A) deletions in relapsed ALL, inhibitors of cyclin dependent kinases (CDKs) have been

Substance	Synonym	Target	Clinical Trial	Identifier	Study Start	Study end	Condition	Age Eligibility	Combination
AMD3100	plerixafor	CXCR4	I	NCT01319864	03/2011	07/2014	R	3-29 y	eto, ara-c
CMC-544	inotuzumab ozogamicin	CD22	I	NCT01134575	06/2010	06/2013	R	>16 y	rit
			I	NCT01363297	07/2011	01/2015	R	>18 y	-
			I	NCT01371630	11/2011	09/2015	untreated	>60 y	cpm, vin, dex, mtx, ara-c
G3139	oblimersen	BCL-2	I	NCT00004862	completed		R	>16 y	flu, ara-c
PS 341	bortezomib	proteasome	I	NCT01075425	05/2010	02/2012	R	>18 y	berlinostat
			I/II	NCT00410423	01/2006	01/2013	R	>18 y	mit, eto, ara-c
			I	NCT00383474	completed		R	>18 y	tipifarnib
			I/II	NCT00440726	06/2006	02/2011	R	>18 y	asp, dox, vin, dex, mtx, ara-c
			II	NCT01312818	06/2011	06/2012	R	2-30 y	vor, dex, mtx, ima
			I	NCT00077467	01/2004	03/2006	R	1-21 y	-
MK-0752		γ-secretase	I	NCT00100152	07/2005	10/2006	R	>1 y	-
PF-03084014			I	NCT00878189	06/2009	01/2014	R	>16 y	-
STA-9090		Hsp90	I/II	NCT00964873	ongoing		untreated	>18 y	-
PKC412	midostaurin	FLT3	I/II	NCT00866281	09/2009	06/2012	R	3 mo – 18 y	-
CEP-701	lestaurtinib		III	NCT00557193	01/2008	06/2012	untreated	<1 y	asp, dau, vin, dex, mtx, ara-c, eto, mer, cpm, pre
R115777	tipifarnib	FTIs	I	NCT00022451	completed		R	<21 y	-
5-Aza-2'-deoxycytidine	decitabine	DNA	I	NCT00042796	completed		R	<21 y	-
			I	NCT00349596	07/2006	07/2012	R	any age	-
			II	NCT00882206	04/2009	11/2011	R	2-60 y	ara-c, dox, mtx, asp, pre, vin, vor, ima
LBH589	panobinostat	HDAC	I	NCT01321346	03/2011	03/2014	R	8-21 y	ara-c
SAHA	vorinostat		I	NCT00278330	completed		R	>18 y	alvocidib
AY 22989	sirolimus	mTOR	I	NCT01184885	07/2010	01/2013	R	>18 y	cpm, vin, dox, dex
			I/II	NCT00968253	08/2009	03/2011	R	>10 y	cpm, vin, dox, dex, mtx, ara-c
RAD001	everolimus		I	NCT00874562	07/2007	07/2010	R	>1 y	pre
			I	NCT00957320	06/2009	06/2017	R	>21 y	asp
HMR 1274	flavopiridol	p16 (INK4A)	II	NCT00016016	completed		R	>18 y	ara-c, mit

(R= relapse, eto= etoposide, ara-c= cytarabine, rit= rituximab, cpm= cyclophosphamide, vin= vincristine, dex= dexamethasone, flu= fludarabine, mit= mitoxantrone, asp= asparaginase, dau= daunorubicine, dox= doxorubicine, mer= mercaptopurine, vor= vorinostat, pre= predinison, mtx= methotrexate, ima= imatinib)

Table 1. Active and completed clinical trials with novel therapeutic targets for ALL.

investigated for their antileukemic potential. Among them, the synthetic flavone derivative flavopiridol (Alvocidib, L86-8275; Behringwerke) is the first to undergo human trials.

Flavopiridol binds to the adenosine triphosphate (ATP) site of CDK, thereby reducing the activity of CDK1, CDK2, CDK4, CDK6, and CDK7, leading to cell cycle arrest in $G_{0/1}$ and G_2 (Sedlacek et al, 2001). In addition, flavopiridol disrupts the CDK9/cyclin T complex resulting in reduced phosphorylation of the carboxyl-terminal domain of RNA Pol-II and subsequent inhibition of mRNA synthesis (Chao et al, 2000). Consequently, short lived anti-

apoptotic proteins such as MCL-1 and BCL-2 and those that are cell cycle dependent such as cyclin D1 are depleted. This could provide an explanation for increased apoptosis observed following exposure to flavopiridol.
Pre-clinical studies have demonstrated the efficacy of flavopiridol in primary ALL samples. A phase I clinical trial of flavopiridol followed by cytarabine and mitoxantrone in patients with relapsed or refractory adult ALL has shown moderate biological and clinical benefits (Karp et al, 2005). Dose-limiting toxicities include sustained neutropenia, diarrhoea and mucositis. As suggested by a CLL clinical trial, a more sustained schedule of flavopiridol might be needed to improve the clinical response rate, without increasing neutropenia as the dose-limiting toxicity.

15. Conclusion

The future of treatment optimization resides in exploring the molecular pathways involved in the pathogenesis of leukemia and in understanding the pharmacogenomic factors of the host. If successful, new protein products can be generated that are administered as targeted therapy with a narrow therapeutic window. A primary example of such therapy is given by the inhibitor of tyrosine kinase imatinib, which is the first anti-cancer agent that specifically targets the genetic defect underlying Philadelphia positive ALL. Although imatinib is currently implemented in the treatment of BCR/ABL positive ALL and has improved overall survival, its use as single agent should not be overestimated. In fact, imatinib is targeting a specific molecular pathway that regulates gene transcription, cell proliferation or survival, but not the principal genetic lesion. Accordingly, imatinib produces relatively short-lived remission in Ph+ ALL as single agent, but has the potential to improve survival, when combined with current chemotherapy. Similarly, it is likely that the key to the successful use of other molecular targeted therapies will be in the careful combination of novel agents with traditional chemotherapeutic regimes and/or with other molecularly targeted agents. Indeed many agents, including imatinib, flavopiridol and oblimersen are being tested in combination with standard chemotherapy, while imatinib is also being combined with inhibitors of farnesyl transferase, HDAC, cyclin dependent kinases, HSP90 and BCL-2. Ultimately, these combinations need to be based on a thorough understanding of the molecular pathways driving disease in each patient. Additionally, pharmacogenomic information will be essential for the development of optimal effective treatment regimes with minimal side effects.

16. Acknowledgment

This work was supported by the Children's Cancer Aid Society Tirol and Vorarlberg.

17. References

Adams J, Behnke M, Chen SW, Cruickshank AA, Dick LR, Grenier L, Klunder JM, Ma YT, Plamondon L, Stein RL. (1998). Potent and selective inhibitors of the proteasome: Dipeptidyl boronic acids. *Bioorganic & Medicinal Chemistry Letters*, Vol.8, No.4, pp.333-338

Aggarwal BB, Bhardwaj A, Aggarwal RS, Seeram NP, Shishodia S, Takada Y. (2004). Role of resveratrol in prevention and therapy of cancer: Preclinical and clinical studies. *Anticancer Research*, Vol.24, No.5A, pp.2783-2840

Armstrong SA, Staunton JE, Silverman LB, Pieters R, de Boer ML, Minden MD, Sallan SE, Lander ES, Golub TR, Korsmeyer SJ. (2002). MLL translocations specify a distinct gene expression profile that distinguishes a unique leukemia. *Nature Genetics*, Vol.30, No.1, pp.41-47

Armstrong SA, Kung AL, Mabon ME, Silverman LB, Stam RW, den Boer ML, Pieters R, Kersey JH, Sallan SE, Fletcher JA, Golub TR, Griffin JD, Korsmeyer SJ. (2003). Inhibition of FLT3 in MLL: Validation of a therapeutic target identified by gene expression based classification. *Cancer Cell*, Vol.3, No.2, pp.173-183

Armstrong SA, Mabon ME, Silverman LB, Li AH, Gribben JG, Fox EA, Sallan SE, Korsmeyer SJ. (2004). FLT3 mutations in childhood acute lymphoblastic leukemia. *Blood*, Vol.103, No.9, pp.3544-3546

Barr RD, Sala A. Osteonecrosis in children and adolescents with cancer. (2008). Pediatric Blood & Cancer, Vol.50, No.2, pp.483-485

Bernhard D, Tinhofer I, Tonko M, Hubl H, Ausserlechner MJ, Greil R, Kofler R, Csordas A. (2000). Resveratrol causes arrest in the S-phase prior to Fas-independent apoptosis in CEM-C7H2 acute leukemia cells. *Cell Death and Differentiation*, Vol.7, No.9, pp.834-842

Bernhard D, Skvortsov S, Tinhofer I, Hubl H, Greil R, Csordas A, Kofler R. (2001). Inhibition of histone deacetylase activity enhances Fas receptor-mediated apoptosis in leukemic lymphoblasts. *Cell Death and Differentiation*, Vol.8, No.10, pp.1014-1021

Bhojwani D, Kang HN, Moskowitz NP, Min DJ, Lee H, Potter JW, Davidson G, Willman CL, Borowitz MJ, Belitskaya-Levy I, Hunger SP, Raetz EA, Carroll WL. (2006). Biologic pathways associated with relapse in childhood acute lymphoblastic leukemia: a Children's Oncology Group study. *Blood*, Vol.108, No.2, pp.711-717

Borthakur G, Kantarjian H, Daley G, Talpaz M, O'Brien S, Garcia-Manero G, Giles F, Faderl S, Sugrue M, Cortes J. (2006). Pilot study of lonafarnib, a farnesyl transferase inhibitor, in patients with chronic myeloid leukemia in the chronic or accelerated phase that is resistant or refractory to imatinib therapy. *Cancer*, Vol.106, No.2, pp.346-352

Broxmeyer HE, Orschell CM, Clapp DW, Hangoc G, Cooper S, Plett PA, Liles WC, Li XX, Graham-Evans B, Campbell TB, Calandra G, Bridger G, Dale DC, Srour EF. (2005). Rapid mobilization of murine and human hematopoietic stem and progenitor cells with AMD3100, a CXCR4 antagonist. *Journal of Experimental Medicine*, Vol.201, No.8, pp.1307-1318

Brown P, Levis M, Shurtleff S, Campana D, Downing J, Small D. (2005). FLT3 inhibition selectively kills childhood acute lymphoblastic leukemia cells with high levels of FLT3 expression. *Blood*, Vol.105, No.2, pp.812-820

Byrd JC, Marcucci G, Parthun MR, Xiao JJ, Klisovic RB, Moran M, Lin TS, Liu SJ, Sklenar AR, Davis ME, Lucas DM, Fischer B, Shank R, Tejaswi SL, Binkley P, Wright J, Chan KK, Grever MR. (2005). A phase 1 and pharmacodynamic study of depsipeptide (FK228) in chronic lymphocytic leukemia and acute myeloid leukemia. *Blood*, Vol.105, No.3, pp.959-967

Bueso-Ramos C, Xu YL, McDonnell TJ, Brisbay S, Pierce S, Kantarjian H, Rosner G, Garcia-Manero G. (2005). Protein expression of a triad of frequently methylated genes, p73, p57(Kip2), and p15, has prognostic value in adult acute lymphocytic leukemia independently of its methylation status. *Journal of Clinical Oncology*, Vol.23, No.17, pp.3932-3939

Burger JA, Tsukada N, Burger M, Zvaifler NJ, Dell'Aquila M, Kipps TJ. (2000). Blood-derived nurse-like cells protect chronic lymphocytic leukemia B cells from spontaneous apoptosis through stromal cell-derived factor-1. *Blood*, Vol.96, No.8, pp.2655-2663

Calne RY, Lim S, Samaan A, Collier DSJ, Pollard SG, White DJG, Thiru S. (1989). Rapamycin for Immunosuppression in Organ Allografting. *Lancet*, Vol.2, No.8658, pp.227

Carow CE, Levenstein M, Kaufmann SH, Chen J, Amin S, Rockwell P, Witte L, Borowitz MJ, Civin CI, Small D. (1996). Expression of the hematopoietic growth factor receptor FLT3 (STK-1/Flk2) in human leukemias. *Blood*, Vol.87, No.3, pp.1089-1096

Cecchinato V, Chiaramonte R, Nizzardo M, Cristofaro B, Basile A, Sherbet GV, Comi P. (2007). Resveratrol-induced apoptosis in human T-cell acute lymphoblastic leukaemia MOLT-4 cells. *Biochemical Pharmacology*, Vol.74, No.11, pp.1568-1574

Chao SH, Fujinaga K, Marion JE, Taube R, Sausville EA, Senderowicz AM, Peterlin BM, Price DH. (2000). Flavopiridol inhibits P-TEFb and blocks HIV-1 replication. *Journal of Biological Chemistry*, Vol.25, No.37, pp.28345-28348

Cortes J, Thomas D, Koller C, Giles F, Estey E, Faderl S, Garcia-Manero G, McConkey D, Patel G, Guerciolini R, Wright J, Kantarjian H. (2004). Phase I study of bortezomib in refractory or relapsed acute leukemias. *Clinical Cancer Research*, Vol.10, No.10, pp.3371-3376

Crazzolara R, Kreczy A, Mann G, Heitger A, Eibl G, Fink FM, Mohle R, Meister B. (2001). High expression of the chemokine receptor CXCR4 predicts extramedullary organ infiltration in childhood acute lymphoblastic leukaemia. *British Journal of Haematology*, Vol.115, No.3, pp.545-553

Crazzolara R, Cisterne A, Thien M, Hewson J, Bradstock KF, Bendall LJ. (2009). The mTOR inhibitor RAD001 (Everolimus) improves survival in preclinical models of primary human ALL. *Blood*, Vol.113, No.14, pp.3297-3306

Dann SG, Thomas G. (2006). The amino acid sensitive TOR pathway from yeast to mammals. *Febs Letters*, Vol.580, No.12, pp.2821-2829

DeAngelo DJ, Stone RM, Silverman LB, Stock W, Attar EC, Fearen I, Dallob A, Matthews C, Stone J, Freedman SJ, Aster J. (2006). A phase I clinical trial of the notch inhibitor MK-0752 in patients with T-cell acute lymphoblastic leukemia/lymphoma (T-ALL) and other leukemias. *Journal of Clinical Oncology*, Vol.24, No.18, pp.357S

DiJoseph JF, Armellino DC, Boghaert ER, Khandke K, Dougher MM, Sridharan L, Kunz A, Hamann PR, Gorovits B, Udata C, Moran JK, Popplewell AG, Stephens S, Frost P, Damle NK. (2004). Antibody-targeted chemotherapy with CMC-544: a CD22-targeted immunoconjugate of calicheamicin for the treatment of B-lymphoid malignancies. *Blood*, Vol.103, No.5, pp.1807-1814

DiJoseph JF, Dougher MM, Armellino DC, Evans DY, Damle NK. (2007). Therapeutic potential of CD22-specific antibody-targeted chemotherapy using inotuzumab ozogamicin (CMC-544) for the treatment of acute lymphoblastic leukemia. *Leukemia*, Vol.21, No.11, pp.2240-2245

Dorrie J, Gerauer H, Wachter Y, Zunino SJ. (2001). Resveratrol induces extensive apoptosis by depolarizing mitochondrial membranes and activating caspase-9 in acute lymphoblastic leukemia cells. *Cancer Research;* , Vol.61, No.12, pp.4731-4739

Evin G, Sernee MF, Masters CL. (2006). Inhibition of gamma-secretase as a therapeutic intervention for Alzheimer's disease - Prospects, limitations and strategies. *Cns Drugs*, Vol.20, No.5, pp.351-372

Fiedler W, Serve H, Dohner H, Schwittay M, Ottmann OG, O'Farrell AM, Bello CL, Allred R, Manning WC, Cherrington JM, Louie SG, Hong W, Brega NM, Massimini G, Scigalla P, Berdel WE, Hossfeld DK. (2005). A phase 1 study of SU11248 in the treatment of patients with refractory or resistant acute myeloid leukemia (AML) or not amenable to conventional therapy for the disease. *Blood*, Vol.105, No.3, pp.986-993

Fontecave M, Lepoivre M, Elleingand E, Gerez C, Guittet O. (1998). Resveratrol, a remarkable inhibitor of ribonucleotide reductase. *Febs Letters*, Vol.421, No.3, pp.277-279

Freycon F, Trombert-Paviot B, Casagranda L, Bertrand Y, Plantaz D, Marec-Berard P. (2008). Trends in treatment-related deaths (TRDs) in childhood cancer and leukemia over time: A follow-up of patients included in the childhood cancer registry of the Rhone-Alpes Region in France (ARCERRA). *Pediatric Blood & Cancer*, Vol.50, No.6, pp.1213-1220

Furuichi Y, Goi K, Inukai T, Sato H, Nemoto A, Takahashi K, Akahane K, Hirose K, Honna H, Kuroda I, Zhang X, Kagami K, Hayashi Y, Harigaya K, Nakazawa S, Sugita K. (2007). Fms-like tyrosine kinase 3 ligand stimulation induces MLL-rearranged leukemia cells into quiescence resistant to antileukemic agents. *Cancer Research*, Vol.67, No.20, pp.9852-9861

Garcia-Manero G, Yang H, Bueso-Ramos C, Ferrajoli A, Cortes J, Wierda WG, Faderl S, Koller C, Morris G, Rosner G, Loboda A, Fantin VR, Randolph SS, Hardwick JS, Reilly JF, Chen C, Ricker JL, Secrist JP, Richon VM, Frankel SR, Kantarjian HM. (2008). Phase 1 study of the histone deacetylase inhibitor vorinostat (suberoylanilide hydroxamic acid [SAHA]) in patients with advanced leukemias and myelodysplastic syndromes. *Blood*, Vol.111, No.3, pp.1060-1066

Gelb MH. (1997). Protein biochemistry - Protein prenylation, et cetera: Signal transduction in two dimensions. *Science*, Vol.275, No.5307, pp.1750-1751

Goetz MP, Toft D, Reid J, Ames M, Stensgard B, Safgren S, Adjei AA, Sloan J, Atherton P, Vasile V, Salazaar S, Adjei A, Croghan G, Erlichman C. (2005). Phase I trial of 17-allylamino-17-demethoxygeldanamycin in patients with advanced cancer. *Journal of Clinical Oncology*, Vol.23, No.6, pp.1078-1087

Gorre ME, Ellwood-Yen K, Chiosis G, Rosen N, Sawyers CL. (2002). BCR-ABL point mutants isolated from patients with imatinib mesylate-resistant chronic myeloid leukemia remain sensitive to inhibitors of the BCR-ABL chaperone heat shock protein 90. *Blood*, Vol.100, No.8, pp.3041-3044

Hawkins LM, Jayanthan AA, Narendran A. (2005). Effects of 17-allylamino-17-demethoxygeldanamycin (17-AAG) on pediatric acute lymphoblastic leukemia (ALL) with respect to Bcr-Abl status and imatinib mesylate sensitivity. *Pediatric Research*, Vol.57, No.3, pp.430-437

Hogarth LA, Hall AG. (1999). Increased BAX expression is associated with an increased risk of relapse in childhood acute lymphocytic leukemia. *Blood*, Vol.93, No.8, pp.2671-2678

Hoover RR, Mahon FX, Melo JV, Daley GQ. (2002). Overcoming STI571 resistance with the farnesyl transferase inhibitor SCH66336. *Blood*, Vol.100, No.3, pp.1068-1071

Horton TM, Gannavarapu A, Blaney SM, D'Argenio DZ, Plon SE, Berg SL. (2006). Bortezomib interactions with chemotherapy agents in acute leukemia in vitro. *Cancer Chemotherapy and Pharmacology*, Vol.58, No.1, pp.13-23

Inoue S, MacFarlane M, Harper N, Wheat LMC, Dyer MJS, Cohen GM. (2004). Histone deacetylase inhibitors potentiate TNF-related apoptosis-inducing ligand (TRAIL)-induced apoptosis in lymphoid malignancies. *Cell Death and Differentiation*, Vol.11, pp.S193-S206

Isaacs JS, Xu WP, Neckers L. (2003). Heat shock protein 90 as a molecular target for cancer therapeutics. *Cancer Cell*, Vol.3, No.3, pp.213-217

Jabbour E, O'Brien SM, Thomas DA, Ravandi F, York S, Kwari M, Faderl S, Kadia TM, Wilson C, Tarnai R, Advani AS, Garcia-Manero GC, Cortes JE, Kantarjian H. (2011) Inotuzumab ozogamicin (IO; CMC544), a CD22 monoclonal antibody attached to calicheamycin, produces complete response (CR) plus complete marrow response (mCR) of greater than 50% in refractory relapse (R-R) acute lymphocytic leukemia (ALL). *Journal of Clinical Oncology*, Vol.29, Suppl; abstr 6507

Jang MS, Cai EN, Udeani GO, Slowing KV, Thomas CF, Beecher CWW, Fong HHS, Farnsworth NR, Kinghorn AD, Mehta RG, Moon RC, Pezzuto JM. (1997). Cancer chemopreventive activity of resveratrol, a natural product derived from grapes. *Science*, Vol.275, No.5297pp. 218-220

Juarez J, Bradstock KF, Gottlieb DJ, Bendall LJ. (2003). Effects of inhibitors of the chemokine receptor CXCR4 on acute lymphoblastic leukemia cells in vitro. *Leukemia*, Vol.17, No.7, pp.1294-1300

Juarez J, Dela Pena A, Baraz R, Hewson J, Khoo M, Cisterne A, Fricker S, Fujii N, Bradstock KF, Bendall LJ. (2007). CXCR4 antagonists mobilize childhood acute lymphoblastic leukemia cells into the peripheral blood and inhibit engraftment. *Leukemia*, Vol.21, No.6, pp.1249-1257

Khan RB, Raizer JJ, Malkin MG, Bazylewicz KA, Abrey LE. (2002). A phase II study of extended low-dose temozolomide in recurrent malignant gliomas. *Neuro-Oncology*, Vol.4, No.1, pp.39-43

Klisovic MI, Maghraby EA, Parthun MR, Guimond M, Sklenar AR, Whitman SP, Chan KK, Murphy T, Anon J, Archer KJ, Rush LJ, Plass C, Grever MR, Byrd JC, Marcucci G. (2003). Depsipeptide (FR 901228) promotes histone acetylation, gene transcription, apoptosis and its activity is enhanced by DNA methyltransferase inhibitors in AML1/ETO-positive leukemic cells. *Leukemia*, Vol.17, No.2, pp.350-358

Laney JD, Hochstrasser M. (1999). Substrate targeting in the ubiquitin system. *Cell*, Vol.97, No.4, pp.427-430

Lebowitz PF, Prendergast GC. (1998). Non-Ras targets of farnesyltransferase inhibitors: focus on Rho. *Oncogene*, Vol.17, No.11, pp.1439-1445

Levis M, Pham R, Smith BD, Small D. (2004). In vitro studies of a FM inhibitor combined with chemotherapy: sequence of administration is important to achieve synergistic cytotoxic effects. *Blood*, Vol.104, No.4, pp.1145-1150

Maki CG, Huibregtse JM, Howley PM. (1996). In vivo ubiquitination and proteasome-mediated degradation of p53. *Cancer Research*, Vol.56, No.11, pp.2649-2654

Marcucci G, Byrd JC, Dai GW, Klisovic MI, Kourlas PJ, Young DC, Cataland SR, Fisher DB, Lucas D, Chan KK, Porcu P, Lin ZP, Farag SF, Frankel SR, Zvviebel JA, Kraut EH, Balcerzak SP, Bloomfield CD, Grever MR, Caligiuri MA. (2003). Phase 1 and pharmacodynamic studies of G3139, a Bcl-2 antisense oligonucleotide, in combination with chemotherapy in refractory or relapsed acute leukemia. *Blood*, Vol.101, No.2, pp.425-432

Messinger Y, Reaman GH, Ek O, Uckun FM. (1999). Evaluation of temozolomide in a SCID mouse model of human B-cell precursor leukemia. *Leukemia & Lymphoma*, Vol.33, No.3-4, pp.289-293

Mizuki M, Fenski R, Halfter H, Matsumura I, Schmidt R, Muller C, Gruning R, Kratz-Abers K, Serve S, Steur C, Buchner T, Kienast J, Kanakura Y, Berdel WE, Serve H. (2000). Flt3 mutations from patients with acute myeloid leukemia induce transformation of 32D cells mediated by the Ras and STAT5 pathways. *Blood*, Vol.96, No.12, pp.3907-3914

Muller A, Homey B, Soto H, Ge NF, Catron D, Buchanan ME, McClanahan T, Murphy E, Yuan W, Wagner SN, Barrera JL, Mohar A, Verastegui E, Zlotnik A. (2001). Involvement of chemokine receptors in breast cancer metastasis. *Nature*, Vol.410, No.6824, pp.50-56

Nagasawa T, Hirota S, Tachibana K, Takakura N, Nishikawa S, Kitamura Y, Yoshida N, Kikutani H, Kishimoto T. (1996). Defects of B-cell lymphopoiesis and bone-marrow myelopoiesis in mice lacking the CXC chemokine PBSF/SDF-1. *Nature*, Vol.382, No.6592, pp. 635-638

Pelicano H, Carew JS, McQueen TJ, Plunkett M, Keating MJ, Huang P. (2006). Targeting Hsp90 by 17-AAG in leukemia cells: mechanisms for synergistic and antagonistic drug combinations with arsenic trioxide and Ara-C. *Leukemia*, Vol.20, No.4, pp.610-619

Piloto O, Nguyen B, Huso D, Kim KT, Li YW, Witte L, Hicklin DJ, Brown P, Small D. (2006). IMC-EB10, an anti-FLT3 monoclonal antibody, prolongs survival and reduces nonobese diabetic/severe combined immunodeficient engraftment of some acute lymphoblastic leukemia cell lines and primary leukemic samples. *Cancer Research*, Vol.66, No.9, pp.4843-4851

Pinto A, Attadia V, Fusco A, Ferrara F, Spada OA, Difiore PP. (1984). 5-Aza-2'-Deoxycytidine Induces Terminal Differentiation of Leukemic Blasts from Patients with Acute Myeloid Leukemias. *Blood*, Vol.64, No.4, pp.922-929

Pui CH, Evans WE. (2006). Drug therapy - Treatment of acute lymphoblastic leukemia. *New England Journal of Medicine*, Vol.354, No.2, pp.166-178

Pui CH, Robison LL, Look AT. (2008). Acute lymphoblastic leukaemia, *Lancet*, Vol.371, No.9617, pp. 1030-1043

Reed JC. (1995). Bcl-2 - Prevention of Apoptosis As A Mechanism of Drug-Resistance. *Hematology-Oncology Clinics of North America*, Vol.9, No.2, pp.451-473

Richel DJ, Colly LP, Kluinnelemans JC, Willemze R. (1991). The Antileukemic Activity of 5-Aza-2 Deoxycytidine (Aza-Dc) in Patients with Relapsed and Resistant Leukemia. *British Journal of Cancer*, Vol.64, No.1, pp.144-148

Scuto A, Kirschbaum M, Kowolik C, Kretzner L, Juhasz A, Atadja P, Pullarkat V, Bhatia R, Forman S, Yen Y, Jove R. (2008). The novel histone deacetylase inhibitor, LBH589, induces expression of DNA damage response genes and apoptosis in Ph- acute lymphoblastic leukemia cells. *Blood*, Vol.110, No.10, pp.5093-5100

Sedlacek HH. (2001). Mechanisms of action of flavopiridol. *Critical Reviews in Oncology Hematology*, Vol.38, No.2, pp.139-170

Seiter K, Liu D, Loughran T, Siddiqui A, Baskind P, Ahmed T. (2002). Phase I study of temozolomide in relapsed/refractory acute leukemia. *Journal of Clinical Oncology*, Vol.20, No.15, pp.3249-3253

Smith MCP, Luker KE, Garbow JR, Prior JL, Jackson E, Piwnica-Worms D, Luker GD. (2004). CXCR4 regulates growth of both primary and metastatic breast cancer. *Cancer Research*, Vol.64, No.23, pp.8604-8612

Smith BD, Levis M, Beran M, Giles F, Kantarjian H, Berg K, Murphy KM, Dauses T, Allebach J, Small D. (2004). Single-agent CEP-701, a novel FLT3 inhibitor, shows biologic and clinical activity in patients with relapsed or refractory acute myeloid leukemia. *Blood*, Vol.103, No.10, pp.3669-3676

Sutheesophon K, Kobayashi Y, Takatoku MA, Ozawa K, Kano Y, Ishii H, Furukawa Y. (2006). Histone deacetylase inhibitor depsipeptide (FK228) induces apoptosis in leukemic cells by facilitating mitochondrial translocation of Bax, which is enhanced by the proteasome inhibitor bortezomib. *Acta Haematologica*, Vol.115, No.1-2, pp.78-90

Takeshita A, Yamakage N, Shinjo K, Ono T, Hirano I, Nakamura S, Shigeno K, Tobita T, Maekawa M, Kiyoi H, Naoe T, Ohnishi K, Sugimoto Y, Ohno R. (2009), CMC-544 (inotuzumab ozogamicin), an anti-CD22 immunoconjugate of calicheamicin, alters the levels of target molecules of malignant B-cell. *Leukemia*, Vol.33, No.7, pp.1329-1336

Teachey DT, Obzut DA, Cooperman J, Fang JJ, Carroll M, Choi JK, Houghton PJ, Brown VI, Grupp SA. (2006). The mTOR inhibitor CCI-779 induces apoptosis and inhibits growth in preclinical models of primary adult human ALL. *Blood*, Vol.107, No.3, pp.1149-1155

Viana MB, Vilela MNP. (2008). Height deficit during and many years after treatment for acute lymphoblastic leukemia in children: A review. *Pediatric Blood & Cancer*, Vol.50, No.2, pp.509-516

Vitale A, Guarini A, Chiaretti S, Foa R. (2006). The changing scene of adult acute lymphoblastic leukemia. *Current Opinion in Oncology*, Vol.18, No.6, pp.652-659

Vignot S, Faivre S, Aguirre D, Raymond E. (2005). MTOR-targeted therapy of cancer with rapamycin derivatives. *Annals of Oncology*, Vol.16, No.4, pp.525-537

Webb A, Cunningham D, Cotter F, Clarke PA, diStefano F, Ross P, Corbo M, Dziewanowska Z. (1997). BCL-2 antisense therapy in patients with non-Hodgkin lymphoma. *Lancet*, Vol.349, No.9059, pp.1137-1141

Weng AP, Ferrando AA, Lee W, Morris JP, Silverman LB, Sanchez-Irizarry C, Blacklow SC, Look AT, Aster JC. (2004). Activating mutations of NOTCH1 in human T cell acute lymphoblastic leukemia. *Science*, Vol.306, No. 5694, pp.269-271

9

Aberrant Proliferative and Apoptotic Pathways in Acute Lymphoblastic Leukemia (ALL): Molecular Therapies to Overcome Chemo-Resistance

Agostino Tafuri[1], Michele Milella[2], Stefano Iacovelli[1], Fabiana De Cave[1], Chiara Gregorj[3], Paola Bergamo[2], Andrea Miele[1], Roberto Licchetta[1], Marina Konopleva[4], James A. McCubrey[5], Alberto M. Martelli[6,7], Robin Foà[1], Maria Teresa Petrucci[1] and Maria Rosaria Ricciardi[1*]

1. Introduction

Adult acute lymphoblastic leukemia (ALL) is characterized by a high relapse rate, with the majority of patients developing chemo-resistance and ultimately dying of the disease with a 5-year survival rate of 40% (Faderl et al., 2010). Significant advances, however, have been made in cases carrying the acquired genetic alteration BCR-ABL (ALL-Ph+) targeted by tyrosine-kinase inhibitors (Ottmann & Pfeifer, 2009). Therefore, several studies have recently been carried out to look for additional, therapeutically exploitable, genetic lesions. Aberrant activation of signal transduction pathways (STP) implicated in proliferation and survival mechanisms are generally involved in leukemogenesis and drug resistance (Zhao et al., 2010). Genes in the PI3K/PTEN/AKT/mTOR, RAS/RAF/MEK/ERK, and Jak/STAT pathways are frequently mutated and their expression is often altered in hematopoietic malignancies, including ALL (McCubrey et al., 2011; Steelman et al. 2008). In addition, deregulation of survival mechanisms may confer chemo-resistance to leukemic cells, particularly involving alterations of the Bcl-2 signaling cascade, which may represent one of the most important, potentially druggable, pathways for therapeutic intervention in ALL.
Starting from our studies on chemo-resistance in ALL, particularly on multidrug resistance (MDR1) expression and prognostic significance, in this chapter we will illustrate the major pathways aberrantly activated in ALL - PI3K/PTEN/AKT/mTOR, RAF/RAS/MEK/ERK, and the Bcl-2 family of proteins - with the ultimate goal of summarizing novel targets for

*[1]*Hematology, Department of Cellular Biotechnologies and Hematology, Sapienza University of Rome, Italy*
[2]*Medical Oncology A, Regina Elena National Cancer Institute, Rome, Italy*
[3]*Hematology Unit, Campus Bio-Medico University Hospital, Rome, Italy*
[4]*Section of Molecular Hematology and Therapy, Department of Leukemia, University of Texas, M.D. Anderson Cancer Center, Houston, Texas, USA*
[5]*Department of Microbiology and Immunology, Brody School of Medicine, East Carolina University, Greenville, NC, USA*
[6]*Department of Human Anatomical Sciences, University of Bologna, Bologna, Italy &* [7]*IGM-CNR, c/o IOR, Bologna, Italy*

molecular therapies, especially in resistant/refractory cases. Controversies on and potential benefits of novel approaches based on STP inhibitors will be discussed. Epigenetic changes will be examined to address their importance in association with post-translational modifications. Future perspectives will encompass review of Reverse Phase Protein Arrays (RPPA) as a promising new tool for translational studies in clinical sample series, helping define the functional proteomic profile at steady-state; this approach may lead to the identification of aberrant molecular target(s), possibly guiding the choice of specific molecular therapies, on one hand, and leading to the elucidation of post-treatment changes, on the other, with the overall objective of improving the strategies currently employed to counteract leukemia chemo- and targeted drug-resistance.

2. Multidrug resistance

Chemo-resistance has been one of the major problems in cancer treatment, contributing to therapeutic failure, particularly in leukemia patients treated with regimens containing drugs such as anthracyclines, vinca alkaloids, or epipodophyllins, all modulated in their intracellular retention by the P-glycoprotein 170 (P-gp) product of the mdr-1 gene (Longley et al., 2005). An expanding number of proteins with a prominent role in MDR-dependent mechanisms of accelerated drug efflux and potentially implicated in leukemia drug resistance have been described: the multidrug resistance-associated protein 1 (MRP1), the lung-resistance protein (LRP) and the transporter breast cancer resistance protein (BCRP) (Chen, 2010). MRP1 is a protein distinct from MDR1, with different substrate specificity (amphophilic anions or glutathione-conjugated) and different susceptibility to drugs that can restore chemotherapy sensitivity (butathionine, which depletes intracellular glutathione content). LRP is a component of the major vault protein complex that appears to be involved in nuclear-cytoplasmic trafficking and in promoting drug redistribution away from the nucleus. BCRP is another member of the ATP-binding cassette protein involved in the MDR phenotype. In our previous studies (Tafuri et al., 2002) we have established the frequency and biologic–clinical significance of MDR1 expression and function and of MDR-associated proteins in *de novo* adult ALL. Our analysis was performed in the context of the ALL0496 study of the GIMEMA (Gruppo Italiano Malattie EMatologiche dell'Adulto) cooperative group. This prospective multicenter study enrolled a large series of uniformly treated *de novo* adult ALL patients, providing a unique opportunity to investigate the prognostic influence of MDR1 on CR achievement and clinical outcome, in context with other clinical and biological factors. Our results indicate that MDR1 is expressed in approximately 20% of patients enrolled in the study, playing a statistically significant unfavorable prognostic role on CR achievement at both univariate and multivariate analysis; in addition, together with age and CD34 expression, MDR1 expression significantly predicted response failure. Since MDR1 expression was described as an independent predictor of CR in patients with *de novo* adult ALL, additional studies (Gregorj et al., 2005) were performed by our group to investigate the prognostic role of other proteins implicated in drug efflux mechanisms in ALL. Analysis of primary ALL samples evaluated for the expression of MRP1 and BCRP found these proteins expressed in 51.3% and 72.9% of the cases, respectively. BCRP expression was associated with age ($P=0.027$), but not with MDR1 expression. Neither BCRP nor MRP1 individually influenced CR achievement. In contrast, when their simultaneous co-expression was analyzed, the majority of double negative patients achieved CR ($P=0.034$). Alterations in drug-efflux due to aberrant ABC transporter protein expression in cancer cells

led to the development of P-gp inhibitors, tested in clinical trials with discouraging results. In fact, the combined use of the MDR-reversal agent cyclosporine was associated with unacceptable toxicity, while a second generation-drug, vaslapodar (PSC-833), had unpredictable pharmacokinetic interactions. Third-generation inhibitors (tariquidar XR9576, zosuquidar LY335979, laniquidar R101933, and ONT-093) have high potency and specificity for P-gp but no appreciable impact on cytochrome P450 3A4 drug metabolism and no clinically significant drug interactions with common chemotherapy agents. Overall, the proposed chemo-sensitizing activity of MDR-reversal agents evaluated in clinical trials failed to improve either response rate or survival in leukemia patients (Molnár et al., 2010).
Since advances in microarray and proteomic technologies, in conjunction with the development of novel small molecules therapeutically targeting molecular determinants of resistance in cancer cells, have opened new opportunities to combat chemo-resistance, studies have explored and characterized the signaling pathways involved in the regulation of tumor cell response to chemotherapy, mostly those involved in aberrant proliferation and prolonged survival.

3. Signal transduction pathways

Leukemic cells are frequently characterized by the constitutive activation of multiple signaling cascades, which ensures a proliferative and survival advantage over normal hematopoietic cells. In fact, several studies have shown that the PI3K/PTEN/AKT/mTOR, RAS/RAF/MEK/ERK, Notch1, and JAK/STAT pathways are frequently up-regulated in ALL (Brown et al., 2008). Herein, some of these key signaling are reviewed as potential molecular targets for specific therapeutic interventions in ALL (Fig.1).

3.1 PI3K/PTEN/AKT/mTOR pathway

The phosphoinositide 3-kinase (PI3K)/PTEN/AKT/mTOR pathway is a crucial signaling cascade involved in the control of cell growth, survival, proliferation, motility, apoptosis and autophagy (Fig. 1). This pathway plays a pivotal role in maintaining numerous physiological processes, such as nutrient uptake, ribosomal biogenesis and cellular metabolism (Brown et al., 2008). PI3K is activated by a variety of extracellular stimuli, including receptor tyrosine kinases (i.e. FLT3, EGFR, HER-2/neu) (Fathi et al., 2010). The activation of PI3K catalyzes the phosphatidylinositol-4,5-bisphosphate (PIP2) conversion to the phosphatidylinositol-3,4,5-trisphosphate (PIP3) at the inner surface of the cell membrane, allowing for the recruitment of PDK1 and AKT to the membrane. AKT is an important mediator of the intracellular cascade, acting on multiple downstream targets to regulate proliferation and apoptotic signals. Downstream of AKT, a key protein is represented by mTOR, which regulates translation in response to nutrient levels (Fig.1). The major negative regulator of the PI3K/AKT/mTOR pathway is the lipid phosphatase PTEN (Phosphatase and tensin homologue deleted on chromosome 10).
The PI3K/PTEN/AKT/mTOR pathway is deregulated in several human cancers, including ALL. First, Barata et al. (2004) demonstrated that the PI3K pathway is essential for IL-7–mediated survival, activation, proliferation, and growth of T-ALL cells indicating the existence of a functional IL-7–mediated PI3K signaling cascade in T-ALL cells. Additional reports showed that the constitutive activation of PI3K/PTEN/AKT/mTOR pathway occurs frequently in childhood ALL and is crucial for blast survival (Avellino et al., 2005; Jotta et al., 2010). Aberrant activation of this signaling cascade can be induced by overproduction of

growth factors or chemokines, by loss of PTEN expression, or by mutations in PTEN or in other mediators downstream of growth factor receptors (RAS and PI3K itself). PTEN mutations, deletions or inactivation are found in many ALL cell lines and are particularly frequent in human T-ALL cell lines derived from relapsed patients (Jotta et al., 2010). Conversely, PTEN gene mutations have been reported in a small but significant subset of *de novo* T-ALL patients (Silva et al., 2008). The NOTCH1 receptor, which is activated by mutations in about 50% of T-ALL, inhibits PTEN expression that, in turn, leads to AKT activation and resistance to glucocorticoids. Additionally, the PI3K/PTEN/AKT/mTOR pathway has been proposed to be involved in the regulation of MDR-1 expression and drug resistance in ALL, as suggested by cleavage of the 170-kDa P-gp during PI3K inhibitor-induced apoptosis of VBL100 human T-lymphoblastoid CEM cells (Mantovani et al., 2006).
All these findings lend significant support to the development of therapies targeting the PI3K/PTEN/AKT/mTOR pathway in ALL, particularly in T-ALL.

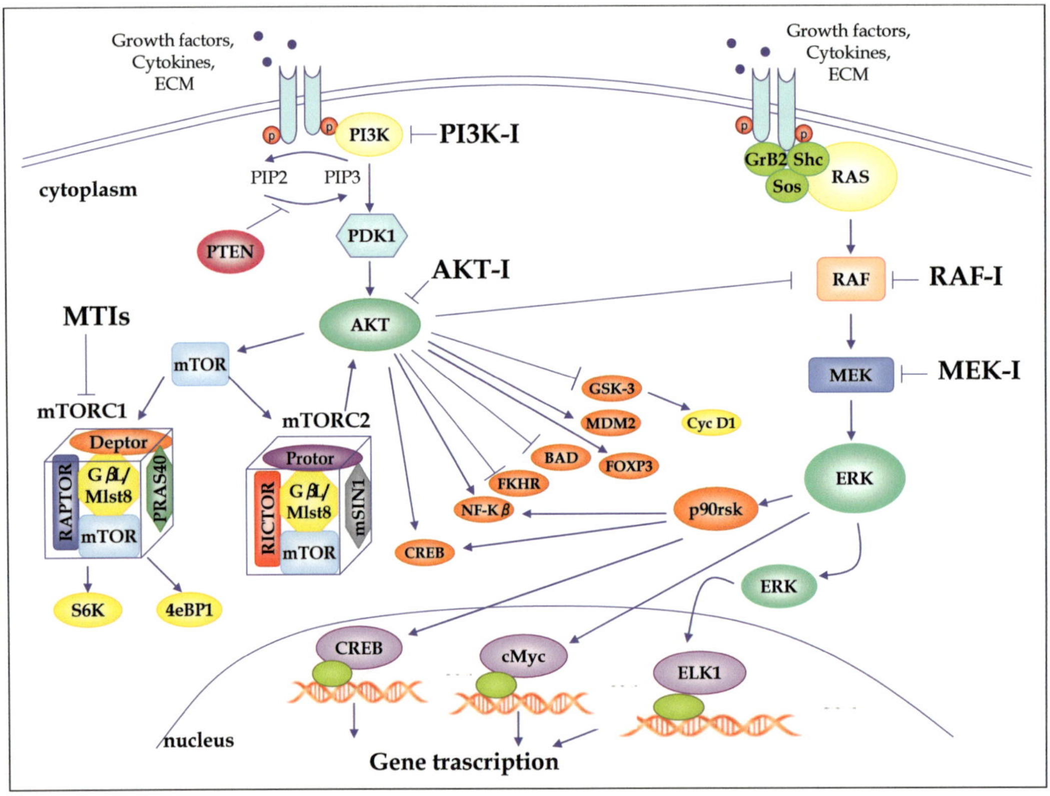

Fig. 1. PI3K/PTEN/AKT/mTOR and RAS/RAF/MEK/ERK pathways and their sites of interaction.

Inhibition of the PI3K signaling cascade can be achieved by targeting the pathway at different levels or simultaneously at multiple sites. In addition, however, these effects could be enhanced by also inhibiting crosstalking pathways. Specific inhibitors of PI3K, AKT and mTOR have shown significant promise in preclinical studies and are now under evaluation in clinical trials (Tab. 1) (Fathi et al., 2010; Levitzki & Klein, 2010; Zhao, 2010). Levy et al. (2009) reported that GSK690693, a pan-AKT kinase inhibitor, induces growth inhibition and

Inhibitor	Targets	Cancer Examined	Clinical Trials	Company
AR-12	PDK-1, PI3K, Akt	breast, colon, lung, prostate, lymphoma	Phase I	Arno Therapeutics
LY294002	PI3K, other related kinases	advanced hematological and advanced solid cancers	Preclinical	Lilly
CAL-101	PI3K (p110δ)	leukemias, lymphomas, myeloma	Phase I	Calistoga Pharmaceuticals
GDC-0941	PI3K (p110α), Flt3	lymphoma, NSCLC, breast, solid tumors	Phase I	PIramed Pharma/Roche/ Genetech
Wortmannin	PI3K, mTOR, DNA-PK, MAPK	advanced hematological and advanced solid cancers	Preclinical	
Perifosine (KRX- 0401)	Akt, MEK 1/2, ERK 1/2, JNK	multiple myeloma, leukemias, NSCLC, advance solid tumors	Phase I, II	Æterna Zentaris Inc./Keryx Biopharmaceuticals
triciribine (API-2)	Akt 1, 2, 3	AML, advanced hematological cancer	Phase I	VioQuest Pharmaceuticals
GSK690693	Akt1, 2, 3	leukemia, lymphoma	Phase I	GlaxoSmithKline
KP372-1	Akt, PDK-1, Flt3	leukemia, thyroid, H&N, glioma	Preclinical	QLT Inc.
VQD-002 (API-2)	Akt	NSCLC, leukemias, lymphomas, prostate	Phase I, II	VioQuest Pharmaceuticals
A-443654	Akt	hematological and solid cancers	Preclinical	Abbott Laboratories
Rapamycin (Sirolimus)	mTORC1	advanced hematological, advanced solid tumors, HIV, AIDS related malignancies	Phase I, II	Wyeth/Pfizer
CCI-779 (Torisel®, Temsirolimus)	mTORC1	leukemia, lymphoma, NSCLC, prostate, colorectal, renal	Phase I, II	Wyeth/Pfizer
RAD001 (Afinitor®, Everolimus)	mTORC1 mTORC2	cervical, renal, HCC, leukemia, lymphoma	Phase I, II	Novartis
AP-23573 (Ridaforolimus, Deforolimus)	mTORC1	advanced hematological cancer, prostate, endometrial	Phase I, II	Ariad/Merck
AZD-8055	mTORC1 mTORC2	advanced solid tumors, lymphomas, HCC	Phase I, II	AstraZeneca
OSI-027	mTORC1 mTORC2	advanced solid tumors, lymphomas	Phase I	OSI Pharmaceuticals
INK-128	mTORC1 mTORC2	advanced cancers, multiple myeloma, Waldenstrom macroglobulinemia	Phase I	Intellikine
PP-242	mTORC1 mTORC2		Phase I	UCSF

Table 1. PI3K/PTEN/AKT/mTOR inhibitors in hematological malignancies.

apoptosis of most of the ALL cell lines tested (89%), and exerts a selective antiproliferative effect on malignant cells (lack of effects on normal human CD4+ peripheral T lymphocytes). Much attention has been recently focused on blocking mTOR. This component of PI3K signaling cascade can form two distinct complexes termed mTORC1 and mTORC2 (Bjornsti & Houghton, 2004; Ciuffreda et al., 2010; Steelman et al., 2008). The first complex, composed of mTOR, GβL/Mlst8, PRAS40, RAPTOR and Deptor, is sensitive to the mTOR inhibitors (MTIs), such as rapamycin and its analogs RAD001, CCI-779 and AP23573 (rapalogs). Conversely, mTORC2 complex is generated when mTOR is associated with GβL, mSIN1, RICTOR, and PROTOR/PRR5. Rapamycin and its analogs are in this case unable to disrupt mTORC2 activity. However, it has been demonstrated that prolonged exposure and/or higher concentrations of MTIs may inhibit mTORC2. MTIs are currently in various stages of development for treatment of human cancer, as they showed great preclinical promise in the treatment of many cancer types, including ALL (Chappell et al., 2011). A recent ongoing phase I/II study from Amadori et al. performed in acute myeloid leukemia (AML) by combining the RAD001 with clofarabine, has been preliminary reported with encouraging results in a poor prognosis patient population overexpressing the drug-target (Amadori et al., 2010). It has been reported that inhibition of mTOR by rapamicin leads to apoptosis of blasts from ALL patients of both B-cell and T-cell origin (Avellino et al., 2005). The efficacy of CCI-779 (temsirolimus) in primary human ALL was also evaluated by Teachey et al. (2006), who demonstrated its activity using both NOD/SCID xenograft models and bone marrow-derived stromal cell co-culture systems. They observed that CCI-779 induced a dramatic decrease in cell proliferation and an increase of apoptosis in lymphoblasts from adult B-ALL patients cultured on bone marrow stroma. Moreover, in a NOD/SCID xenograft model they found that CCI-779 showed a decrease in peripheral blood blast counts and in splenomegaly. More recently, Batista et al. (2011) reported that inhibition of mTOR by CCI-779 markedly potentiated the anti-leukemic effects of dexamethasone and doxorubicin in primary T-ALL cells, showing in addition highly synergistic interactions in combination with other specific inhibitors of the PI3K cascade or with inhibitors of JAK3 signaling. According to the observation that ALL cells are frequently characterized by the deregulation of the apoptotic machinery, we explored *in vitro* a novel therapeutic strategy for ALL cells based on the combined inhibition of mTOR signaling and Bcl-2 activity, using CCI-779 and ABT-737, a small molecule BH3-mimetic that inhibits Bcl-2/Bcl-xL proteins (Iacovelli et al., 2010). We demonstrated that the simultaneous inhibition of Bcl-2 and mTOR pathways results in higher apoptotic effects and decreased proliferation in ALL cell lines and primary cells. Nevertheless, the evidence of a phenotype resistant to the ABT-737/CCI-779 combination prompts further studies on the simultaneous interruption of multiple pathways in ALL.

3.2 RAS/RAF/MEK/ERK pathway

In the last decades, the RAS/RAF/MEK/ERK pathway (Fig. 1) has emerged as one of the key components of the signaling network that regulates several cellular processes, such as cell growth, proliferation, survival, and, under certain conditions, also differentiation, migration and apoptosis (Tortora et al., 2007; Steelman et al., 2011). The RAS cascade is activated by a large number of extracellular stimuli and various internal processes. At the intracellular level, through a sequential phosphorylation and activation of protein kinases, regulates a wide array of substrates, including transcription factors and other protein kinases (Steelman et al., 2011; Wang et al., 2007).

Deregulation of RAS signaling is commonly found in cancer cells and is often caused by mutations in the RAS family of genes or by endogenous receptor-ligand interactions, resulting in a constitutive activation of G proteins. Mutations in NRAS and KRAS2 have been demonstrated in 15% and 22%, respectively, of childhood ALL (Case et al., 2008). A persistently active form of RAS signaling can also arise from mutations in genes encoding others proteins that impinge on this signaling pathway and that have recently been shown to be mutated in childhood ALL, such as FLT3, PTPN11, and BRAF (Taketani et al., 2004; Tartaglia et al., 2004). By a complete mutational screen of key exons of NRAS, KRAS2, PTPN11, FLT3, and BRAF in a large cohort of unselected ALL cases at diagnosis and at relapse, Case et al. (2008) showed that somatic mutations of these genes represent a common genetic aberration in childhood ALL and are related to disease progression, thus providing the rational base for including RAS inhibitors as novel targeted therapy for childhood ALL. Evidences provided by our group and others, indicate that the RAS/RAF/MEK/ERK pathway is an extremely promising therapeutic target in hematological malignancies. Studies performed in ALL have shown constitutive ERK phosphorylation in 30% of clinical samples and higher ERK kinase activity in ALL primary cells, compared to normal BM cells (Meng et al., 2003; Towatari et al., 1997). During the past years, we have described the incidence and prognostic impact of constitutive ERK activation in a large series of ALL clinical samples taken at diagnosis from 131 patients uniformly treated according to the GIMEMA LAL 2000 study protocol (Gregorj et al., 2007). One third (34,5%) of these samples showed constitutive activation of ERK, as evaluated using a flow cytometric assay that quantifies phosphoprotein expression in individual cells. We found that constitutive ERK activation was associated with higher WBC counts ($p=0.013$); most importantly, ERK phosphorylation was an independent predictor of failure to achieve CR ($P=0.027$) in multivariate analysis. Consequently, strategies aimed at inhibiting MEK activity have been investigated experimentally.

Potent small-molecules that selectively inhibit different molecular targets of the RAS/RAF/MEK/ERK pathway have been developed (Wang et al., 2007). These compounds have shown promising anticancer activity *in vitro* and *in vivo* by suppressing tumor growth and/or inducing apoptosis in a broad spectrum of solid tumors and in hematological malignancies including AML, multiple myeloma (MM), lymphomas and ALL. Some of them are currently under investigation in early-phase clinical trials (Chappell et al., 2011).

We have investigated the molecular and functional consequences of the pharmacological disruption of the MEK/ERK module by selective inhibitors of MEK. However, discouraging preliminary results were observed in both ALL primary cells and cell lines exposed *in vitro* to the MEK inhibitors PD98059 and PD0325901, with significant inhibition of ERK phosphorylation in a proportion of samples, but neither occurrence of cell cycle changes nor induction of apoptosis (Tafuri et al, unpublished results). These data may suggest that in ALL pro-survival signals could be mediated by additional pathways. Nevertheless, since one of the most exciting features of MEK inhibitors as potential anticancer agents is their ability to lower cancer cells' apoptotic threshold, sensitizing tumor cells to the proapoptotic action of other agents, they represent useful tools for building up pharmacological combinations with synergistic proapoptotic effects (Milella et al., 2005; Tortora et al., 2007).

4. Apoptosis modulators

In order to maintain cells homeostasis, a correct balance between cell proliferation and survival is preserved by several mechanisms, including the physiologic cell death program, called "apoptosis". During this process, old, mutated or irreparably damaged cells are removed from the organism in a properly regulated fashion, without eliciting an inflammatory response (Danial & Korsmeyer, 2004). In mammalian cells, apoptosis can be triggered by a broad variety of stimuli such as developmental signals, cellular stress or DNA damage, cytotoxic insults or environmental factors, resulting in activation of two different apoptotic signaling pathways: the extrinsic and the intrinsic pathway. The extrinsic pathway is activated in response to the binding of extracellular signals to cell surface death receptors (Ashkenazi et al., 1999) and it is independent of mitochondrial involvement. Instead, the intrinsic pathway is activated by intracellular events that involve the release of apoptotic factors from mitochondria (Danial & Korsmeyer, 2004). In particular, the intrinsic pathway involves a mechanism called "mitochondrial outer membrane permeabilization" (MOMP) by which several apoptotic factors such as cytochrome c, AIF and Smac-DIABLO, are released into the cytoplasm (Green & Reed, 1998; Wang et. al, 2001). MOMP following cell-intrinsic apoptotic stimuli is to a large extent regulated by the Bcl-2 family of proteins (van Loo et al., 2002), which thus constitute a critical checkpoint of the intrinsic pathway. Bcl-2 was first identified at the chromosomal breakpoint of t(14;18)-bearing human follicular B-cell lymphoma (Tsujimoto et al., 1985) and its oncogenic potential has been demonstrated through a gene transfer approach (Reed et al., 1988). The Bcl-2 family is an evolutionarily-conserved family of proteins that consists of more than 20 members which can be divided into three subgroups based on their function and on the presence of conserved Bcl-2 homology (BH) regions (Fig. 2). The most important members of the Bcl-2 antiapoptotic repertoire contain four Bcl-2 homology domains (BH1–4) and are generally integrated within the outer mitochondrial membrane (OMM), including Bcl-2, Bcl-2 related gene A1 (A1) and the long isoform Bcl-xL, Bcl-w and myeloid cell leukemia 1 (Mcl-1). Their function is to preserve and maintain OMM integrity by direct inhibition of the proapoptotic members of the family (Green & Evan, 2002). The proapoptotic proteins are divided into two groups: effector proteins and BH3-only proteins. The multi-region proapoptotic effector proteins, Bax and Bak, were conventionally thought to share BH 1–3 regions; however, by structure-based alignment of globular Bcl-2 family proteins, a conserved BH4 motif was recently observed (Kvansakul et al., 2008). Following activation, Bak and Bax undergo homo-oligomerization thus promoting MOMP by formation of proteolipid pores within the OMM. The BH3-only proteins, sharing the homology with Bcl-2 in the BH3 region only, are divided based on their ability to interact either with the antiapoptotic members or with both the antiapoptotic and the effector proteins. BH3-only proteins such as Bad (Bcl-2 antagonist of cell death) and Noxa are referred to as "sensitizer" and/or "derepressor" and interact, through the BH3 region, only with the antiapoptotic members of the family. The BH3-only proteins that are referred as "direct activators", such as Bid (Bcl-2-interacting domain death agonist) and BIM (Bcl-2-interacting mediator of cell death), can interact with the antiapoptotic repertoire as well as with the effectors, and can directly induce Bak and Bax oligomerization and MOMP (Chipuk et. al, 2010). Correct interactions between pro and antiapoptotic Bcl-2 family members are crucial for the normal activation of the intrinsic pathway and apoptosis regulation.

Resistance to apoptosis, frequently caused by overexpression of antiapoptotic proteins, is a common feature of cancer. In fact, it has been demonstrated that deficiency in apoptosis is one of the key hallmarks of cancer (Hanahan & Weinberg, 2000). High levels of Bcl-2 expression have been found in many cancers, such as follicular lymphoma (Gaulard et al., 1992), chronic lymphocytic leukemia (CLL) (Schena et al., 1992), AML (Andreeff et al., 1999), MM (Harada et al., 1998), small cell lung cancer (Ben-Ezra et al., 1994) and melanoma (Leiter et al., 2000). Elevated expression of the antiapoptotic proteins Bcl-2, Bcl-xL and Mcl-1 has been reported also in ALL cell lines and primary samples (Campana et al., 1993; Coustan-Smith et al. 1996; Del Gaizo Moore et al., 2008; Hogarth & Hall, 1999). In particular, several studies have shown that higher Bcl-2 levels are associated with improved ability of ALL cells to survive under very unfavorable culture conditions, such as the absence of stromal-derived growth factors. Therefore, Bcl-2 overexpression may contribute to leukemogenesis and influences the survival ability of leukemic lymphoblasts. Moreover, Bcl-2 overexpression may provide an explanation of the ability of leukemic lymphoblasts to expand outside the bone marrow microenvironment (Campana et al., 1993; Coustan-Smith et al., 1996). To test the hypothesis that the apoptotic defects are essential for tumor maintenance, Letai et al. (2004) have generated a transgenic mouse model expressing a conditional Bcl-2 gene and constitutive c-myc that develop lymphoblastic leukemia. They have shown that Bcl-2 elimination yielded rapid loss of leukemic cells and significantly prolonged mouse survival, formally validating Bcl-2 as a rational target for a targeted cancer therapy (Letai et al., 2004). Furthermore, high Bcl-2 levels are observed also in ALL characterized by t(4;11) (Robinson et al., 2008). It has been demonstrated that the equilibrium in the formation of Bcl-2:Bax heterodimers (suppressors of death) and Bax:Bax homodimers (activators of death) appears to be central in the molecular regulation of apoptosis (Coustan-Smith et al, 1996). In fact, high Bax expression alone was shown to be associated with an increased probability of relapse (Hogarth & Hall, 1999) and both Bax expression levels and the Bax/Bcl-2 ratio are significantly lower in samples at relapse, as compared with samples at initial diagnosis (Prokop et al., 2000). Kaufman et al. (1998) have shown that Mcl-1 is highly expressed in ALL at relapse, resulting two times higher as compared to pre-treatment levels. Further studies have correlated increased expression of Bcl-2 antiapoptotic family members to increased tumor cell survival and drug resistance *in vitro* and *in vivo* (Del Gaizo Moore et al., 2008). Holleman et al. (2004) observed overexpression of the antiapoptosis gene Mcl-1 in prednisolone-resistant ALL. Wei et al. (2006) have shown that Mcl-1 is also involved in glucocortocoid (GC) resistance in ALL. In this report, by combining bioinformatic analyses of gene expression profiles of childood ALL (classified as GC-sensitive/resistant by *ex vivo* testing) with functional data obtained from experimental systems, they identified Mcl-1 as the key member of the antiapoptotic Bcl-2 family, responsible for GC resistance (Wei et al., 2006). These observations suggest that inhibition of the antiapoptotic/pro-survival members of Bcl-2 family proteins may represent an attractive approach for the treatment of ALL.

Several strategies have been developed to inhibit the activity of the Bcl-2 family of proteins, including antisense oligonucleotides, peptides derived from the BH3 domain, and small molecule antagonists. While clinical studies with peptides rarely progress to late-stage trials, because of poor pharmacological properties (Lessene et al., 2008), small molecules proved more effective. Small molecule inhibitors are designed to compete with activator and sensitizer molecules for the same binding site on Bcl-2 family members (the BH3 domain) and consequently they are referred to as BH3 mimetics (Richardson & Kaye, 2008). Several molecules has been developed as BH3 mimetics; one the most attractive is ABT-737 (Oltersdorf et al. 2005) and its orally bioactive analog ABT-263. Apoptosis induced by ABT-737 is dependent on Bax and Bak (Van Delft et al., 2006) suggesting that its primary mechanism of action is through the regulation of the intrinsic apoptosis pathway. ABT-737 is a Bcl-2/Bcl-xL inhibitor that specifically binds the hydrophobic groove that normally serves as a binding site for the BH3 domain of activators and sensitizers. ABT-737 binds

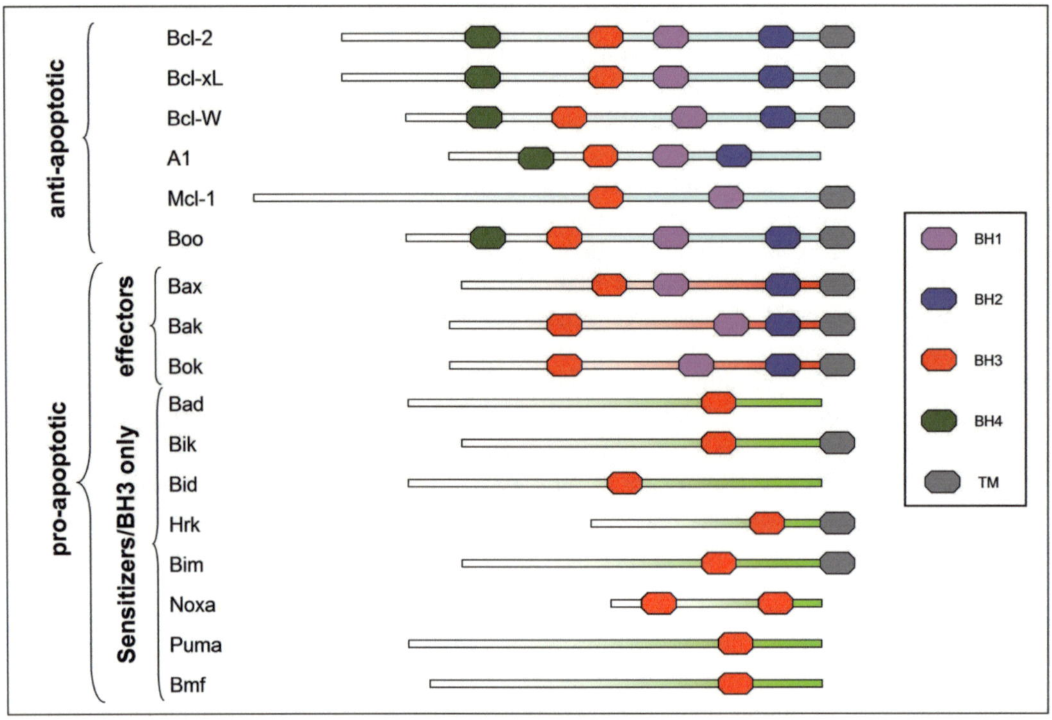

Fig. 2. The Bcl-2 family of proteins (TM: transmembrane domain).

potently Bcl-2, Bcl-xL and Bcl-w, instead only weakly Bfl/A1 or Mcl-1. In fact, Mcl-1 overexpression is reported to be one of the principal factors that may confer resistance to ABT-737 (Konopleva et al., 2006). Pre-clinical studies have shown that ABT-737 displays a potent growth-inhibitory activity in ALL. In particular we and others have evaluated preclinical activity of ABT-737 on a panel of ALL cell lines and primary cells obtained from ALL patients, observing a strong increase in apoptosis induction (Del Gaizo Moore et al., 2008; Tafuri et al., 2007). Furthermore, we employed a combined preclinical strategy to overcome the ABT-737 resistance in ALL cells using the mTOR inhibitor CCI-779. We observed synergistic effects on apoptosis induction between ABT-737 and CCI-779 in both ALL cell lines and in a proportion of primary cells (Iacovelli et al., 2010). Other studies employing ABT-737 in combination with L-asparaginase, topotecan, vincristine and etoposide have shown increased antileukemic effects against drug-resistant ALL xenografts models (High et al., 2010). Since ABT-737 was not orally bio-available, the oral analog ABT-263, capable of initiate apoptosis following 2 hours from administration, has been developed. The dosing flexibility of ABT-263 accomplished by its oral efficacy prompt the clinical investigation of this molecule, both as a single agent and in combination. The ABT-263 is currently employed in phase I clinical trials in both hematological and solid tumors (Gandhi et al., 2011; Wilson et al., 2010). GX15-070 (Obatoclax) is another BH3 mimetic, which binds to Bcl-2, Bcl-xL and Mcl-1 with comparable affinity (Lessene et al., 2008); for this reason, Obatoclax may potentially overcome resistance conferred by high levels of Mcl-1, inhibiting the interaction between Bak and Mcl-1 (Trudel et al., 2007). Several reports have shown that increased Mcl-1 expression is associated with GC resistance (Holleman et al., 2004; Stam et al., 2010) and it has been demonstrated that Obatoclax treatment can resensitizes GC-resistant ALL cells (Bonapace et al., 2010). Other results suggest that Obatoclax could be useful as a therapeutic agent against ALL and that the activity and/or the expression of antiapoptotic proteins could be used as a biomarker to determine the appropriate treatment strategy for ALL patients (Heidari et al., 2010). In particular, Bonapace et al have shown that Obatoclax can overcome the resistance to GC through rapid activation of autophagy-dependent necroptosis, which was able to bypass the apoptotic block in the mitochondrion. This effect required Obatoclax-mediated dissociation of Beclin-1 from Mcl-1 and was associated with inhibition of mTOR activity (Bonapace et al., 2010). Autophagy is a cell death mechanism distinct from apoptosis, also called type 2, non-apoptotic cell death. Autophagy is characterized by the inclusion of cytoplasmic material into vacuoles, leading to degradation mediated by lysosomal enzymes (Klionsky, 2007). Beclin-1 is a novel BH3 domain protein involved in autophagy, which plays an essential role in the activation of this cell death process. Beclin-1 can be activated or inactivated by its interaction with the pro or antiapoptotic members of the Bcl-2 family, respectively, through the BH3 domain. Thus, the cells can regulate autophagy by targeting Beclin-1 through Bcl-2 family members (Levine et al., 2008). Small molecules, such as ABT-737 and Obatoclax, by acting as BH3 inhibitors, can overcome resistance mediated by Bcl-2 antiapoptotic members, thereby restoring the cellular ability to induce autophagy (Bonapace et al., 2010; Levine et al., 2008).

The use of the BH3 mimetics, alone or in combination with other inhibitors or chemotherapy, can be of great importance in customizing an individual patient's therapy especially in cases in which chemotherapy alone is not able to decrease tumor burden.

5. Epigenetic silencing

The term "epigenetic" is generally referred to heritable changes in gene expression not caused by alterations in the DNA coding sequences. Epigenetic changes such as DNA methylation or histone modifications work in concert with each other to regulate gene expression in normal mammalian development (Baylin & Ohm 2006). However, it is now evident that epigenetic modifications considerably contribute to development and progression of carcinogenesis in general, and of leukemogenesis in particular (Baylin & Ohm, 2006; Chen et al., 2010).

5.1 DNA methylation

DNA methylation is mediated by a family of enzymes, DNA methyltransferases (DNMTs), which catalyze the covalent addition of a methyl group at the 5' carbon of cytosine residues that precede guanosine (CpG) islands (Herman & Baylin, 2003). The resulting 5-methylcytosines protrude into the major groove of DNA, inhibiting gene transcription.

In mammalian cells, 5-methylcytosine is found in approximately 5% of the whole genome. Compared to normal cells, cancer cells display aberrant methylation of cytosine residues both in gene promoters or coding regions, leading to a transcriptional silencing of tumor suppressor gene. Cyclin-dependent kinase inhibitors, such as CDKN2B, which encodes the tumor suppressor p15 (INK4B), and CDKN2A, which encodes the tumor suppressors p16 (INK4A) are, among other genes, frequently methylated in their promoter regions (Garcia-Manero et al., 2009; Roman-Gomez et al., 2004). This epigenetic modification has been described also in ALL. Results obtained by Roman-Gomez at al. (2004) in 251 consecutive ALL patients demonstrated that promoter hypermethylation of multiple genes is a common phenomenon in ALL and is a strong independent prognostic factor in predicting the clinical outcome of ALL patients. In particular, they observed that methylation in ALL cells mostly participate to inactivation of genes involved in: 1) cell growth regulation by controlling directly (p15, p16 and p57) or indirectly (p73, PTEN, NES-1) cell cycle check-points; 2) apoptosis inhibition (p14, TMS1, APAF-1 and DAPK); 3) cell adhesion (some members of cadherin family). However, the relationship between aberrant DNA methylation and protein expression of tumor suppression genes has not yet been extensively evaluated in adult ALL series. Bueso-Ramos et al. (2005) showed that methylation of more than one gene of the pathway composed of p73, p15 and p57 was associated with a worse outcome of adult ALL patients. However, lack of association was reported between p73 protein expression and clinical-biologic characteristic. We analyzed the promoter methylation status of p73, p21, p15 and p16, evaluating in addition the p21, p15 and p16 protein expression, in primary cells from newly diagnosed adult ALL patients, uniformly treated according to the GIMEMA LAL2000 protocol. Our results indicate that in vivo p15 and p21 protein expression plays an unfavorable prognostic role in adult ALL patients independently of the p73, p21, p15 and p16 gene promoter methylation status (De Cave et al. 2007). Data reported by Yang et al. (2009) demonstrated that detection of epigenetic alterations allows the identification of ALL patients with poor prognosis within the standard-risk group. More recently, Milani L et al. (2010), analyzing the methylation patterns of CpG sites in 416 genes, have found a striking difference in the methylation patterns within a large number of samples from ALL patients. Notably, they observed a correlation between the methylation level and clinical outcome within major subgroups of ALL patients, identifying 20 genes with DNA methylation levels capable to predict leukemia relapse. These observations suggest that methylation analysis should be explored to identify ALL patients at different risk.

5.2 Histone modifications

Structural studies have demonstrated that histones easily undergo post-translational modifications in their long amino-teminal tails that project outward from the nucleosome. These tail modifications, which include acetylation, methylation, phosphorylation, ubiquitination, ADP-ribosylation, are involved in several biological processes related to the chromatin structure, i.e. gene regulation, DNA repair, DNA replication, chromatin condensation etc. (Bhaumik et al., 2007).

Histone acetylation acts in concert with DNA methylation to regulate gene expression. Several data have demonstrated that histone acetylation, catalysed by histone acetyltransferases (HATs), is involved in maintaining chromatin structure in a transcriptionally active form (Chen et al., 2010). In contrast, histone deacetylation (HDAC), removing acetyl groups from histone tails, permits the histones to wrap more tightly around the DNA and thus maintains genes inactivated and silenced. High level of HDAC expression is a common finding in cancer cells (Moreno et al, 2010) and accounts for the aberrant expression and activity of numerous proteins involved in proliferation, differentiation, apoptosis, adhesion and migration (Lane & Chabner, 2009). A high expression of HDAC has also been described in hematological malignancies, particularly in lymphomas (Marquard et al, 2009) and in AML (Cimino et al, 2006). Thus far, very few data are available about HDAC expression in ALL.

In a recent study conducted by Moreno and colleagues (2010) on childhood ALL samples, the authors observed a differential HDACs expression between clinical samples.

Particularly, they found a higher expression of HDAC1 and HDAC4 and a lower expression of HDAC5 in T-ALL. Moreover, they reported that higher expression of HDAC7 and HDAC9 is associated with poor prognosis both in the overall group of childhood ALL and in B-lineage CD10-positive cases suggesting the use of HDAC inhibitors as a promising therapeutic intervention for the treatment of refractory childhood ALL.

5.3 Epigenetic therapy

Because of the key role of epigenetic modifications in the pathogenesis of cancer, pharmacological agents that target components of the epigenetic machinery are become promising elements of the therapeutic arsenal for cancer treatment.

Several data have indicated that DNA methyltransferase inhibitors (DNMTi), such as azacitidine, decitabine, and other derivative, are able to restore tumor suppressor gene expression and exert antitumor effects *in vitro* and *in vivo* by inhibiting hypermethylation (Chen et al., 2010). Clinical studies have clearly demonstrated that DNMTi, used alone or in combination, may convey clinical benefit to patients with hematological malignancies, especially myelodysplastic syndrome and AML. In contrast, the application of this therapeutic strategy to ALL patients is so far limited. Recent data reported by Schafer et al. (2010) have demonstrated that MLL rearranged (MLL-r) infant ALL samples, compared with other childhood leukemias and normal controls, are characterized by promoter hypermethylation of several genes. Notably, they showed that decitabine preferentially kills MLL-r lymphoblastic leukemia cell lines and also that this response correlates with the upregulation of several of the identified silenced genes, suggesting predictable efficacy of demethylating agents in this category of infant ALL that is reported as the most aggressive type of childhood leukemia. More recently, studying the same category of MLL-r infant ALL patients, Stumpel et al. (2011) observed that in samples from infant ALL patients carrying the t(4;11), eleven miRNAs were downregulated as a consequence of hypermethylation and seven of these were re-activated after exposure to a demethylating agent, thus providing additional evidence that demethylating agents should be tested for their efficacy in MLL-r infant ALL patients.

HDAC inhibitors (HDAC-Is) are a class of agents with the capacity to induce acetylation of histone and non-histone proteins (Lee et al. 2010). These molecules have been intensively investigated in preclinical models as well as in clinical trials for a variety of malignancies, because of their ability to inhibit proliferation, induce differentiation, and cause apoptosis in tumor cells (Bolden et al. 2006; Lee et al., 2010). Since only a portion of patients has a therapeutic response, a very important issue is the need to identify markers of potential response or resistance to HDAC-Is. Currently, there is great interest in the HDAC-Is field, as several new and more effective compounds are being developed and entering clinical trials. In ALL, HDAC-Is have been used only for *in vitro* studies. It has been demonstrated that HDAC-Is induce apoptosis in ALL cell lines (Moreno et al., 2010; Romanski et al., 2004), including those resistant to glucocorticoid, and in *ex vivo*-cultured samples. Our preliminary results *in vitro* show that novel HDAC-Is are potent growth inhibitors and inducers of apoptosis in human leukemia cells, including ALL cell lines, and suggest their potential therapeutic use for patients with leukemias.

Future research will definitely suggest additional therapeutic targets regulating epigenetic pathways and continued clinical trials with demethylating agents and HDAC inhibitors, alone or in combination, will undoubtedly provide further advance in the treatment of hematological malignancies, including ALL cases.

6. Bone marrow microenvironment

Bone marrow (BM) is a complex and dynamic network of hematopoietic and stromal cells, blood vessels, proteins and others microenvironmental factors, such as growth factors and cytokines that compose the extracellular matrix (ECM) (Ayala et al., 2009). The interaction between hematopoietic and stromal or mesenchymal cells, as well as between cellular and soluble components of BM microenvironment, sustains normal hematopoiesis by promoting cell growth, regulating differentiation, and importantly maintaining a pool of undifferentiated pluripotent and long-lived stem cells (Ayala et al., 2009; Rizo et al., 2006). The BM microenvironment is critical for B-cell lymphopoiesis.

Similar to normal hematopoiesis, the survival and growth of leukemic cells largely depend on the support provided by the BM microenvironment, which also contributes to blunt the effects of chemotherapy and provides a sanctuary for minimal residual disease. Notably, several data have demonstrated the key role of BM microenvironment in supporting the survival of leukemic stem cells (LCS), also known as "leukemia initiating cells", i.e. the subpopulation of cells within a tumor that are long lived, has the potential to self-renew, can generate the original tumor in xenograft models (Konopleva & Jordan, 2011; Moore & Lyle, 2011) and are therefore thought to be the cause of relapse in patients treated with traditional drugs. The emerging concept of LSC niche as a dynamic entity in which interactions between the LCS and its microenvironment take place are now becoming a hot topic highlighting the relevance of BM microenvironment for leukemia initiation, progression and drug resistance and opening up opportunities for therapeutic intervention (Ayala et al., 2009; Rizo et al., 2006).

The mechanism by which the BM stroma modulates growth, progression and response to chemotherapy of ALL cells is not fully elucidated. In vitro studies of primary ALL cells usually demonstrate a large amount of spontaneous ALL cell apoptosis which could be reduced by co-culturing them with BM stromal cells, increasing survival and proliferation and blunting the cytotoxic effects of chemotherapeutic agents (Brown et al., 2008). There are evidences that interactions of ALL cells with BM stroma are mediated by different members of the integrin family of proteins, constitutively expressed on leukemic cells (LFA-1 on T-ALL and VLA-4 on B-ALL), with their respective ligands exposed on the surface of BM stromal cells or secreted in the ECM (fibronectin) (Ayala et al., 2009; Tabe et al., 2007). These interactions lead to the activation of tyrosine kinases, and consequently of downstream pathways which regulate cell growth, survival, adhesion, migration, angiogenesis, apoptosis and autophagy (Tabe et al., 2007; Veiga et al., 2006). The PI3K/PTEN/AKT/mTOR cascade is a critical pathway in stromal/leukemic cells interactions mediated by integrins, chemokines (such as CXCR4/CXCL12), angiogenic factors and interleukins (Konopleva & Jordan, 2011).

It is well known that interleukins, such as IL-7 and IL-3, have a critical role in regulation proliferation and survival of T- (Scupoli et al., 2007) and B-ALL (Juarez et al., 2007) cells by activating stroma interactions. Addition of IL-7 to co-cultures of BM stromal cells and ALL cells has been reported to increase ALL cell survival through phosphorylation of AKT, ERK1/2, and p38 (Juarez et al., 2007). Crosstalk between BM microenvironment and leukemic cells has also been demonstrated by upregulation of IL-8 in leukemic cells promoted by CXCR4/CXCL12-induced activation of the NF-kB and JNK/AP-1 pathways (Scupoli et al., 2008). High levels of IL-8 could in turn enhance angiogenesis in the BM microenvironment and indirectly sustain tumor growth (Scupoli et al., 2008). Ultimately, it has been demonstrated that CXCR4 has a role in homing and migration of ALL blasts in BM and in other organs (Konopleva & Jordan, 2011; Sipkins et al., 2005).

Increased neovascularization, which effectively contributes to growth and progression of cancer, has been described in ALL as a result of autocrine and/or paracrine loops of the main proangiogenic mediators (bFGF, VEGF and angiopoietin) promoted by BM stroma/leukemic blast interactions (Ayala et al., 2009). Beside marked neovascularisation, extensive endothelial cell proliferation represents one of the most pronounced microenvironmental changes observed in BM of ALL patients (Veiga et al., 2006). Several studies have demonstrated the existence of a crosstalk between the endothelium and leukemic cells, in which leukemia cells stimulate BM endothelium and promote de novo angiogenesis and neovascularisation, while BM endothelium promoted leukemia cell survival through modulation of antiapoptotic bcl-2 family members (Veiga et al., 2006). Another study by Aref et al. (2007) described in B-ALL an abnormal expression of matrix metalloproteinases (MMP), which is a further class of angiogenesis and tumor progression regulators produced by both stromal and leukemic cells (Aref et al., 2007)

A further interesting aspect related to BM microenvironment and leukemia cells interactions regards the role of BM microenvironment on lineage commitment and differentiation. Several studies have indeed demonstrated that BM microenvironment can drive lineage-specific differentiation in leukemia by modulating different cytokines and other soluble components (Kankuri et al., 2008; Wei et al., 2008). In an elegant study performed on a human MLL-AF9 leukemia model transplanted into immunodeficient mice, Wei J et al. (2008) showed that ALL, AML or mixed-lineage leukemia were generated by altering the cytokine milieu of human CD34+ cells expressing MLL-AF9, thus demonstrating the importance of the microenvironment in driving leukemia phenotype.

Finally, a translationally relevant concept is that the BM microenvironment can also regulate the response of leukemic cells to chemotherapy through a variety of mechanisms. According to the evidences described before, BM microenvironment mainly contributes to protection of leukemic cells from drug effects participating in induction of a chemo-resistant phenotype. For instance, high levels of asparagine synthetase produced by BM-derived mesenchymal cells have been demonstrated as one of the mechanisms participating in the resistance to asparaginase in ALL samples (Iwamoto et al., 2007). Moreover, it has been reported that IL-7 and TSLP protect ALL cells in vitro from MTI-induced effects suggesting that stromal cell-derived cytokines can contribute to MTI resistance (Brown et al, 2007).

In conclusion, these evidences demonstrate the importance of interaction between BM stromal cells and ALL blasts and chemoresistance, the role of BM microenvironment and ultimately the potential of therapeutic approaches based on disrupting this interaction in ALL patients.

7. From personalized proteomic profiles to personalized medicine in ALL

In order to tailor a personalized therapy, it is mandatory that research is aimed at identifying specific targets on the malignant cells in order to dissect groups of patients with different risks and to develop new drugs with selective activity against the tumor cell. The characterization of molecular profiles of cancer cells, compared to their normal counterparts, requires the continuous development of comprehensive molecular analysis technologies. It is particularly crucial to implement and support the development of novel technologies that allow high-throughput analysis of genetic alterations, expression of genome products and monitoring the STP in cancers. Although a complete description of these new technologies is beyond the scope of this chapter, some observations regarding the most promising techniques that may allow to further decipher the molecular profile of leukemia samples at the post-translational level are herein reported.

Understanding cancer cell physiopathology at the protein level requires the development of reliable proteomics. In addition, profiling and classification of several components of multiple aberrant STP would be expected to accurately predict disease behavior and prognosis. Moreover, the challenge of translating proteomic pathway profiling to the bedside would require a technique capable of efficiently processing small numbers of cancer cells by routinely assessing multiple STP simultaneously. Traditional protein assay techniques like Western blotting (WB) and ELISA assay can assess the level of protein phosphorylation. WB can evaluate a limited number of proteins and samples in a semi-quantitative way requiring large amounts of cellular material. The ELISA assay gives quantitative information but is extremely expensive. Further attempts have been made by MALDI-TOF (matrix assisted laser desorption/ionization-time of flight) and by two-dimensional gel-electrophoresis. However, both methods cannot be performed on a large scale on clinical samples and, more importantly, they require large numbers of cells (Petricoin et al., 2005)

The Reverse Phase Protein Arrays (RPPA) is an emerging, sensitive, high-throughput technology that allows profiling the STP working state of large clinical populations, examining the functional proteomic profile of each sample. By quantitative analysis of minuscule amounts of proteins (nanoliters of protein lysates equivalent to picograms of proteins), RPPA permits the measurements of proteins and their corresponding phosphoproteins by using high-quality monoclonal antibodies. At the same time, cell lysates collected from hundred of samples are spotted on a single slide, making this methods highly effective in retrospective clinical sample analysis or in prospectively collected sets of samples. Compared to WB, which uses proteins from 5×10^5 cells for each antibody analysis, RPPA requires proteins from only 5.000-20.000 cells per sample preparation and a protein amount equivalent to 200 cells is spotted per slide for a single antibody. Therefore, 20.000 cells would be sufficient to analyze 100 different protein targets and the amount of material previously used for single WB will be now used for 2500 antibodies by RPPA. This will thus be particularly useful for protein detection of rare populations (stem cells, residual cells surviving after chemotherapy) (Kornblau et al., 2009). RPPA has been successfully applied in a number of basic and clinical studies (Accordi et al., 2010; Kornblau et al., 2009; Petricoin et al., 2007). In a very recent study published by Accordi et al. (2011) the RPPA technique was applied to analyze the activation/expression status of 92 key signaling proteins in 118 pediatric B-ALL patients. The authors found an aberrant activation and/or increased expression of several pathways involved in cell proliferation (such as Bcl-2 hyperphosphorylation, LCK and cyclin E up-modulation) in patients with poor prognosis. Our group has applied RPPA on adult and pediatric ALL patients, identifying B- and T-lineage ALL by the proteomic profile, showing in addition a prognostic role of cell cycle and apoptotic molecule over-expression in ALL patients (Tafuri et al. unpublished results).

Alternatively to the phospho-proteomic array technology, it is possible to perform a "single-cell proteomic" analysis by using flow cytometry (Irish et al., 2006). The powerful multi-parametric single cell analysis platforms nowadays available allow simultaneously determining and quantifying the active or inactive state of multiple signaling components in individual cancer cells using fluorophore-conjugated antibodies. A "single-cell signaling signature" can be obtained for each cell in a mixed population and compared either with other features on the same cell or with normal cells present in patient samples. Therefore, single-cell analysis by flow cytometry is particularly useful to analyze samples for rare (HCS or LCS) and/or heterogeneous cell type populations. Recent data published by Gibbs et al (2011) demonstrated the biochemical and functional heterogeneity of human HSCs by using single-cell phospho-specific flow cytometric analysis. Analyzing the response profile of human HSCs to a broad range of hematopoietic cytokines the authors demonstrated that the HSC compartment is composed of biochemically distinct subsets, and that cellular proliferation can be directly regulated by G-CSF.

8. Concluding remarks

Comprehensive molecular analysis of cancer over the past decades has clearly shown that most malignancies are composed of several molecular subgroups, each defined by specific genetic/epigenetic alterations and with different prognosis. In the past years, diagnostic and prognostic achievements obtained through molecular genetics have improved patient follow-up, addressing treatment choice and anticipating treatment failure. In the post-genomic era, the translational approach to diseases, especially to hematologic and solid malignancies, must exceed including new tools for dissecting the functional proteomic and metabolomic profiling. Future clinical technologies may expand studies on protein arrays helping to define in large clinical population the functional proteomic profile at steady-state; this approach may lead to the identification of aberrant molecular target(s), possibly guiding the choice of specific molecular therapies, on one hand, and leading to elucidate of post-treatment changes, on the other hand, with the overall objective of improving the strategies currently employed to counteract leukemia chemo- and targeted drug-resistance. The ongoing new challenge will be to manage the enormous amount of data often produced by these technologies, approaching statistical methods that may accurately identify the most important clinical and biological variables.

9. Acknowledgments

The research was supported by the Italian Ministry of Education,University and Scientific Research (MIUR), PRIN 2008 (2008NYJZXB_005) and the Sapienza, University of Rome, Ricerche Universitarie (C26A10SW9X)

10. References

Accordi, B., Espina, V., Giordan, M., VanMeter, A., Milani, G., Galla, L., Ruzzene, M., Sciro, M., Trentin, L., De Maria, R., te Kronnie, G., Petricoin, E., Liotta, L. & Basso, G. (2010). Functional protein network activation mapping reveals new potential molecular drug targets for poor prognosis pediatric BCP-ALL. *PLoS One*, Vol. 5,No. 10, (Oct 2010), e13552, ISSN 1932-6203

Amadori, S., Venditti, A., Ammatuna, E., Martelli, A.M., et al. (2010). Temsirolimus, An mTOR Inhibitor, In Combination with Low-Dose Clofarabine in Older Patients with Advanced Acute Myeloid Leukemia: Results of a Phase 2 GIMEMA Study

(AML-1107) *Blood* (ASH Annual Meeting Abstracts), Vol. 116, (Nov 2010), 510, ISSN 0006-4971

Andreeff, M., Jiang, S., Zhang, X., Konopleva, M., Estrov, Z., Snell, V.E., Xie Z., Okcu, M.F., Sanchez-Williams, G., Dong, J., Estey, E.H., Champlin, R.C., Kornblau, S.M., Reed, J.C.& Zhao, S., (1999). Expression of Bcl-2-related genes in normal and AML progenitors: changes induced by chemotherapy and retinoic acid. *Leukemia,* Vol. 13, No.11, (Nov 1999), pp. 1881-92, ISSN 0987-6924

Aref, S., Osman, E., Mansy, S., Omer, N., Azmy, E., Goda, T. & El-Sherbiny, M. (2007). Prognostic relevance of circulating matrix metalloproteinase-2 in acute myeloid leukaemia patients. *Hematol Oncol.* Vol. 25, No. 3, (Sep 2007), pp. (121-6), ISSN 0278-0232

Ashkenazi, A., Pai, R.C., Fong, S., Leung, S., Lawrence, D.A., Marsters, S.A. et al. (1999). Safety and antitumor activity of recombinant soluble Apo2 ligand. *J Clin Invest,* Vol. 104, No. 3, (Sep 1999), pp. 155–162, ISSN 0021-9738

Avellino, R., Romano, S., Parasole, R., Bisogni, R., Lamberti, A., Poggi, V., Venuta, S. & Romano. M.F. (2005). Rapamycin stimulates apoptosis of childhood acute lymphoblastic leukemia cells. *Blood,* Vol. 106, No.4, pp. 1400-1406, ISSN 0006-4971

Ayala, F., Dewar, R., Kieran, M. & Kalluri, R. (2009) Contribution of bone microenvironment to leukemogenesis and leukemia progression. *Leukemia,* Vol. 23, No. 12, (Dec 2009), pp. 2233–2241, ISSN 0987-6924

Barata, J.T., Silva, A., Brandao, J.G., Nadler, L.M., Cardoso, A.A. & Boussiotis, V.A. (2004). Activation of PI3K Is Indispensable for Interleukin 7–mediated Viability, Proliferation, Glucose Use, and Growth of T Cell Acute Lymphoblastic Leukemia Cells. *J Exp Med.,* Vol. 200, No. 5, (Sep 2004), pp. 659-969, ISSN 0022-1007.

Batista, A., Barata, J.T., Raderschall, E., Sallan, S.E., Carlesso, N., Nadler, L.M. & Cardoso, A.A. (2011). Targeting of active mTOR inhibits primary leukemia T cells and synergizes with cytotoxic drugs and signaling inhibitors. *Exp Hematol.,* Vol 39, No. 4, (Apr 2011), pp. 457-472, ISSN 0301-472X

Baylin, S.B. & Ohm, J.E. (2006). Epigenetic gene silencing in cancer - a mechanism for early oncogenic pathway addiction? *Nat Rev Cancer* , Vol. 6, No. 2, (Feb 2006), pp. 107-16, ISSN 1474-178X

Ben-Ezra, J.M., Kornstein, M.J., Grimes, M.M. & Krystal G. (1994). Small cell carcinomas of the lung express the Bcl-2 protein. *Am J Patho.,* Vol. 145, No. 5, (Nov 1994), pp. 1036-1040

Bhaumik, S. R., Smith, E. & Shilatifard, A. (2007). Covalent modifications of histones during development and disease pathogenesis. *Nature Struct. Mol. Biol.,* Vol. 14, No. 11, (Nov 2007), pp. 1008–1016

Bjornsti, M.A. & Houghton PJ. (2004). The TOR pathway: a target for cancer therapy. *Nat. Rev. Cancer,* Vol 4, No. 5, (May 2004), pp. 335-348, ISSN 1474-178X

Bolden, J.E., Peart, M.J. & Johnstone, R.W. (2006). Anticancer activities of histone deacetylase inhibitors. *Nat Rev Drug Discov.,* Vol. 5, No. 9, (Sep 2006), pp. 769-784, ISSN 1474-1776

Bonapace, L., Bornhauser, B.C., Schmitz, M., Cario, G., Ziegler, U., Niggli, F.K., Schäfer, B.W., Schrappe, M., Stanulla, M. & Bourquin, J.P. (2010). Induction of autophagy-dependent necroptosis is required for childhood acute lymphoblastic leukemia cells to overcome glucocorticoid resistance. *J Clin Invest.*, Vol 1;120, No. 4, (Apr 2010), pp. 1310-1323, ISSN 0021-9738

Brown, V.I., Hulitt, J., Fish, J., Sheen, C., Bruno, M., Xu, Q., Carroll, M., Fang, J., Teachey, D. & Grupp, S.A. (2007). Thymic stromal-derived lymphopoietin induces proliferation of pre-B leukemia and antagonizes mTOR inhibitors, suggesting a role for interleukin-7Ralpha signaling. *Cancer Res.*, Vol. 67, No. 20, (Oct 2007), pp. 9963-9970, ISSN 0008-5472

Brown, V.I., Seif, A.E., Reid, G.S., Teachey, D.T. & Grupp S.A. (2008). Novel molecular and cellular therapeutic targets in acute lymphoblastic leukemia and lymphoproliferative disease. *Immunol Res.*, Vol. 42, No. 1-3, (2008), pp. 84-105, ISSN 0257-277X

Bueso-Ramos, C., Xu, Y., McDonnell, T.J., Brisbay, S., Pierce, S., Kantarjian, H., Rosner, G. & Garcia-Manero, G. (2005). Protein expression of a triad of frequently methylated genes, p73, p57Kip2, and p15, has prognostic value in adult acute lymphocytic leukemia independently of its methylation status. *J Clin Oncol.*, Vol. 23, No. 17, (Jun 2005) pp. 3932-3939, ISSN 0732-183X

Campana, D., Coustan-Smith, E., Manabe, A., Buschle, M., Raimondi, S.C., Behm, F.G., Ashmun, R., Aricò, M., Biondi, A. & Pui CH. (1993). Prolonged survival of B-lineage acute lymphoblastic leukemia cells is accompanied by overexpression of bcl-2 protein. *Blood*, Vol. 81, No. 4, (Feb 1993), pp. 1025-1031, ISSN 0006-4971.

Case, M., Matheson, E., Minto, L., Hassan, R., Harrison, C.J., Bown, N., Bailey, S., Vormoor, J., Hall, A.G. & Irving, .JA. (2008). Mutation of genes affecting the RAS pathway is common in childhood acute lymphoblastic leukemia. *Cancer Res.*, Vol. 68, No. 16, (Aug 2008), pp. 6803-6809, ISSN 0008-5472

Cimino, G., Lo-Coco, F., Fenu, S., Travaglini, L., Finolezzi, E., Mancini, M., Nanni, M., Careddu, A., Fazi, F., Padula, F., Fiorini, R., Spiriti, M.A., Petti, M.C., Venditti, A., Amadori, S., Mandelli, F., Pelicci, P.G. & Nervi, C. (2006). Sequential valproic acid/all-trans retinoic acid treatment reprograms differentiation in refractory and high-risk acute myeloid leukemia. *Cancer Res.*, Vol. 66, No. 17, (Sep 2006), pp. 8903-8911, ISSN 0008-5472

Ciuffreda, L., Di Sanza, C., Incani, U.C. & Milella, M. (2010). The mTOR pathway: a new target in cancer therapy. *Curr Cancer Drug Targets.*, Vol. 10, No. 5, (Aug 2010), pp. 484-495, ISSN 1568-0096

Chappell, W.H., Steelman, L.S., Long, J.M., et al. (2011). Ras/Raf/MEK/ERK & PI3K/PTEN/Akt/mTOR inhibitors: rationale and importance to inhibiting these pathways in human health. *Oncotarget.*, Vol. 2, No.3 (Mar 2011), pp. 135-64.

Chen, J., Odenike, O. & Rowley J.D. (2010). Leukaemogenesis: more than mutant genes. *Nat Rev Cancer*, Vol. 10, No. 1, (Jan 2010), pp. 23-36, ISSN 1474-178X

Chen, T. (2010). Overcoming drug resistance by regulating nuclear receptors. *Advanced Drug Delivery Reviews*, Vol. 62, No. 13, (Oct 2010), pp. 1257–1264, ISSN 0169-409X

Chipuk, J.E., Moldoveanu, T., Llambi, F., Parsons, M.J. & Green DR. (2010). The BCL-2 family reunion. *Mol Cell*, Vol. 37 No. 3, (Feb 2010), pp. 299-310, ISSN 1097-2765

Coustan-Smith, E., Kitanaka, A., Pui, C.H., McNinch, L., Evans, W.E., Raimondi, S.C., Behm, F.G., Aricò, M. & Campana D. (1996) Clinical relevance of BCL-2 overexpression in childhood acute lymphoblastic leukemia. *Blood*, Vol. 87, No. 3, (Feb 1996), pp. 1140-1146, ISSN 0006-4971

Danial, N.N. & Korsmeyer S.J. (2004). Cell death: critical control points. *Cell*, Vol. 116, No. 2, (Jan 2004), pp. 205–219, ISSN 0029-8674

De Cave, F., Petrucci, M.T., Gregorj, C., et al. (2007). Protein Expression of p15 and p21 Plays an Unfavorable Prognostic Role in Adult Acute Lymphoblastic Leukemia (ALL) Patients Independently of Their Gene Promoter Methylation Status. *Blood* (ASH Annual Meeting Abstracts), (Nov 2007) 110:2802, ISSN 0006-4971

Del Gaizo Moore, V., Schlis, K.D., Sallan, S.E., Armstrong, S.A., Letai, A. (2008) BCL-2 dependence and ABT-737 sensitivity in acute lymphoblastic leukemia. *Blood*, Vol. 111, No. 4, (Feb 2008), pp. 2300-2309, ISSN 0006-4971

Faderl, S., O'Brien, S., Pui, C.H., Stock, W., Wetzler, M., Hoelzer, D. & Kantarjian, H.M. (2010). Adult acute lymphoblastic leukemia: concepts and strategies. *Cancer*, Vol. 116, No. 5, (Mar 2010) , pp. 1165-1176, ISSN 0008-543X

Fathi, A.T., Grant, S. & Karp, J.E. (2010). Exploiting cellular pathways to develop new treatment strategies for AML. *Cancer Treatment Reviews*, Vol. 36, No. 2, (Apr 2010), pp. 142–150, ISSN 0305-7372

Gandhi, L., Camidge, D.R., Ribeiro de Oliveira, M., et al. (2011). Phase I study of Navitoclax (ABT-263), a novel Bcl-2 family inhibitor, in patients with small-cell lung cancer and other solid tumors. *J Clin Oncol.*, Vol. 29, No. 7, (Mar 2011), pp. 909-916, ISSN 0732-183X

Garcia-Manero, G., Yang, H., Kuang, S.Q., O'Brien, S., Thomas, D. & Kantarjian, H. (2009). Epigenetics of acute lymphocytic leukemia. *Semin Hematol.*, Vol. 46,No. 1, (Jan 2009), pp. 24-32, ISSN 0037-1963

Gaulard, P., d'Agay, M.F., Peuchmaur, M., Brousse, N., Gisselbrecht, C., Solal-Celigny, P., Diebold, J., & Mason, D.Y. (1992). Expression of the bcl-2 gene product in follicular lymphoma. *Am J Pathol*, Vol. 140, No. 5, (May 1992), pp. 1089–1095, ISSN 0002-9440

Gibbs, K.D. Jr, Gilbert, P.M., Sachs, K., Zhao, F., Blau, H.M., Weissman, I.L., Nolan, G.P. Majeti, R. (2011). Single-cell phospho-specific flow cytometric analysis demonstrates biochemical and functional heterogeneity in human hematopoietic stem and progenitor compartments. *Blood*, Vol. 117, No 16, (Apr 2011), pp. 4226-4233, ISSN 0006-4971

Green, D.R. & Reed, J.C. (1998). Mitochondria and apoptosis. *Science*, Vol. 281, No. 5381, (Aug 1998), pp. 1309–1312, ISSN 0036-8075

Green, D.R., & Evan, G.I. (2002). A matter of life and death. *Cancer Cell*, Vol. 1, No. 1, (Feb 2002), pp. 19–30, ISSN 1535-6108

Gregorj, C., Petrucci, M.T., De Cave, F., et al. (2005). Breast Cancer Resistance Protein (BCRP) expression affects event-free survival in Adult Acute Lymphoblastic Leukemia Patients uniformly treated according to the GIMEMA LAL 2000 protocol. *Blood* (ASH Annual Meeting Abstracts), Vol. 106, (Dec 2005), 252a, ISSN 0006-4971.

Gregorj, C., Ricciardi, M.R., Petrucci, M.T., Scerpa, M.C., De Cave, F., Fazi, P., Vignetti, M., Vitale, A., Mancini, M., Cimino, G., Palmieri, S., Di Raimondo, F., Specchia, G.,

Fabbiano, F., Cantore, N., Mosna, F., Camera, A., Luppi, M., Annino, L., Miraglia, E., Fioritoni, G., Ronco, F., Meloni, G., Mandelli, F., Andreeff, M., Milella, M., Foà, R. & Tafuri, A. GIMEMA Acute Leukemia Working Party. (2007). ERK1/2 phosphorylation is an independent predictor of complete remission in newly diagnosed adult acute lymphoblastic leukemia. *Blood,* Vol. 109, No. 12, (Jun 2007), pp. 5473-5476, ISSN 0006-4971

Hanahan, D. & Weinberg, R.A. (2000). The hallmarks of cancer. *Cell,* Vol. 100, No. 1, (Jan 2000), pp. 57–70, ISSN 0092-8674

Harada, N., Hata, H., Yoshida, M., Soniki, T., Nagasaki, A., Kuribayashi, N., Kimura, T., Matsuzaki, H., & Mitsuya, H. (1998). Expression of Bcl-2 family of proteins in fresh myeloma cells. *Leukemia,* Vol.12, No. 11, (Nov 1998), pp. 1817–1820, ISSN 0987-6924

Heidari, N., Hicks, M.A. & Harada, H. (2010). GX15-070 (obatoclax) overcomes glucocorticoid resistance in acute lymphoblastic leukemia through induction of apoptosis and autophagy. *Cell Death Dis.,* (Sep 2010), 1:e76, ISSN 2041-4889

Herman, J.G. & Baylin, S.B. (2003). Gene silencing in cancer in association with promoter hypermethylation. *N Engl J Med,* Vol. 349, No. 21, (Nov 2003), pp. 2042-2054, ISSN 0028-4793

High, L.M., Szymanska, B., Wilczynska-Kalak, U., Barber, N., O'Brien, R., Khaw, S.L., Vikstrom, I.B., Roberts, A.W. & Lock, R.B. (2010). The Bcl-2 homology domain 3 mimetic ABT-737 targets the apoptotic machinery in acute lymphoblastic leukemia resulting in synergistic in vitro and in vivo interactions with established drugs. *Mol Pharmacol.,* Vol.77 , No. 3, (Mar 2010), pp. 483-494, ISSN 0026-895X

Hogarth, L.A. & Hall, A.G. (1999). Increased BAX Expression Is Associated With an Increased Risk of Relapse in Childhood Acute Lymphocytic Leukemia. *Blood,* Vol. 93, No. 8, (Apr 1999) , pp. 2671-2678, ISSN 0006-4971

Holleman, A., Cheok, M.H., den Boer, M.L., Yang, W., Veerman, A.J., Kazemier, K.M., Pei, D., Cheng, C., Pui, C.H., Relling, M.V., Janka-Schaub, G.E., Pieters, R. & Evans, W.E. (2004). Gene-expression patterns in drug-resistant acute lymphoblastic leukemia cells and response to treatment. *N Engl J Med.,* Vol. 5, No. 351(6), (Aug 2004), pp. 533-542, ISSN 0028-4793

Iacovelli, S., Ricciardi, M.R., Miele, A., Bergamo, P., Licchetta, R., Vitale, A., Testi, A.M., Petrucci, M.T., Milella, M., Foà, R. & Tafuri A. (2010). Bcl-2 and mTOR as Effective Targets for Molecular Therapy of Acute Lymphoblastic Leukemia. *Blood* (ASH Annual Meeting Abstracts), Vol. 116, (Dec 2010), 3228, ISSN 0006-4971.

Irish, J.M., Kotecha, N. & Nolan, G.P. (2006). Mapping normal and cancer cell signalling networks: towards single-cell proteomics. *Nat Rev Cancer.,* Vol. 6, No. 2, (Feb 2006), pp. 146-155, ISSN 1474-178X

Iwamoto, S., Mihara, K., Downing, J.R., Pui, C.H. & Campana, D. (2007). Mesenchymal cells regulate the response of acute lymphoblastic leukemia cells to asparaginase. *J Clin Invest.,* Vol. 117, No. 4, (Apr 2007), pp. 1049-1057, ISSN 0021-9738

Jotta, P.Y., Ganazza, M.A., Silva, A., Viana, M.B., da Silva, M.J., Zambaldi, L.J., Barata, J.T, Brandalise, S.R. & Yunes, J.A. (2010). Negative prognostic impact of PTEN mutation in pediatric T-cell acute lymphoblastic leukemia. *Leukemia,* Vol. 24, No. 1, (Jan2010), pp. 239-242, ISSN 0987-6924

Juarez, J., Baraz, R., Gaundar, S., Bradstock, K. & Bendall L. (2007). Interaction of interleukin-7 and interleukin-3 with the CXCL12-induced proliferation of B-cell progenitor acute lymphoblastic leukemia. *Haematologica.*, Vol. 92, No. 4, (Apr 2007), pp. 450-459, ISSN 0390-6078

Kankuri, E., Babusikova, O., Hlubinova, K., Salmenperä, P., Boccaccio, C., Lubitz, W., Harjula, A. & Bizik, J. (2008). Fibroblast nemosis arrests growth and induces differentiation of human leukemia cells. *Int J Cancer.*, Vol. 122, No. 6, (Mar 2008), pp. 1243-1252, ISSN 0020-7136

Kaufmann, S.H., Karp, J.E., Svingen, P.A., Krajewski, S., Burke, P.J., Gore, S.D. & Reed, J.C. (1998) Elevated Expression of the Apoptotic Regulator Mcl-1 at the Time of Leukemic Relapse. *Blood,* Vol. 91, No. 3, (Feb 1998), pp. (991-1000), ISSN 0006-4971

Klionsky, D.J. (2007). Autophagy: from phenomenology to molecular understanding in less than a decade. *Nat Rev Mol Cell Biol,* Vol. 8, No. 11, (Nov 2007) , pp. 931-937, ISSN 0270-7306

Konopleva, M.Y., Contractor, R., Tsao, T., et al. (2006) Mechanisms of apoptosis sensitivity and resistance to the BH3 mimetic ABT-737 in acute myeloid leukaemia. *Cancer Cell.*, Vol. 10, No. 5, (Nov 2006), pp. 375-388, ISSN 1535-6108

Konopleva, M.Y. & Jordan, C.T. (2011). Leukemia Stem Cells and Microenvironment: Biology and Therapeutic Targeting. *J Clin Oncol.*, Vol. 29, No. 5, (Feb 2011), pp. 591-599, ISSN 0732-183X

Kornblau, S.M., Tibes, R., Qiu, Y.H., Chen, W., Kantarjian, H.M., Andreeff, M, Coombes, K.R. & Mills, G.B. (2009). Functional proteomic profiling of AML predicts response and survival. *Blood,* Vol. 113, No. 1, (Jan 2009), pp. 154-164, ISSN 0006-4971

Kvansakul, M., Yang, H., Fairlie, W.D., Czabotar, P.E., Fischer, S.F., Perugini, M.A., Huang, D.C., & Colman, P.M. (2008). Vaccinia virus anti-apoptotic F1L is a novel Bcl-2-like domain-swapped dimer that binds a highly selective subset of BH3-containing death ligands. *Cell Death Differ.*, Vol. 15, No. 10, (Oct 2008), pp. 1564–1571, ISSN 1350-9047

Lane, A.A. & Chabner, B.A. (2009). Histone deacetylase inhibitors in cancer therapy. *J Clin Oncol,* Vol. 27, No. 32, (Nov 2009), pp. 5459–5468, ISSN 0732-183X

Lee, J.H., Choy, M.L., Ngo, L., Foster, S.S. & Marks, P.A. (2010). Histone deacetylase inhibitor induces DNA damage, which normal but not transformed cells can repair. *Proc Natl Acad Sci U S A.,*Vol. 107, No. 33, (Aug 2010), pp. 14639-14644, ISSN 0027-8424

Leiter, U., Schmid, R.M., Kaskel, P., Peter, R.U., & Krahn, G. (2000). Antiapoptotici bcl-2 and bcl-xL in advanced malignant melanoma. *Arch Dermatol Res.,* Vol. 292, No. 5, (May 2000), pp. 225–232, ISSN 0340-3696

Lessene, G., Czabotar, P.E. & Colman, P.M. (2008) BCL-2 family antagonists for cancer therapy. *Nat Rev Drug Discov.*, Vol. 7, No. 12, (Dec 2008), pp. 989-1000, ISSN 1474-1776

Letai, A., Sorcinelli, M.D., Beard, C. & Korsmeyer, S.J. (2004) Antiapoptotic BCL-2 is required for maintenance of a model leukemia. *Cancer Cell.,* Vol. 6, No. 3, (Sep 2004), pp. 241-249, ISSN 1535-6108

Levine, B. Sinha, S. & Kremer, G. (2008) Bcl-2 family members Dual regulators of apoptosis and autophagy. *Autophagy*, Vol. 4, No. 5,(Jul 2008) , pp. 600-606, ISSN 1554-8627

Levitzki, A. & Klein, S. (2010). Signal transduction therapy of cancer. *Molecular Aspects of Medicine*, Vol. 31, No. 4, (Aug 2010), pp. 287–329, ISSN 0098-2997

Levy, D.S., Kahana, J.A. & Kumar R. (2009). AKT inhibitor, GSK690693, induces growth inhibition and apoptosis in acute lymphoblastic leukemia cell lines. *Blood*, Vol.113, No. 8, (2009), pp. 1723-1729, ISSN 0006-4971

Longley, D.B. & Johnston, P.G. (2005). Molecular mechanisms of drug resistance. *J Pathol*, Vol. 205, No. 2, (Jan 2005), pp. 275-292, ISSN 0022-3417

Mantovani, I., Cappellini, A., Tazzari, P.L., Papa, V., Cocco, L. & Martelli, A.M. (2006). Caspase-dependent cleavage of 170-kDa P-glycoprotein during apoptosis of human T-lymphoblastoid CEM cells. *J Cell Physiol.*, Vol.207, No. 3, (Jun 2006), pp. 836-844, ISSN 0021-9541

Marquard, L., Poulsen, C.B., Gjerdrum, L.M., de Nully Brown, P., Christensen, I.J., Jensen, P.B., Sehested, M., Johansen, P. & Ralfkiaer, E. (2009). Histone deacetylase 1, 2, 6 and acetylated histone H4 in B- and T-cell lymphomas. *Histopathology*, Vol. 54, No. 6, (May 2009), pp. 688–698, ISSN 0309-0167

McCubrey, J.A., Steelman, L.S., Kempf, C.R., Chappell, W., Abrams, S.L., Stivala, F., Malaponte, G., Nicoletti, F., Libra, M., Bäsecke, J., Maksimovic-Ivanic, D., Mijatovic, S., Montalto, G., Cervello, M., Cocco, L. & Martelli, A.M. (2011). Therapeutic Resistance Resulting from Mutations in Raf/MEK/ERK and PI3K/PTEN/Akt/mTOR Signaling Pathways. *J Cell Physiol.* (Feb 2011), [Epub ahead of print] doi: 10.1002/jcp.22647, ISSN 0021-9541

Meng, X.W., Chandra, J., Loegering, D., Van Becelaere, K., Kottke, T.J., Gore, S.D., Karp, J.E., Sebolt-Leopold, J. & Kaufmann, S.H. (2003). Central role of Fas-associated death domain protein in apoptosis induction by the mitogen-activated protein kinase linase inhibitor CI-1040 (PD184352) in acute lymphoblastic leukemia cells in vitro. *J Biol Chem.*, Vol.278, No. 47, (Nov 2003), pp. 47326-47339, ISSN 0021-9258

Milani, L., Lundmark, A., Kiialainen, A., et al. (2010). DNA methylation for subtype classification and prediction of treatment outcome in patients with childhood acute lymphoblastic leukemia. *Blood.*, Vol.115, No. 6,(Feb 2010), pp. 1214-1225, ISSN 0006-4971.

Milella, M., Precupanu, C.M., Gregorj, C., Ricciardi, M.R., Petrucci, M.T., Kornblau, S.M., Tafuri, A. & Andreeff, M. (2005). Beyond single pathway inhibition: MEK inhibitors as a platform for the development of pharmacological combinations with synergistic anti-leukemic effects. *Curr Pharm Des.*, Vol.11, No. 21, (2005), pp. 2779-2795, ISSN 1381-6128

Molnár, J., Engi, H., Hohmann, J., Molnár, P., Deli, J., Wesolowska, O., Michalak, K. & Wang, Q. (2010). Reversal of multidrug resistance by natural substances from plants. *Curr Top Med Chem.*, Vol. 10, No. 17, (2010), pp. 1757-1768, ISSN 1568-0266

Moore N, Lyle S. Quiescent, slow-cycling stem cell populations in cancer: a review of the evidence and discussion of significance. *J Oncol.* (2011); 2011. pii: 396076.

Moreno, D.A., Scrideli, C.A., Cortez, M.A., de Paula Queiroz, R., Valera, E.T., da Silva Silveira, V., Yunes, J.A., Brandalise, S.R. & Tone, L.G. (2010). Differential expression of HDAC3, HDAC7 and HDAC9 is associated with prognosis and survival in childhood acute lymphoblastic leukaemia. *Br J Haematol.*, Vol. 150, No. 6, (Sep 2010), pp. 665-73, ISSN 0007-1048

Oltersdorf, T., Elmore, S.W., Shoemaker, A.R., et al. (2005). An inhibitor of Bcl-2 family proteins induces regression of solid tumours. *Nature*, Vol. 435, No. 7042, (Jun 2005), pp. 677-681, ISSN 0028-0836

Ottmann, O.G. & Pfeifer, H. (2009). First-line treatment of Philadelphia chromosome-positive acute lymphoblastic leukaemia in adults. *Curr Opin Oncol.*, Vol.21, (Jun 2009) Suppl 1:S43-6, ISSN 1040-8746

Petricoin, E.F. 3rd, Bichsel, V.E., Calvert, V.S., Espina, V., Winters, M., Young, L., Belluco, C., Trock, B.J., Lippman, M., Fishman, D.A., Sgroi, D.C., Munson, P.J., Esserman, L.J. & Liotta, L.A. (2005). Mapping molecular networks using proteomics: a vision for patient-tailored combination therapy. *J Clin Oncol.*, Vol. 23, No. 15, (May 2005), pp. 3614-3621 ISSN 0732-183X

Petricoin, E.F. 3rd, Espina, V., Araujo, R.P., Midura, B., Yeung, C. et al. (2007). Phosphoprotein pathway mapping: Akt/mammalian target of rapamycin activation is negatively associated with childhood rhabdomyosarcoma survival. *Cancer Res.*,Vol. 67, No. 7, (Apr 2007), pp. 3431–3440, ISSN 0008-5472

Prokop, A., Wieder, T., Sturm, I., Essmann, F., Seeger, K., Wuchter, C., Ludwig, W.D., Henze, G., Dörken, B. & Daniel, P,T. (2000) Relapse in childhood acute lymphoblastic leukemia is associated with a decrease of the Bax/Bcl-2 ratio and loss of spontaneous caspase-3 processing in vivo. *Leukemia*, Vol. 14, No.9, (Sep2000), pp. 1606-1613, ISSN 0987-6924

Reed, J.C., Cuddy, M., Slabiak, T., Croce, C.M. & Nowell, P.C. (1988). Oncogenic potential of bcl-2 demonstrated by gene transfer. *Nature*, Vol. 336, No.6196 (Nov 1988), pp. 259-261, ISSN 0028-0836

Richardson, A. & Kaye, S.B. (2008). Pharmacological inhibition of the Bcl-2 family of apoptosis regulators as cancer therapy. *Curr Mol Pharmacol.*, Vol. 1, No. 3, (Nov 2008), pp. 244-254

Rizo, A., Vellenga, E., de Haan, G. & Schuringa, J.J. (2006). Signaling pathways in self-renewing hematopoietic and leukemic stem cells: do all stem cells need a niche? *Hum Mol Genet*. Vol.15 Spec, No 2, (Nov 2006) R210-219, ISSN 0964-6906

Robinson, B.W., Behling, K.C., Gupta, M., Zhang, A.Y., Moore, J.S., Bantly, A.D., Willman, C.L., Carroll. A.J., Adamson, P.C., Barrett, J.S. & Felix, C.A. (2008). Abundant anti-apoptotic BCL-2 is a molecular target in leukaemias with t(4;11) translocation. *Br J Haematol.*, Vol. 141, No. 6, (Jun 2008), pp. 827-839, ISSN 0007-1048

Roman-Gomez, J., Jimenez-Velasco, A., Castillejo, J.A., Agirre, X., Barrios, M., Navarro, G., Molina, F.J., Calasanz, M.J., Prosper, F., Heiniger, A. & Torres, A. (2004). Promoter hypermethylation of cancer-related genes: a strong independent prognostic factor in acute lymphoblastic leukemia. *Blood*, Vol. 104, No. 5, (Oct 2004), pp. 2492-2498, ISSN 0006-4971

Romanski, A., Bacic, B., Bug, G., Pfeifer, H., Gul, H., Remiszewski, S., Hoelzer, D., Atadja, P., Ruthardt, M. & Ottmann, O.G. (2004). Use of a novel histone deacetylase inhibitor to induce apoptosis in cell lines of acute lymphoblastic leukemia. *Haematologica,* Vol. 89, No. 4, (Apr 2004), pp. 419–426, ISSN 0390-6078

Schafer, E., Irizarry, R., Negi, S., McIntyre, E., Small, D., Figueroa, M.E., Melnick, A. & Brown, P. (2010). Promoter hypermethylation in MLL-r infant acute lymphoblastic leukemia: biology and therapeutic targeting. *Blood,* Vol. 115, No. 23, (Jun 2010), pp. 4798-4809, ISSN 0006-4971

Schena, M., Larsson, L.G., Gottardi, D., Gaidano, G., Carlsson, M., Nilsson, K. & Caligaris-Cappio F. (1992) Growth- and differentiation-associated expression of bcl-2 in B-chronic lymphocytic leukemia cells. *Blood,* Vol. 79, No. 11, (Jun 1992), pp. 2981-2989, ISSN 0006-4971

Scupoli, M.T., Perbellini, O., Krampera, M., Vinante, F., Cioffi, F. & Pizzolo, G. (2007). Interleukin 7 requirement for survival of T-cell acute lymphoblastic leukemia and human thymocytes on bone marrow stroma. *Haematologica.,* Vol. 92, No. 2, (Feb 2007), pp. 264-266, ISSN 0390-6078

Scupoli, M.T., Donadelli, M., Cioffi, F., Rossi, M., Perbellini, O., Malpeli, G., Corbioli, S., Vinante, F., Krampera, M., Palmieri, M., Scarpa, A., Ariola, C., Foà, R. & Pizzolo, G. (2008). Bone marrow stromal cells and the upregulation of interleukin-8 production in human T-cell acute lymphoblastic leukemia through the CXCL12/CXCR4 axis and the NF-kappaB and JNK/AP-1 pathways. *Haematologica,* Vol. 93, No. 3, (Apr 2008), pp. 524-532, ISSN 0390-6078

Silva, A., Yunes, J.A., Cardoso, B.A., Martins, L.R., Jotta, P.Y., Abecasis, M., Nowill, A.E., Leslie, N.R., Cardoso, A.A. & Barata, J.T. (2008). PTEN posttranslational inactivation and hyperactivation of the PI3K/Akt pathway sustain primary T cell leukemia viability. *J Clin Invest.,* Vol. 118, No. 11, (Nov 2008), pp. 3762-3774, ISSN 0021-9738

Sipkins, D.A., Wei, X., Wu, J.W., Runnels, J.M., Côté, D., Means, T.K., Luster, A.D., Scadden, D.T. & Lin, C.P. (2005). In vivo imaging of specialized bone marrow endothelial microdomains for tumour engraftment. *Nature,* Vol. 435, No. 7044, (Jun 2005), pp. 969-973, ISSN 0028-0836

Stam, R.W., Den Boer, M.L., Schneider, P., de Boer, J., Hagelstein, J., Valsecchi, M.G., de Lorenzo, P., Sallan, S.E., Brady, H.J., Armstrong, S.A. & Pieters, R. (2010) Association of high-level MCL-1 expression with in vitro and in vivo prednisone resistance in MLL-rearranged infant acute lymphoblastic leukemia. *Blood,* Vol. 115, No. 5, (Feb 2010), pp. 1018-1025, ISSN 0006-4971

Steelman, L.S., Abrams, S.L., Whelan, J., Bertrand, F.E., Ludwig, D.E., Bäsecke, J., Libra, M., Stivala, F., Milella, M., Tafuri, A., Lunghi, P., Bonati, A., Martelli, A.M. & McCubrey, J.A. (2008). Contributions of the Raf/MEK/ERK, PI3K/PTEN/Akt/mTOR and Jak/STAT pathways to leukemia. *Leukemia,* Vol. 22, No. 4 (Apr 2008), pp. 686-707, ISSN 0987-6924

Steelman, L.S., Franklin, R.A., Abrams, S.L., Chappell, W., Kempf, C.R., Bäsecke, J., Stivala, F., Donia, M., Fagone, P., Nicoletti, F., Libra, M., Ruvolo P.P., Ruvolo, V., Evangelisti, C., Martelli, A.M. & McCubrey, J.A. (2011). Roles of the Ras/Raf/MEK/ERK pathway in leukemia therapy. *Leukemia,* Vol. 35, No. 7, (Apr 2011), pp. 1080-1094, ISSN 0987-6924

Stumpel, D.J., Schotte, D., Lange-Turenhout, E.A., Schneider, P., Seslija, L., de Menezes, R.X., Marquez, V.E., Pieters, R., den Boer, M.L. & Stam, R.W. (2011). Hypermethylation of specific microRNA genes in MLL-rearranged infant acute lymphoblastic leukemia: major matters at a micro scale. *Leukemia*, Vol. 25, No. 3, (Mar 2011), pp. 429-439, ISSN 0987-6924

Tabe, Y., Jin, L., Tsutsumi-Ishii, Y., Xu, Y., McQueen, T., Priebe, W., Mills, G.B., Ohsaka, A., Nagaoka, I., Andreeff, M. Konopleva, M.Y. (2007). Activation of integrin-linked kinase is a critical prosurvival pathway induced in leukemic cells by bone marrow derived stromal cells. *Cancer Res*, Vol. 67, No. 2, (Jan 2007), pp. 684-694, ISSN 0008-5472

Tafuri, A., Gregorj, C., Petrucci, M.T., et al. (2002). MDR1 protein expression is an independent predictor of complete remission in newly diagnosed adult acute lymphoblastic leukemia. *Blood*, Vol. 1, No. 100(3), (Aug 2002),pp. 974-81, ISSN 0006-4971.

Tafuri, A., Ricciardi, M.R., Gregorj, C., De Cave, F., Santinelli, S., Bergamo, P., Decandia, S., Vitale, A., Petrucci, M.T., Milella, M. & Foà, R. (2007). Effective cell killing of primary acute lymphoblastic leukemia cells by the Bcl-2 antagonist ABT-737. *Haematologica/the Hematology journal* 2007; 92[suppl. 1]:abstract n. 0015, ISSN 0390-6078

Taketani, T., Taki, T., Sugita, K., , Furuichi, Y., Ishii, E., Hanada, R., Tsuchida, M., Sugita, K., Ida, K. & Hayashi, Y. (2004) FLT3 mutations in the activation loop of tyrosine kinase domain are frequently found in infant ALL with MLL rearrangements and pediatric ALL with hyperdiploidy. *Blood*, Vol. 103, No. 3, (Feb 2004), pp. 1085–1088, ISSN 0006-4971

Tartaglia, M., Martinelli, S., Cazzaniga, G., Cordeddu, V., Iavarone, I., Spinelli, M., Palmi, C., Carta, C., Pession, A., Aricò, M., Masera, G., Basso, G., Sorcini, M., Gelb, B.D. & Biondi, A. (2004) Genetic evidence for lineage-related and differentiation stage-related contribution of somatic PTPN11 mutations to leukemogenesis in childhood acute leukemia. *Blood*, Vol. 104, No. 2, (Jul 2004), pp. 307–313, ISSN 0006-4971.

Teachey, D.T., Obzut, D.A., Axsom, K., Choi, J.K., Goldsmith, K.C., Hall, J., Hulitt, J., Manno, C.S., Maris, J.M., Rhodin, N., Sullivan, K.E., Brown, V.I. & Grupp, S.A. (2006). Rapamycin improves lymphoproliferative disease in murine autoimmune lymphoproliferative syndrome (ALPS). *Blood*, Vol. 108, No. 6, (Sep 2006), pp. 1965-1971, ISSN 0006-4971

Tortora, G., Bianco, R., Daniele, G., Ciardiello, F., McCubrey, J.A., Ricciardi, M.R., Ciuffreda, L., Cognetti, F., Tafuri, A. & Milella, M. (2007). Overcoming resistance to molecularly targeted anticancer therapies: Rational drug combinations based on EGFR and MAPK inhibition for solid tumours and haematologic malignancies. *Drug Resist Updat.*, Vol. 10, No. 3 (Jun 2007), pp. 81-100, ISSN 1368-7646

Towatari, M., Iida, H., Tanimoto, M., Iwata, H., Hamaguchi, M. & Saito, H. (1997). Constitutive activation of mitogen-activation protein kinase pathway in acute leukemic leukemia cells. *Leukemia*, Vol. 11, No. 4, (Apr 1997), pp. 479-484, ISSN 0987-6924

Trudel, S., Li, Z.H., Rauw, J., Tiedemann, R.E., Wen, X.Y. & Stewart, A.K. (2007) Preclinical studies of the pan-Bcl inhibitor obatoclax (GX015-070) in multiple myeloma. *Blood*, Vol. 109, No. 12, (Jun 2007), pp. 5430-5438, ISSN 0006-4971

Tsujimoto, Y., Cossman, J., Jaffe, E. & Croce, C.M. (1985). Involvement of the bcl-2 gene in human follicular lymphoma. *Science*, Vol. 228, No. 4706, (Jun 1985), pp. 1440-1443, ISSN 0036-8075

van Delft, M.F., Wei, A.H., Mason, K.D., Vandenberg, C.J., Chen, L., Czabotar, P.E., Willis, S.N., Scott, C.L., Day, C.L., Cory, S,, Adams, J.M., Roberts, A.W. & Huang, D.C. (2006). The BH3 mimetic ABT-737 targets selective Bcl-2 proteins and efficiently induces apoptosis via Bak/Bax if Mcl-1 is neutralized. *Cancer Cell.*, Vol. 10, No. 5, (Nov 2006), pp. 389-399, ISSN 1535-6108

van Loo, G., Saelens, X., van Gurp, M., MacFarlane, M., Martin, S.J. & Vandenabeele, P. (2002). The role of mitochondrial factors in apoptosis: a Russian roulette with more than one bullet. *Cell Death Differ*, Vol. 9, No. 10, (Oct 2002), pp. 1031-1042, ISSN 1350-9047

Veiga, J.P., Costa, L.F., Sallan, S.E., Nadler, L.M. & Cardoso, A.A. (2006)Leukemia stimulated bone marrow endothelium promotes leukemia cell survival. *Exp Hematol.*, Vol. 34, No. 5, (May 2006), pp. 610-621, ISSN 0301-472X

Wang, D., Boerner, S.A., Winkler, J.D. & LoRusso, P.M. (2007). Clinical experience of MEK inhibitors in cancer therapy. *Biochim Biophys Acta*, Vol. 1773, No. 8, (Aug 2007), pp. 1248-1255, ISSN 0167-4889

Wang, J., Chun, H.J., Wong, W., Spencer, D.M. & Lenardo, M.J. (2001). Caspase-10 is an initiator caspase in death receptor signaling. *Proc Natl Acad Sci USA*. Vol. 98, No. 24, (Nov 2001), pp. 13884-13888, ISSN 0027-8424

Wei, G., Twomey, D., Lamb, J., Schlis, K., Agarwal, J., Stam, R.W., Opferman, J.T., Sallan, S.E., den Boer, M.L., Pieters, R., Golub, T.R. & Armstrong, S.A. (2006). Gene expression-based chemical genomics identifies rapamycin as a modulator of MCL1 and glucocorticoid resistance. *Cancer Cell.*, Vol. 10, No. 4, (Oct 2006), pp. 331-342, ISSN 1535-6108

Wei, J., Wunderlich, M., Fox, C., Alvarez, S., Cigudosa, J.C., Wilhelm, J.S., Zheng, Y., Cancelas, J.A., Gu, Y., Jansen, M., Dimartino, J.F. & Mulloy, J.C. (2008). Microenvironment determines lineage fate in a human model of MLL-AF9 leukemia. *Cancer Cell.*, Vol. 13, No. 6, (Jun 2008), pp. 483-495, ISSN 1535-6108

Wilson, W.H., O'Connor, O.A., Czuczman, M.S., LaCasce, A.S., Gerecitano, J.F., Leonard, J.P., Tulpule, A., Dunleavy, K., Xiong, H., Chiu, Y.L., Cui, Y., Busman, T., Elmore, S.W., Rosenberg, S.H., Krivoshik, A.P., Enschede, S.H. & Humerickhouse, R.A. (2010). Navitoclax, a targeted high-affinity inhibitor of BCL-2, in lymphoid malignancies: a phase 1 dose-escalation study of safety, pharmacokinetics, pharmacodynamics, and antitumour activity. *Lancet Oncol.*, Vol. 11, No. 12, (Dec 2010), pp. 1149-1159, ISSN 1470-2045

Yang, H., Kadia, T., Xiao, L., Bueso-Ramos, C.E., et al.. (2009). Residual DNA methylation at remission is prognostic in adult Philadelphia chromosome-negative acute lymphocytic leukemia. *Blood*, Vol. 113, No. 9, (Feb 2009), pp. 1892-1898, ISSN 0006-4971

Zhao, W.L. (2010). Targeted therapy in T-cell malignancies: dysregulation of the cellular signaling pathways. *Leukemia*, Vol. 24, No. 1, (Jan 2010), pp. 13–21, ISSN 0987-6924

10

The Role of PAX5 in ALL

Grazia Fazio, Andrea Biondi and Giovanni Cazzaniga
Centro Ricerca M. Tettamanti, Clinica Pediatrica Università di Milano-Bicocca, Ospedale S. Gerardo - Fondazione MBBM, Monza
Italy

1. Introduction

It is now widely acknowledged that, like other cancers, acute lymphoblastic leukaemia is caused by the acquisition of mutations in somatic cells. The first hit in childhood ALL has been documented to occur in most (if not all) cases before birth (Golub, 2007). The progress in genomics technology holds the promise of making the complete characterization of the 'cancer genome' possible by a systematic search for submicroscopical mutations.

Molecular studies on recurrent chromosomal translocations in ALL have indicated that, beside the constitutive activation of tyrosine kinases, the aberrant expression of transcription factors plays a central role in the pathobiology of lymphoid leukaemia. This aberrant expression leads to abnormal proliferation and differentiation arrest of lymphoid progenitors (O'Neil & Look, 2007). In some cases, recurrent chromosomal translocations generate fusion transcription factors with new functions, enabling them to target genes other than those recognized by the endogenous factors.

In the past few years, the *PAX5* gene has been demonstrated to be a recurrent target of genetic alterations in B-lineage ALL, both in adult and paediatric patients (Mullighan et al., 2007). The role of these aberrancies in human leukemogenesis is still, however, poorly understood (Cobaleda et al., 2007a).

This chapter will review the role of *PAX5* gene involvement in B-lineage ALL to outline the biological and functional effects of different genetic aberrations affecting this new master gene in leukaemia. Moreover, we will address whether *PAX5* alterations are driver or passenger lesions and finally what their potential prognostic impact can be.

2. Role of the *PAX5* transcription factor in normal B-cell precursor development

The *PAX5* gene, located on 9p13, belongs to the paired box (*PAX*) gene family of transcription factors, essential for B lymphoid cell commitment (Cobaleda et al., 2007a). Nine mammalian PAX transcription factors have been described, but PAX5 is the only PAX protein expressed in the haematopoietic system. In addition, *PAX5* is expressed in the nervous system at the midbrain–hindbrain boundary and in adult testes.

In B-cells, PAX5 fulfils a unique function by controlling the identity of B lymphocytes throughout B-cell development, from the pro-B to the mature B-cell stage. It functions both as a transcriptional activator and as a repressor on different target genes, which are involved in lineage development (Busslinger, 2004; Matthias & Rolink, 2005).

2.1 B-cell development

Haematopoiesis is an ideal system for investigating the developmental relationships between cells of an organ system. All lineages can be reconstituted from a single bone marrow-derived haematopoietic stem cell (HSC) (Ceredig et al., 2009). According to the classical "tree model" by Weissman, (Akashi et al., 2000; Manz et al., 2002) the haematopoietic system constantly generates a large number of specialized cell types from pluripotent haematopoietic stem cells (PHSCs), which have a self-renewal potential and give rise to different progenitors with a more restricted differentiation capacity (Busslinger, 2004; Matthias & Rolink, 2005).

One of the earliest differentiated precursors is the multipotential progenitor (MPP), which is at the junction between the myeloid and lymphoid lineages. MPPs can differentiate into common myeloid progenitors (CMPs), common lymphoid progenitors (CLPs) or, as recently identified, early lymphoid progenitors (ELPs) (Matthias & Rolink, 2005).

It is generally thought that CLPs have the potential to develop into lymphoid cells (B cells, T cells and NK cells), while the CMPs differentiate either 1) into granulocyte-monocyte progenitors (GMPs), (which subsequently produce mature granulocytes (neutrophils, basophils and eosinophils) and monocyte/macrophages,) or 2) into megakaryocyte-erythrocyte progenitors (MEPs), which give rise to platelets and red erythrocytes (Akashi et al., 2000; Manz et al., 2002).

However, the idea that CLPs have exclusively lymphoid but not myeloid potential has been questioned by several studies (Akashi et al., 2000; Adolfsson et al., 2005; Balciunaite et al., 2005; Benz & Bleul, 2005). It has been suggested that immune-cell progenitors have both lymphoid and myeloid potential and a "circular model" has been proposed accordingly (Ceredig et al., 2009). These cells have been called early progenitors with lymphoid and myeloid potential (EPLMs), and they express B220, cKit (also known as CD117), IL-7 receptor α-chain (IL-7rα; also known as CD127), FLT3 (FmS-related tyrosine kinase 3, also known as CD135 and FlK2) and CD93, but do not express CD19 or NK1.1.

Indeed, *CD19* expression is completely controlled by PAX5, whose expression starts later in precursor B-cells. Research on the specific role of the *PAX5* gene in haematopoietic development has demonstrated its requirement exclusively in B-cell development. A knock out mouse model has shown a complete block in B-cell differentiation, which is immediately downstream of the block that is seen in the absence of E2A or EBF (Nutt et al., 1999). Remarkably, $PAX5^{-/-}$ pre-BI cells have extraordinary developmental plasticity showing haematopoietic stem cell features such as multipotency and a self renewing capacity (Rolink et al., 2002a). In fact, it has been reported that EPLMs resemble $PAX5^{-/-}$ pro-B cells, since they can both differentiate *in vitro* into myeloid cells (macrophages and dendritic cells), NK cells and T cells (Balciunaite et al., 2005).

The plasticity of EPLMs is greater than that of $PAX5^{-/-}$ pro-B cells because EPLMs can express *PAX5* and thereby generate B-cells. It is possible that EPLMs are a mixture of committed progenitors and their fate is directed by signals and growth factors (Ceredig et al., 2009).

Overall, these features support the key role of PAX5 in B-cell commitment and differentiation. Further details on its function will be discussed in paragraph 2.2.3.

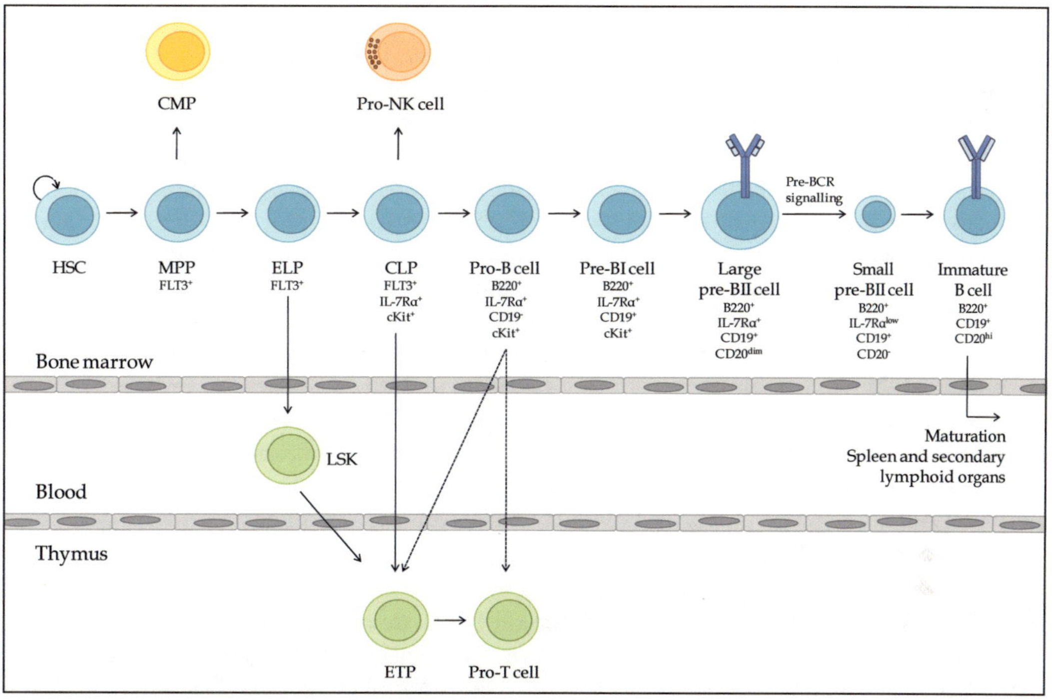

Fig. 1. B-cell development. HSC, haematopoietic stem cell; MPP, multipotential progenitor; ELP, early lymphoid progenitor; CLP, common lymphoid progenitor; CMP, common myeloid progenitor; LSK, Lin^{-} Sca^{hi} $cKit^{hi}$; ETP, early T progenitor.

Schematically, B-cell development initiates in progenitors when they start expressing the recombination-activating gene 1 (Rag1) and Rag2 and the process of rearrangement at the immunoglobulin heavy chain (IgH) locus occurs. Indeed, the stages in primary B-cell development are defined by the sequential rearrangement and expression of heavy- and light-chain immunoglobulin genes. Intermediate differentiation stages have been distinguished on the basis of the expression of other cell-surface proteins, together with direct DNA analysis of the state of the immunoglobulin gene loci (Janeway et al., 2001). More specifically, expression of the B-cell marker B220 by a subset of progenitors, known as pro-B cells, coincides with their entry into the B-cell differentiation pathway. Subsequently, CD19 is expressed and the IgH diversity (DH)-to-joining (JH) gene-segment rearrangement is completed, identifying pre-BI cells. The IgH locus then continues to rearrange its variable (V)-region gene segments until productive VH–DJH alleles are generated in large pre-BII cells. These cells cease to express Rag1 and Rag2, and they display the product of the rearranged *IgH* gene at the cell surface. There, they assemble with the surrogate immunoglobulin light chains (IgLs), VpreB and λ5, together with the signalling molecules Igα (which is encoded by the *MB-1* gene) and Igβ (which is encoded by the *B29* gene) to form a pre-B-cell receptor (pre-BCR). The expression of the pre-BCR is a crucial check-point in early B-cell development, and its signalling stimulates a proliferative clonal expansion of large pre-BII cells, which is followed by the re-expression of RAGs and rearrangement at the IgL locus in small pre-BII cells.

Once an immature B cell expresses IgM on its surface (sIgM), its fate is guided by the nature of the signals it receives through its antigen receptor. Binding to self molecules in the bone marrow can lead to the death or inactivation of immature B cells; otherwise they leave the bone marrow, enter the periphery and reach the spleen (Janeway et al., 2001). There they further differentiate through three transitional stages T1, T2 and T3, on the basis of the expression of various cell-surface markers, their short half-life (2–4 days) and their sensitivity to apoptosis induced by antibodies specific for IgM. Indeed transitional B cells can be negatively selected in the periphery. The tumour-necrosis-factor family member B-cell-activating factor (BAFF; also known as BLYS) and its receptor play a crucial role in regulating the transition of immature B cells into mature B cells (Rolink & Melchers, 2002b; Rolink et al., 2002c). Transitional, follicular and even memory B cells can give rise to marginal-zone B cells (responsible for antibody response to blood pathogens) and/or be recruited into this compartment. In mice, most mature B cells are follicular B cells. These cells are mainly responsible for generating humoral immune responses to protein antigens. With the help of T cells, they form germinal centres. Germinal-centre B cells proliferate rapidly, undergo somatic hypermutation of their immunoglobulin variable gene segments and undergo isotype-switch recombination of immunoglobulin genes. Subsequently, germinal centres slowly vanish, and memory B cells and effector plasma cells are generated (Matthias & Rolink, 2005).

2.1.1 Comparison between mouse and human B-cell development

Most of our understanding of the initiation and regulation of Ig gene rearrangements in precursor B-cell differentiation comes from studies on mouse models. Genome-wide gene expression profiling has been performed in human precursor B-cells, contributing enormously to the understanding of lymphocyte differentiation. Therefore, Van Dongen and colleagues (van Zelm et al., 2005) purified cells in the five main stages of human precursor B-cell differentiation, pro-B, pre-BI, pre-BII large and small, and immature B-cells. In correspondence with each stage, the authors characterized the IGH and IGK/IGL rearrangements independently from each other and independently from the selection processes. Altogether they have deepened the knowledge about the different stages of human B-cell development, which seems to follow mechanisms similar to that of mice.

This confirms the previous studies reviewed by Ghia (Ghia et al., 1998), in which they concluded that the main mechanisms of selection and the key events during B lymphopoiesis appear to be strikingly similar in murine and human bone marrow.

There are some differences in surface marker expression (e.g. the absence of CD10 and CD34 in mouse pre-BI cells and the absence of CD25 in human pre-BI cells) as well as different growth requirements. Human pre-BI cells are mainly unresponsive to IL-7; they can be grown only 3-4 weeks *in vitro* in presence of IL-7 and do not show a proliferative expansion comparable to mouse cells (Ghia et al., 1998).

2.1.2 Transcription factors in B-cell precursor development

The comprehension of the different stages of B-cell development is based on results from multiple levels of analysis including immunophenotype, status of immunoglobulin gene rearrangement, *in vitro* or *in vivo* cell differentiation properties (Matthias & Rolink, 2005) as well as gene-targeting studies of many regulatory molecules in mice. By these studies, B lymphopoiesis has emerged as one of the leading models for research on lineage specification (induction of a lineage-specific gene-expression program) and commitment (repression of alternative gene expression programs).

Transcription factors play a central role in this process. B-cell development, maturation and function are coordinated by a 'battery' of transcription factors and signal-transduction molecules that regulate the sequential execution of the different steps (Matthias & Rolink, 2005; Nutt & Kee, 2007).

The generation of lymphoid progenitors depends on signalling through the c-Kit, FLT3 and IL-7 receptors; in their absence, early B cell progenitors in the bone marrow are severely affected (Nutt & Kee, 2007).

In addition, developmental control of early B lymphopoiesis is exerted by a regulatory network of key transcription factors that include PU.1 (an Ets-family member), Ikaros, Bcl11a (a zinc finger transcription factor), E2A (a helixloop-helix protein), EBF (early B-cell factor) and PAX5 (Fuxa & Skok, 2007).

In particular, three transcription factors have been found to be essential for the differentiation of CLPs into specified pro-B cells: transcription factor E2A, early B-cell factor (EBF; also known as OLF1) and paired box protein 5 (PAX5; also known as BSAP). Absence of any one of these factors leads to an early block in B-cell development at the pro-B-cell or pre-B-cell stage. These three factors seem to work in collaboration, and together, they form a master control switch for engaging B-cell differentiation (Matthias & Rolink, 2005). E2A and EBF are considered primary B-cell fate determinants and co-ordinately activate the expression of B-cell specific genes (e.g. both can initiate the remodelling of MB-1 promoter chromatin) (Fuxa & Skok, 2007). In the absence of E2A or EBF, B-cell development was blocked at early progenitor stages of development, however, EBF can activate the B-cell lineage program in absence of E2A or PU.1. Conversely, in the absence of EBF, B-cell development was not rescued by enforced expression of PAX5 (Hagman & Lukin, 2006).

The ability of EBF to mediate activation of the B-cell program suggests that it has the properties of a 'pioneer' factor (i.e. a protein capable of initiating the activation of transcriptional quiescent genes) (Hagman & Lukin, 2005).

However, the mere activation of the B lymphocyte transcription program is not sufficient to commit B cell progenitors to the B lymphoid lineage in the absence of the paired domain protein PAX5 (Fuxa & Skok, 2007).

2.2 PAX5, the sentinel of B cells: identity and function

The *PAX5* gene is a member of the paired box (PAX) gene family of transcription factors and it is essential for B lymphoid lineage commitment (Morrison et al., 1998; Nutt et al., 1999; Souabni et al., 2002; Cotta et al., 2003) since it controls the identity of B lymphocytes throughout B-cell development from the pro-B to the mature B-cell stage (Busslinger, 2004; Matthias & Rolink, 2005).

This factor has been implicated in the direct transcriptional regulation of several B-cell-specific genes, such as those encoding *CD19*, *Iga* and *BLNK/SLP-65* (Matthias & Rolink, 2005).

2.2.1 Cloning of *PAX5*

PAX5 or the B-cell specific activator protein (BSAP) was independently discovered as a DNA-binding protein with the same DNA sequence specificity as the sea urchin transcription factor TSAP. Biochemical purification and cDNA cloning showed that BSAP is encoded by the *PAX5* gene and is expressed in B lymphocytes, the developing CNS, and adult testes (Cobaleda et al., 2007a).

The human *PAX5* gene is located on chromosome 9p13, is organized in 10 exons and encodes for a transcript of 8536 bp, giving rise to a coding sequence of 1176 bp, which in turn gives rise to a protein of 391 aa, a protein completely homologous to the Mus musculus *PAX5* gene. Indeed, *PAX5* retains a high degree of homology between humans and mice (Ghia et al., 1998).

2.2.2 PAX5 protein structure

PAX5 is a homeodomain protein, which is a member of a class of transcription factors that contains a DNA-binding domain with homology to Drosophila melanogaster homeodomain regulatory proteins. This DNA-binding domain contains a helix–turn–helix motif, which binds to a distinct half-site of the PAX5 recognition sequence in adjacent major grooves of the DNA helix (Cobaleda et al., 2007a).

The defining feature of the PAX protein family is the conserved 'paired' domain, which functions as a bipartite DNA-binding region consisting of an N- and a C-terminal domain. The bipartite nature of the paired domain is responsible for its degenerate consensus recognition sequence, as each half-site independently contributes to the overall affinity of a given binding site (Czerny, 1995).

The transcriptional activity of PAX5, which is responsible for regulating its target genes, is determined by the interaction of distinct partner proteins with the central and C-terminal protein interaction motifs of PAX5. The partial homeodomain of PAX5 associates with the TATA-binding protein of the basal transcription machinery, while a C-terminal transactivation domain regulates gene transcription most likely by interacting with histone acetyltransferases (HAT), such as the co-activator CBP or SAGA complex.

In parallel, PAX5 acts as a repressor, and not as a transcriptional activator, through the binding of its conserved octapeptide motif to co-repressors of the Groucho protein family, which are part of a larger histone deacetylase (HDAC) complex (Cobaleda et al., 2007a).

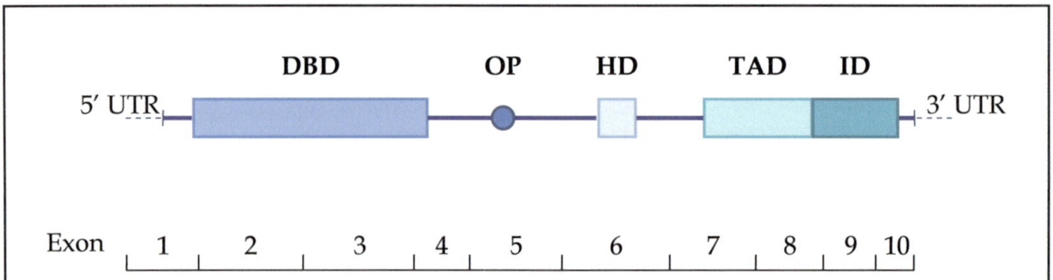

Fig. 2. PAX5 structure, showing functional domains and corresponding exons. DBD, DNA-binding paired domain; OP, conserved octapepetide; HD, partial homeodomain; TAD, transactivation domain; ID, inhibitory domain.

2.2.3 PAX5 is essential in B-cell development

PAX5 is a transcription factor and localizes in the nucleus. In the haematopoietic system it is expressed exclusively in the B-cell compartment, where it is essential for the development of the specific lineage (Matthias & Rolink, 2005; Cobaleda et al., 2007a).

The *PAX5* knock out mouse model leads to a complete block in B-cell differentiation, immediately downstream of the block that is seen in the absence of E2A or EBF (their expression is normal in $PAX5^{-/-}$ B cells) (Nutt et al., 1999). The rearrangement at the IgH locus has already been initiated (Matthias & Rolink, 2005); although DJ gene segments are rearranged normally in these cells, rearrangement of VH gene segments is severely impaired. PAX5 is required not only for rearrangement of VH gene segments and for expression of genes that are required for progression to the pre-B-cell stage but also for commitment to and maintenance of the B-cell differentiation pathway.

Both *in vitro* and *in vivo* studies have demonstrated that, in the absence of PAX5, pre-BI cells show an extraordinary degree of plasticity demonstrating multipotency and a self renewing capacity. After stimulation with the appropriate cytokines, they can in fact differentiate *in vitro* into macrophages, osteoclasts, DCs, granulocytes or NK cells. *In vivo,* however, they develop into all the lineages, even into T cells, and erythrocytes (Rolink et al., 2002a).

From these studies, PAX5 fulfils a dual role in B lineage commitment by activating B cell specific genes while simultaneously repressing lineage-inappropriate genes (Nutt et al., 1998).

More recently, Cobaleda and colleagues (Cobaleda et al., 2007b) showed that conditional *PAX5* deletion in mice allows mature B cells from peripheral lymphoid organs to de-differentiate *in vivo* back to early uncommitted progenitors in the bone marrow, which rescues T lymphopoiesis in the thymus of T-cell-deficient mice. These B-cell-derived T lymphocytes carry immunoglobulin heavy- and light-chain gene rearrangements but also participate as functional T cells in immune reactions. The mice lacking PAX5 in mature B cells in the study also developed aggressive lymphomas, which were identified by their gene expression profile as progenitor cell tumours. Hence, they concluded that the loss of PAX5, in the context of strong BCR signalling results in forward differentiation of mature B cells into plasma cells, whereas PAX5 inactivation initiates the reversal of differentiation into uncommitted progenitors, in the absence of BCR signalling.

Thus, in summary, the PAX5 protein is essentially required from pre-B cells to mature B cells, as schematically represented in Fig 1.

2.2.4 PAX5 target genes

The PAX5 transcription factor represses B lineage-inappropriate genes and activates B-cell specific genes in B lymphocytes, functioning both as a transcriptional activator and as a repressor on different target genes (Nutt et al., 1998).

While screening for PAX5-repressed genes, Delogu et al. (Delogu et al., 2006) recently estimated that PAX5 represses 44% and activates 56% of the genes, which are differentially expressed in $PAX5^{+/+}$ and $PAX5^{-/-}$ pro-B cells.

Examples of PAX5-activated genes are co-receptors CD21 (Horcher et al., 2001) and CD19 (Kozmik et al., 1992), MB-1/CD79a (Maier et al., 2003) and BLNK (Schebesta et al., 2002). PAX5-repressed genes are MCSFR (Morrison et al., 1998), NOTCH1 (Souabni et al., 2002) and FLT3 (Holmes et al., 2006). Among them, one of the most important targets is CD19, which is expressed by B lymphocytes starting from pre-BI cells and lasting to mature B cells (Horcher et al., 2001). Its expression is directly controlled by the *PAX5* gene; indeed it has been demonstrated that a sequence consensus for PD of PAX5 is present in the CD19 promoter region (Kozmik et al., 1992).

Delogu and colleagues (Delogu et al., 2006) identified 110 PAX5-repressed genes, demonstrating that PAX5 regulates diverse biological activities including receptor signalling, cell adhesion, migration, transcriptional control, and cellular metabolism during

B-cell commitment. The T lymphoid or myeloid expression of these genes demonstrates that PAX5-/- pre-BI cells and common lymphoid progenitors display lymphoid and myeloid promiscuity of gene expression. These lineage-inappropriate genes require continuous PAX5 activity for their repression because they are reactivated in committed pro-B cells and mature B cells following conditional PAX5 deletion (Cobaleda et al., 2007b).
More recently, Schebesta and colleagues (Schebesta et al., 2007) have identified 170 PAX5-activated genes, of which 66 (some, already known and some, newly identified) were further confirmed to be expressed under PAX5 control. The PAX5-activated genes code for key regulatory and structural proteins involved in B cell signalling, adhesion, migration, antigen presentation, and germinal-centre B cell formation. Thus they reveal a complex regulatory network that is activated by PAX5 to control B-cell development and function. Six PAX5-activated genes (*CD157, CD44, CD55, CD97, Sdc4,* and *Tnfrsf19*) code for cell-surface molecules, and nine genes (*Bcar3, Capn2, Eps8, Fhod3, Gsn, Myh10, Mylip, Nedd9,* and *Pard3*) code for intracellular proteins, which have been implicated in cell migration and adhesion. PAX5 has been implicated in the control of pre-BCR signalling by the previously characterized PAX5 target genes (*CD19, CD79a/Iga, BLNK,* etc...) already mentioned above. The identification of the PAX5-activated genes *Vpreb3, Igk, Slamf6, Siglecg/CD22, Lcp2, Plekha2, Prkd2, Ikzf2,* and *Spib2* has now extended the notion that PAX5 controls signalling from the pre-BCR on the cell surface to transcription in the nucleus at multiple levels. Comparing T lymphoid and myeloid genes repressed by PAX5 in a specular manner, the PAX5-activated genes require continuous PAX5 activity for normal expression in pro-B and mature B cells (conditional mutagenesis experiments). Expression of the PAX5-activated genes is either absent or significantly reduced upon PAX5 loss in plasma cells.
In conclusion, target genes that are activated by PAX5 code for essential components of pre-B- and B-cell receptor (pre-BCR and BCR, respectively) signalling pathways; and when PAX5 acts as a transcriptional repressor, its function is to limit lineage choices that differ from B cells (Fuxa & Skok, 2007). However, conditional deletion of *PAX5* in pro-B and mature B cells causes the aberrant reactivation of these repressed targets, thus creating the need for continuous repression by PAX5. Surprisingly, even at the transition to the plasma cell stage, when PAX5 is physiologically lost during terminal differentiation, repressed genes are reactivated and contribute to the plasma cell transcriptional program (Fuxa & Skok, 2007).

3. The *PAX5* gene in haematological tumours

In haematological malignancies, *PAX5* was initially described as involved in lymphomas, as a target either of mutation in diffuse large B cell lymphomas (DLBCL) (Busslinger et al., 1996) or of translocation t(9;14)(p13;q32) in non-Hodgkin's lymphoma (Lida et al., 1996).
As recently reviewed (Cobaleda et al., 2007a), in DLBCL, which are germinal-centre B-cell–derived tumours, exon 1B of *PAX5* is the target of misdirected class-switch recombination and somatic hypermutations (SHM). SHMs are essential for the affinity maturation of immunoglobulins in germinal-centre B cells, but can be potentially misdirected to generate oncogenic mutations or chromosomal translocations involved in lymphomagenesis. However, the alternatively transcribed exon 1A, as well as the second *PAX5* allele, are normally expressed; indeed they escape SHMs. The generation of the t(9;14)(p13;q32) translocation is due to a misguided class-switch recombination, which is mainly associated with aggressive B cell non-Hodgkin's lymphoma (Souabni et al., 2007). This translocation

brings one allele of the *PAX5* gene under the control of strong enhancers from the IGH locus, leading to its increased expression. The consequence is tumour formation when the PAX5-dependent gene expression program alters, due to increased *PAX5* transcription in B cells or failed *PAX5* repression at the onset of plasma cell differentiation. The human t(9;14) translocation was recently reconstructed in a knock-in mouse by inserting a *PAX5* minigene into the mouse's IgH locus. IgH-PAX5 knock-in mice develop aggressive T-lymphoblastic lymphomas, demonstrating that even the T cell lineage is particularly sensitive to the oncogenic action of PAX5 (Souabni et al., 2007).

3.1 PAX5 role in leukaemia

Abnormalities of the short arm of chromosome 9 (9p) have been described in approximately 10% of childhood ALL, with a higher incidence in T-ALL (Harrison, 2001). The majority of 9p abnormalities results in wide-spread (frequently complete) deletion of the chromosome's short arm, which usually includes the cell cycle regulatory genes *p14, p15* and *p16*. More specifically, deletions of *p16*, also known as *CDKN2A*, have been detected by molecular analysis and FISH in approximately 80% of childhood T-ALL and 20% of common-pre-B ALL.

More recently, thanks to technological improvements, a new genetic lesion has been identified on 9p, affecting the *PAX5* gene in about 30% of BCP-ALL cases (Mullighan et al., 2007), which can be considered one of the most common alterations. In addition to deletion, the *PAX5* gene has been reported as a recurrent target of mutation (about 7%) and translocation (2-3%), both in adult and in childhood B-Cell Precursor-ALL (BCP-ALL) cases with similar incidence (Familiades et al., 2009).

Both in adult and childhood cases, *PAX5* deletions seem to be secondary events, since they are frequently associated with other lesions, such as ETV6/AML1 (Mullighan et al., 2007), BCR/ABL1 or TCF3/PBX1 (Paulsson et al., 2008; Den Boer et al., 2009; Familiades et al., 2009; Iacobucci et al., 2010).

To further confirm the similar PAX5 genetic profile of adult and paediatric BCP-ALL, translocations were found in both cohorts, even with the same fusion gene, such as *PAX5/ELN, PAX5/FOXP1* and *PAX5/ETV6*, the last, being the most frequent translocation compared to the others. Details about the different cohorts and the frequency of partner genes are reported in table 1.

Although the role of these aberrancies is still poorly understood, a different biological consequence for mutations/deletions and translocations can be hypothesized.

3.1.1 Deletions, point mutations and amplifications

Deletion is the most frequent *PAX5* aberrancy, occurring in about 25% of patients. Three types of deletions have been found: a) wide-range deletions, involving the full length *PAX5* gene and flanking genes, or even the whole short arm of chromosome 9, extended over *CDKN2A-2B*; b) focal deletions involving a subset of *PAX5* exons extending to its 3' region, thus leading to a prematurely truncated gene/protein; c) focal deletions involving only a subset of internal *PAX5* exons, determining different *PAX5* isoforms lacking functional domains, such as the DNA binding domain, the octamer or the transcriptional regulatory domain. In the larger study in childhood ALL, deletions were monoallelic in 53/192 of the cases (27.6%), and among them 25 were focal (13%), while the complete *PAX5* was lost in 28 cases (14.6%); only 3/192 (1.6%) were biallelic (Mullighan et al., 2007). In addition, in the study of adult BCP-ALL, *PAX5* is target of exclusively monoallelic deletions in 27/117 cases (23.1%) (Familiades et al., 2009).

Similarly, aberrant splicing variants have been described as alternative mechanisms of deletion, both in adults and in children (Santoro et al., 2009). Different isoforms have been described, the most frequent lacking either only exon 2, causing frame shift and premature stop; or exon 5, corresponding to the octamer domain; or both exons 8 and 9 which encode the transactivation domain. In leukemic blast cells, these variants are more abundant compared to full length wild type *PAX5*, and are predicted to code for less functional or even completely non-functional PAX5 proteins.

Point mutations have been found in about 7% of both adult and paediatric cases. In childhood leukaemia cases, point mutations were hemizygous in 14/192 of the cases (7.3%) while only 1 case was homozygous (1/192, 0.5%) (Mullighan et al., 2007). A recent study reported a higher rate of *PAX5* point mutations compared to the previous investigations. Point mutations were found in 9/50 (18%) adults and in 14/50 (28%) children, showing novel sites of mutations scattered along all the exons (Santoro et al., 2009). Modelling studies using the PAX5 crystal structure suggested that point mutation should either impair DNA binding, alter transcriptional regulation, or cause frame shift, splice site, or missense mutations. A single case with an exon 1B frame shift mutation resulted in a prematurely truncated ten-residue peptide.

Altogether, point mutations are hemizygous, somatically acquired; they result in reduced expression of *PAX5* mRNA, and lost or altered DNA-binding or transcriptional regulatory function (Mullighan et al., 2007; An et al., 2008). Therefore they generate hypomorphic *PAX5* alleles with reduced gene function that could lead to haploinsufficiency.

An overview of point mutations is represented in Fig. 3.

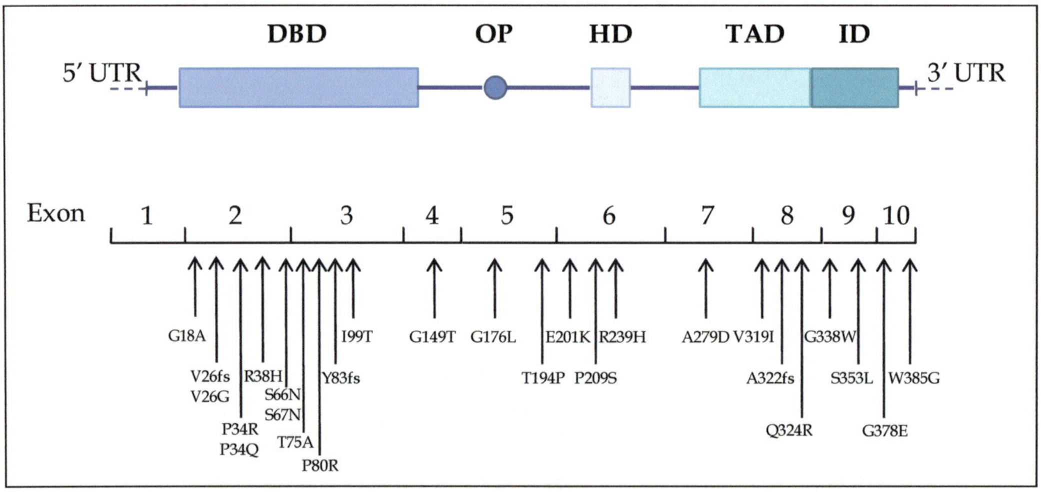

Fig. 3. *PAX5* point mutations. DBD, DNA-binding paired domain; OP, conserved octapepetide; HD, partial homeodomain; TAD, transactivation domain; ID, inhibitory domain.

Amplifications of the *PAX5* gene are less common and include: a) partial amplification, which covers a subset of internal exons (in particular from exon 2 to 5/6); b) complete amplification, which targets the full sequence of the gene (Mullighan et al., 2007; Familiades et al., 2009). It has been proposed that focal amplification of *PAX5* exons 2–5 is predicted to abolish expression of normal *PAX5* from the amplified allele, although further research is required to clarify the importance of this rare genetic lesion.

Epigenetic mechanisms have been investigated to explain lower *PAX5* gene expression, in absence of classical rearrangements (e.g. point mutations and deletions) (Mullighan et al., 2007). However, although high-levels of the *PAX5* promoter methylation were detected in T-ALL, only a minimal methylation level was observed in BCP-ALL, independently by *PAX5* mutational status.

3.1.2 *PAX5* translocations, a new promiscuous gene with several partners

While the t(9;14) translocation in lymphoma gives rise to *PAX5* de-regulated expression, in ALL, *PAX5* is involved in a growing number of chromosomal translocations with several partner genes, resulting in *in frame* fusion genes, with an estimated frequency of 2-3% in paediatric BCP-ALL (Mullighan et al., 2007; Nebral et al., 2009).

A revision of the literature is reported in Table 1.

Since the first case encoding for *PAX5/ETV6* was identified in 2001 (Cazzaniga et al., 2001), as many as 21 known partner genes have been identified in several chromosomes, although chromosomes 7, 12 and 20 are the most frequently involved, with different genes on each chromosome. Interestingly, *PAX5* genetic lesions are typically associated to dicentric chromosomes, although the breakpoint on the short arm of chromosome 9 is very heterogeneous (An et al., 2008). *PAX5* was rearranged in 54 out of 110 paediatric patients carrying a dicentric chromosome: 26/38 of the cases carrying the dic(9;12)(p11~13;p13), 24/59 positive for the dic(9;20)(p11~13;q11) and in 4/13 of the cases harbouring the dic(7;9)(p11;p11~13) (An et al., 2008). Dicentric chromosomes can coexist with established chromosomal changes, for example, dic(7;9) is found in association with t(9;22)(q34;q11) (*BCR/ABL1* fusion), and dic(9;12) occurs with t(12;21)(p13;q22) (*ETV6/RUNX1* fusion), suggesting that these events may cooperate.

A more recent study confirmed the involvement of the *PAX5* gene in dicentric chromosome events in adult and childhood BCP-ALL (Coyaud et al., 2010a). In this study, 40 patients (14 adult and 26 paediatric) harboured a dicentric chromosome involving chromosome 9 with various different partners (such as, 7, 8, 12, 15, 16, 17, 20) and as much as 90% of the cases involved *PAX5* alterations.

The various fusion genes can be classified in different sub-groups according to the molecular function of the PAX5 partner gene, which can encode either for a transcription factor (e.g. ETV6/TEL, PML, FOXP1, ZNF521/EVI3, BRD1, DACH1), for proteins related to transcription regulation (HIPK1, NCOR1), structural proteins (ELN, POM121, LOC39027, KIF3B), kinases (JAK2, TAOK1), carriers of molecules (SLCO1B3) or co-activator proteins (ASXL1). The implicated genes encode less frequently for molecules of unknown function (e.g. C20orf112, AUTS2, GOLGA6). Among this plethora of fusion genes, *PAX5/ETV6* originating from the translocation t(9;12) or dic(9;12) is the most common.

A common feature of *PAX5* translocations is that they result in the fusion of the 5′ N-terminal DNA-binding domain of PAX5 (PAX5-DBD) with the 3′ C-terminal sequences of the partner gene, whose domains therefore substitute PAX5 regulatory domains. The breakpoints are mostly located after exon 5 of *PAX5*, or after exon 4, at the end of the DBD region. Cases with a more distal *PAX5* breakpoint are less common and retain additional domains, including the highly conserved Octamer domain.

Fusion gene	Chromosomal translocation	PAX5 ex-Partner ex	n° pt	Function of partner gene	Literature Reference
PAX5/HIPK1	t(1;9)(p13;p13)	ex5-ex9	1°	*Transcriptional Regulator*	(Nebral et al., 2009)
PAX5/FOXP1	t(3;9)(p14;p13)	ex6-ex7	1°	*Transcription factor*	(Mullighan et al., 2007)
		ex5-ex12	1°		(Kawamata et al., 2008)
		ex6-ex7	2*		(Coyaud et al., 2010a)
PAX5/ELN	t(7;9)(q11;p13)	ex7-ex2	2°*	*Structural protein*	(Bousquet et al., 2007)
			1#		(Coyaud et al., 2010a)
PAX5/AUTS2	t(7;9)(q11.2;p13.2)	ex6-ex4	1°	*Unknown*	(Kawamata et al., 2008)
		ex6-ex6	1°		(Coyaud et al., 2010b)
PAX5/LOC392027	dic(7;9)(p12;p13)	ex4-ex2	1°	*Structural protein*	(An et al., 2008)
PAX5/POM121	t(7;9)(q11;p13)	ex5-ex5	1°	*Structural protein*	(Nebral et al., 2009)
		ex5-ex4	1°		(Coyaud et al., 2010a)
PAX5/JAK2	t(9;9)(p13;p24)	ex5-ex19	2°	*Kinase*	(Nebral et al., 2009)
		ex5-ex19	1°		(Coyaud et al., 2010a)
JAK2/PAX5	t(9;9)(p13;p24)	ex18-ex6	2°	*Kinase*	(Nebral et al., 2009)
PAX5/???	t(9;11)(p13;p?)	?	1°		(Nebral et al., 2009)
PAX5/ETV6	t(9;12)(q11;p13)	ex4-ex3	1*	*Transcription factor*	(Cazzaniga et al., 2001)
	dic(9;12)(p13;p13)	ex4-ex3	2°		(Strehl et al., 2003)
		ex4-ex3	2°		(Mullighan et al., 2007)
		ex4-ex3	2°		(Kawamata et al., 2008)
		ex4-ex3	7°		(An et al., 2008)
		ex4-ex2	1°		(An et al., 2008)
		ex4-ex3	3°*		(Coyaud et al., 2010a)
PAX5/SLCO1B3	dic(9;12)(p13;p12)	ex4-ex2	1°	*Solute carrier transporter*	(An et al., 2008)
PAX5/DACH1	t(9;13)(p13;q24)	ex5-ex5	1°	*Transcription factor*	(Nebral et al., 2009)
PAX5/???	t(9;14)(p13;q32)	?	1°		(Nebral et al., 2009)
PAX5/PML	t(9;15)(p13;q24)	ex6-ex2	2°	*Transcription factor*	(Nebral et al., 2007)
PAX5/GOLGA6	t(9;15)(p13;q24)	ex6-ex3	1*	*Unknown*	(Coyaud et al., 2010a)
PAX5-truncated	dic(9;16)(p13;q11)	intr5/6-?	3°#*	*Unknown partner gene*	(Coyaud et al., 2010a)
PAX5/NCoR1	t(9;17)(p13;p11)	ex5-ex43	1°	*Component of HDAC*	(Coyaud et al., 2010a)
PAX5/TAOK1	t(9;17)(p13;q11)	ex5-intr19	1°	*Kinase*	(Coyaud et al., 2010a)
PAX5-ZNF521	t(9;18)(p13;q11)	ex7-ex4	1°	*Transcription factor*	(Mullighan et al., 2007)
PAX5/C20orf112	dic(9;20)(p13;q11)	ex5-ex8	1°	*Unknown*	(Kawamata et al., 2008)
		ex8-ex3	2°		(Kawamata et al., 2008)
		ex7-ex6	1°		(An et al., 2008)
		ex8-ex8	1°		(Nebral et al., 2009)
PAX5/ASXL1	dic(9;20)(p11;q11)	ex4-ex4	1°	*Co-activator for RA receptor*	(An et al., 2008)
		3'reg-ex1/4	1°		(An et al., 2009)
PAX5/KIF3B	dic(9;20)(p13;q11)	ex7-ex6	1°	*Structural protein*	(An et al., 2008)
PAX5-trunc/PLAGL2	dic(9;20)(p13;q11)	intr6/7-ex3	1°	*Zinc-finger protein*	(Coyaud et al., 2010a)
PAX5/BRD1	t(9;22)(p13;q13)	ex5-ex1	1°	*Transcription factor*	(Nebral et al., 2009)
PAX5/DACH2	t(X;9)(q21;p13)	ex5-ex3	1°	*Transcription factor*	(Coyaud et al., 2010a)

°=paediatric patient (<16 years old) ; #=adolescent patient (16-18 years old); *=adult patient (>18 years old)

Table 1. Reported *PAX5* translocations and corresponding fusion genes.

As a further feature, *PAX5* translocations are unbalanced (An et al., 2008), and therefore the reciprocal fusion gene (5′ partner gene to 3′ *PAX5*) is not preserved, with the sole known exception of the translocation, t(9;9)(p13;p24), encoding for *PAX5/JAK2* (Nebral et al., 2009). *ETV6/TEL*, *ELN* and *FOXP1* are recurrent partner genes, independent of patient age, as well as translocation events giving rise to PAX5-truncated isoforms.

Although the biological significance of PAX5 translocations has not been elucidated yet, it has been demonstrated that patients with dicentric chromosomes carrying either a deletion or a fusion significantly under-expressed the *PAX5* gene, thus indicating that both genetic alterations can result in a similar reduced expression of wild-type *PAX5* (An et al., 2008). These data would suggest that PAX5 haploinsufficiency has a major consequence in patients. However, this is not supported by the *in vivo* studies, B-cell development being normal in heterozygous $PAX5^{+/-}$ mice (Cobaleda et al., 2007b). Moreover, inactivation of one *PAX5* allele in the absence of other oncogenic lesions is not sufficient to induce tumour development in heterozygous Cd19-cre $Pax5^{fl/-}$ mice. Instead, the complete loss of *PAX5* in B cells leads to an aggressive progenitor cell lymphoma, thus identifying *PAX5* as a tumour suppressor gene of the different B-lymphoid lineage malignancies (Cobaleda et al., 2007b).

Furthermore, even though in some cases the translocation events lead only to a truncated form of PAX5, it can be speculated that the role of PAX5 in this setting can be different from deletions or point mutations. The fusion protein could retain the functional activities of the partner genes and therefore it may alter the molecular function of the normal counterparts, affecting both the partner gene and wild type *PAX5* functions. Indeed, many of the PAX5 fusion genes have a dominant negative role on normal PAX5; in fact, in leukemic blasts, expression analysis revealed that its transcriptional targets (e.g. *EBF1, FLT3, ATP9A, ALDH1A1*) are repressed in dicentric cases, indicating a reduced activity of wild type PAX5 (An et al., 2008). Despite these data, *CD19* and *CD79a* expression (direct PAX5 targets) did not correlate with PAX5 altered status (Mullighan et al., 2007).

Comprehensively, several fundamental questions on PAX5 involvement in leukemogenesis are still unresolved. Two points remain to be understood: 1) whether these genetic alterations are responsible for the disruption of PAX5 functions, generating a haploinsufficiency setting; 2) whether these lesions are more generally responsible for the B-cell development block, through deregulation of PAX5 control, which is crucial for normal B lymphopoiesis. A more important role for fusion genes cannot be excluded, in which a gain of function could lead to cell transformation. *In vitro* and *in vivo* studies will be helpful to better elucidate the role of fusion genes.

The molecular and functional role of most relevant fusion genes will be addressed in paragraph 4.

4. Molecular and functional analysis of *PAX5* fusion genes

Although a huge amount of work has to be done to characterize the functional role of the PAX5 fusion proteins, we have revised the functional studies reported in literature to discuss the most corroborated hypothesis, that these fusion proteins could act as aberrant transcription factors, deregulating the physiological pathway of wild type PAX5, and potentially the normal function of the partner gene as well.

Since the availability of patient material is always a limiting factor, human and mouse biological *in vitro* models have been developed to make the functional investigations of PAX5 fusion proteins possible. Among the different models, a common strategy has been

employed to transiently or stably transfect cells by a plasmid that contains the sequence of a variously tagged fusion gene cloned from a patient.
Here, we focus on studies regarding *PAX5/ETV6, PAX5/FOXP1, PAX5/PML, PAX5/ELN* and *PAX5/C20orf112* fusion genes, all of which are in frame genes and are predicted to be translated into protein. These partner genes are representative of different functional classes, being transcription factors (*ETV6, FOXP1, PML*), structural proteins (*ELN*) or unknowns (*C20orf112*).
The *ETV6* (or *TEL*) gene encodes for a transcription factor with suppressor function, belonging to the highly conserved ETS family, which is fundamental for the haematopoietic system. It is widely acknowledged that it is involved in several translocations giving rise to different fusion genes in various haematological malignancies. Among them, ETV6/AML1 is the most recurrent in childhood BCP-ALL (Bohlander, 2005).
Forkhead Box P1 (FOXP1) is a member of the FOX family of evolutionarily conserved transcriptional regulators, which have a broad range of functions. *FOXP1* is widely expressed and has been shown to have a role in cardiac, lung and lymphocyte development, In mice, *FOXP1* deficiency is associated with a block in transition from pro-B cells to mature B cells. *FOXP1* is targeted by recurrent chromosome translocations and its over-expression confers a poor prognosis in a number of types of lymphomas, suggesting that it may function as an oncogene (Koon et al., 2007; Myatt & Lam, 2007).
The *Promyelocytic leukaemia* gene (*PML*) encodes for a protein which is a member of the tripartite motif (TRIM) family. The TRIM motif includes three zinc-binding domains, a RING, a B-box type 1 and a B-box type 2, and a coiled-coil region. This phosphoprotein functions as a transcription factor and tumour suppressor. The gene is often involved in translocation with the *Retinoic Acid Receptor alpha* (*RARa*) gene associated with acute promyelocytic leukaemia (APL), a relatively rare form of acute myelogenous leukaemia (AML) (Gregory & Feusner, 2009).
The *ELN* gene encodes for the protein elastin, an extracellular matrix macromolecule that imparts arterial elasticity and plays a critical role in maintaining vessel integrity and elastic properties under pulsatile flow. Elastin plays an important role in signalling and regulating luminal endothelial cells and smooth muscle cells in the arterial wall (Waterhouse et al., 2011).
The function of *C20orf112* is totally unknown; it is described as involved in translocation events, with the *RUNX1* gene in AML (Guastadisegni et al., 2010) and with the *PAX5* gene in ALL. Kawamata et al. identified two different rearrangements of *PAX5/C20orf112*, which were defined as long or short respectively, since in one case with dic(9;20), exon 5 of *PAX5* was fused to exon 8 of *C20orf112* (*PAX5/C20L*), and in the other case, with dic(9;20), exon 8 of *PAX5* was fused to exon 3 of *C20orf112* (*PAX5/C20S*) (Kawamata et al., 2008).

4.1 Sub-cellular localization, DNA binding ability and transcription activity of *PAX5* fusion genes

PAX5 encodes for a transcription factor, which by definition localizes in the nucleus and regulates several target genes through the binding of a specific consensus sequence on DNA (Delogu et al., 2006; Schebesta et al., 2007). Therefore, the first issues to be addressed are where PAX5 fusion proteins localize in the cell and whether they conserve the ability to bind DNA, with an effect on the transcription process.

By confocal analysis in transfected NIH3T3, PAX5/ELN has been demonstrated to localize exclusively in the nucleus (Bousquet et al., 2007), as we showed for PAX5/ETV6 (Fazio et al., 2008). While PAX5/ELN retains the nuclear localization signal (NLS) of wt-PAX5, this domain is not retained in the PAX/ETV6 fusion protein, but its activity could be exerted by the corresponding ETV6 NLS. By sub-cellular fractionation and western blot analysis in transfected 293T cells, it has been shown that PAX5/ETV6, PAX5/FOXP1 and PAX5/C20S were present mainly in the nucleus and less abundant in the cytoplasm, while PAX5/C20L was exclusively nuclear (Kawamata et al., 2008). In agreement with these data, fluorescent microscopic examination of transiently expressed proteins in HeLa and 293T cells demonstrated that PAX5/PML exhibited a diffuse granular pattern within the nucleus, similar to PAX5 but not to PML (Qiu et al., 2011).

To support the aberrant transcription factor activity, the DNA binding activity of PAX5 fusion genes has been assessed by a direct (through electrophoretic mobility shift assay, EMSA) or indirect (such as the luciferase reporter assay) binding measure. Kawamata demonstrated the specific binding for PAX5/ETV6, PAX5/FOXP1 and PAX5/C20orf112 in parallel to wild type PAX5 (Kawamata et al., 2008). In an analogous setting, it has been demonstrated that PAX5/PML is able to bind to PAX5-responsive elements (Qiu et al., 2011). A formal demonstration of DNA binding by PAX5/ELN is missing in literature, although the transcriptional activity of *PAX5* fusion genes, including the PAX5/ELN, has been proven by reporter gene assays (Bousquet et al., 2007; Mullighan et al., 2007; Kawamata et al., 2008; Kurahashi et al., 2011; Qiu et al., 2011).

4.2 Fusion genes have a dominant effect on wild type PAX5

The PAX5 fusion proteins herewith described retained the DNA-binding domain of PAX5 but substituted its regulatory domains with those of the partner gene, which are mostly responsible for transcription regulation.

PAX5/ETV6 fusion merits a special focus for the central role of the *ETV6/TEL* partner gene in onco-haematology, and because PAX5/ETV6 is the most common PAX5 translocation.

We previously showed that PAX5/ETV6 maintains the transcriptional activity common to both partner genes and it is responsible for the down-regulation of key PAX5-targets, such as *CD19, BLNK/SLP-65* and *MB-1/CD79a* through recruitment of the mSIN3a co-repressor (Fazio et al., 2008). We investigated PAX5/ETV6 function through gene expression profile (GEP) analysis by stable transduction of the PAX5/ETV6 construct in wild type (wt) pre-BI cells, a primary culture of immature B-cells (cKit+/B220+/CD19+) from mouse fetal liver, which express the endogenous wild type PAX5 protein (Fazio et al., 2008). GEP analysis defined a PAX5/ETV6 specific signature, indicating that PAX5/ETV6 acts mainly as a repressor of transcription but, surprisingly, the fusion protein was also able to activate transcription. Among DEGs we identified a reliable number of genes (7%) known to be direct transcriptional targets of PAX5 (Delogu et al., 2006; Schebesta et al., 2007). These results strongly suggest that PAX5/ETV6 primarily affects the PAX5 transcriptional pathway by repressing PAX5-target genes normally activated by wt PAX5 and by up-regulating genes known to be PAX5 wt-repressed. This supports a dual function for PAX5/ETV6 on transcription, which is mainly a repressor but also to a lesser extent, an activator. Therefore, PAX5/ETV6 does not exert a canonical "*dominant negative*" effect on the endogenous protein whilst it does have an "*opposite dominant*" function on wt PAX5 (Fazio et al., 2010).

A canonical *dominant negative* effect of fusion over wt PAX5 was demonstrated for PAX5/ELN, PAX5/FOXP1, PAX5/PML and PAX5/C20orf112. As in the context of PAX5/ETV6, various PAX5 transcriptional targets are repressed by PAX5 fusion proteins, such as *CD19, MB-1/CD79a, BLNK, NEDD9, NEDD5, ATP1B1, TCF7L2,* resulting in reduced PAX5 wild type activity.
Certainly, the molecular mechanism through which repression is achieved includes the competition for binding the consensus sequence on DNA between wt PAX5 and its fusion protein. A novel insight has been provided by the study on PAX5/PML (Qiu et al., 2011), in which they showed that PAX5/PML forms homodimer to bind the PAX5 consensus sequence through the Coiled-Coiled (CC) domain of PML. Furthermore, PAX5/PML can form complexes with PAX5/PML as well as wild-type PML. The intranuclear mobility of PAX5/PML is decreased compared with wild-type PAX5, in analogy to other fusion proteins in leukaemia, such as PML/RARα and AML1/ETO (Dong & Blobe, 2006; Qiu et al., 2011).
Since other PAX5 fusion proteins from ALL patients such as PAX5/FOXP1 and PAX5/EVT6 maintain the dimerization motif of the PAX5 partner, the aberrant molecular mechanism proposed for PAX5/PML can be valid for other *PAX5* fusion genes as well.

4.3 Functional consequences of *PAX5* fusion genes on cellular processes in precursor B cells

Preliminary results indicate that the wt PAX5 protein is present at lower levels in cells positive for translocation (An et al., 2008). In patients with PAX5 translocation, we see that one *PAX5* allele is involved in the translocation event, while the second allele could be partially repressed and also hindered by the fusion protein in its function, by competition and by dynamic deregulation of target genes. Moreover, *PAX5* mutations result in reduced levels of PAX5 protein and corresponding activity (Mullighan et al., 2007).
In the B-cell context, the biological consequences of decreased normal PAX5 function plus the opposite dominance of the fusion protein could be various.
A pathway analysis of GEP results revealed the involvement of several cellular processes, specifically: B-Cell Receptor assembly and B-cell maturation, cell adhesion and migration (our unpublished observations). PAX5/ETV6 cells are impaired to complete the IgM rearrangement, and consequently the precursor B cells are immature and unable to complete the differentiation process (Mullighan et al., 2007; Fazio et al., 2008). This could be due to the direct down-regulation of pre-BCR components, such as the μ chain itself, Igα/MB-1, and BLNK/SLP-65. This incapacity to express a pre-BCR on the cell surface has already been demonstrated in primary leukemic ALL blast cells, in the presence of the BCR/ABL1 fusion gene (Trageser et al., 2009). It is possible to speculate that the survival of precursor B cells carrying a *PAX5* fusion gene could be guaranteed by alternative signalling pathways.
Overall, these data suggest that PAX5 behaves like a tumour suppressor in early B cells, and that impairment of its function can be associated with the development of ALL (Kawamata et al., 2008).

4.4 Future perspective of functional studies

Preliminary results indicate that PAX5/ETV6 cells have a significant advantage over *in vitro* migration to CXCL12 (Fazio et al., 2008). In humans, cells with aberrant PAX5 could therefore have a greater ability to aggressively infiltrate CXCL12-secreting tissues and organs, and thus proliferate and survive better, as described in several tumours (Burger & Burkle, 2007).

In the near future, the *in vivo* mouse models will be crucial for studying the role of translocation on leukemogenesis. Currently, the xenotransplantation of human primary patient cells into immune-deficient mice is the 'gold standard' assay to identify human leukemic stem cells and functionally assess their tumorigenicity *in vivo*. The availability of primary samples from patients carrying a *PAX5* fusion gene will shed light on the human setting.

Among the main questions in leukaemia research is how and in what temporal sequence the genetic lesions lead to abnormal proliferation and differentiation arrest of lymphoid progenitors.

Beside a dissection of the role of PAX5 translocations in leukaemia, several additional questions on PAX5 aberrancies in ALL are still unresolved, namely:

- Are PAX5 translocations responsible for blocking B-cell development?
- Are PAX5 translocations per se sufficient in leukemogenesis?

5. Are PAX5 alterations driver or passenger lesions?

Studies on ALL patients and/or *in vitro* models concentrated the efforts to understand whether PAX5 alterations are part of a complex scenario of cooperating genetic lesions or whether they are a unique genetic aberration event that drives leukemogenesis.

Patients carrying *PAX5* deletion have a more complex karyotype than patients with translocation or dicentric chromosomes. Frequently, classical deletion events or dicentric chromosomes giving rise to prematurely truncated PAX5 transcripts have been described as co-existing in leukemic blast cells together with other PAX5-unrelated genetic lesions, such as *ETV6/AML1* (Mullighan et al., 2007), *BCR/ABL1* and *TCF3/PBX1* fusion genes (Paulsson et al., 2008; Den Boer et al., 2009; Familiades et al., 2009; Iacobucci et al., 2010). This observation led us to hypothesize that there is a cooperative role for *PAX5* deletions over the main genetic lesion. Similarly to micro-deletions on fundamental genes in haematopoiesis (such as *IKZF1, EBF1, TCF3, LEF1*) (Mullighan et al., 2007; Paulsson et al., 2008), *PAX5* aberrancies can contribute to blocking cell development in B cell precursors, as reflected in the mouse model of homozygous *PAX5* deletion, which is characterized by complete blockage at an early stage of differentiation (Nutt et al., 1999).

By contrast, patients with *PAX5* fusion genes (as a consequence of translocations) were mainly reported as negative for the most common genetic aberrations found in childhood (Nebral et al., 2009; Coyaud et al., 2010a).

A high resolution Copy Number Abnormality (CNA) analysis on diagnostic samples with *PAX5* fusion genes revealed that in both childhood and adult ALL, PAX5-translocated cases have a simple karyotype (Coyaud et al., 2010a), with a mean of only three lesions in addition to the translocation event itself (our unpublished observation).

In conclusion, it becomes evident that PAX5 translocations giving rise to fusion genes have a completely different impact on the biology and development of leukaemia compared to *PAX5* deletions. It can be argued that gene fusions occur early, whereas deletions can be regarded as a late/secondary event (Coyaud et al., 2010a). We can therefore presume that *PAX5* fusion genes are driver genetic lesions, whereas *PAX5* deletions can be a cooperative aberrancy, which require further alteration to determine the disease.

The final word on the real impact of PAX5 alterations will come in the near future from robust functional studies, including the development of an appropriate *in vivo* leukemogenesis model.

6. Are PAX5 alterations associated to prognosis and/or outcome? Is PAX5 a new target for leukaemia treatment?

Although the frequency and the molecular nature of PAX5 aberrancies are analogous, the complexity and biological differences between adult and childhood B-ALL may reflect another example of the importance of PAX5 alterations on the disease course.

Gene expression profiling (GEP) of childhood ALL has identified a genetic subtype of childhood ALL with a poor outcome, that clusters close to the subgroup characterized by the *BCR/ABL* fusion gene (thus called '*BCR/ABL* like'). Patients in this group carry mutations in genes that are fundamental in B-cell development, such as *IKZF1, PAX5, VPREB1, TCF3, EBF1* and pre-BCR (Den Boer et al., 2009; Mullighan et al., 2009).

A study by Mullighan et al. showed that *PAX5* abnormalities were not associated with an unfavourable prognosis, in contrast to the *BCR/ABL*-like subtype (Mullighan et al., 2007). Deletions in the *BCR/ABL*-like group not only affect the *PAX5* gene locus but often include larger regions on chromosome 9p and other genes involved in B-cell development. This suggests that the *BCR/ABL*-like group does not exactly overlap with the subgroup of BCP-ALL patients carrying exclusively *PAX5* abnormalities.

A genome-wide DNA copy number analysis on matched diagnosis and relapse samples from paediatric patients with ALL detected an increasing number of additional regions of deletion at relapse, including the *PAX5* and *IKZF1* genes. This suggests that genomic abnormalities contributing to ALL relapse, including *PAX5* alterations, are selected during treatment, paving the way for designing a new therapeutic intervention to target these abnormalities (Mullighan et al., 2008).

Even in adult ALL, *PAX5* alterations are not associated to outcome (Familiades et al., 2009), except for a reported trend toward a higher incidence of relapse in the structural mutant PAX5 subgroup.

Indeed, deletions of *PAX5* were not significantly correlated with overall survival, disease-free survival or cumulative incidence of relapse in BCR/ABL1-positive ALL adult cases treated with conventional or investigational therapy including TKI (imatinib or dasatinib) (Iacobucci et al., 2010).

In conclusion, the state of the art on PAX5 alterations and prognosis gives evidence that no significant correlation exists in paediatric or in adult BCP-ALL. Nevertheless, considering the biology of the different subgroups of genetic lesions (point mutations vs. deletions vs. translocations), we cannot completely exclude the possibility that the sole translocation event may have a different significance and influence on the clinical course of the disease, although the limited number of cases in the reported studies hamper a statistically significant analysis.

We need further clinical data to show whether PAX5 could be a new target for leukaemia treatment, and to inspire the design of a strategy to target the molecule itself or to interfere with its aberrant activity.

7. Conclusion

The *PAX5* gene, encoding for a transcription factor fundamental for B-cell development, is the most recurrent target of genetic lesions in BCP-ALL disease, both in the adult and paediatric population. Its alterations are a hallmark which defines a new molecular subgroup of patients.

Although in general, PAX5 translocations do not influence the prognosis or outcome by themselves but in association to other molecular aberrancies, we can hypothesize that they could play a different role from deletions and point mutations.
Further clinical investigations are needed to assess the real impact of PAX5 alterations on disease progress. In parallel, we believe that *in vitro* and *in vivo* models will help to clarify the biological basis of leukemogenesis driven by PAX5, especially in presence of its fusion genes.
If we are able to fill these biological and clinical gaps, we could recognize the altered PAX5 molecule as a novel target to hit, with the final purpose of eradicating leukaemia.

8. Acknowledgements

We are grateful to Chiara Palmi and Valeria Cazzaniga (Centro Ricerca Tettamanti, Monza) for their collaboration in the experimental work and their continuously stimulating discussion; to Anna Leszl (Padova) and Tiziana Storlazzi (Bari) for detailed cytogenetics and FISH studies; to Antonius Rolink for sharing his vast experience on PAX5 and for providing valuable *in vitro* models; to physicians, nurses and patients from the Italian Association of Pediatric Hemato-Oncology (AIEOP). Our research was supported by grants from the Italian Association for Cancer Research (AIRC), Fondazione Cariplo, the Italian Ministry for Health and the Italian Ministry for University and Research.

9. References

Adolfsson, J., Mansson, R., Buza-Vidas, N., Hultquist, A., Liuba, K., Jensen, C. T., Bryder, D., Yang, L., Borge, O. J., Thoren, L. A., Anderson, K., Sitnicka, E., Sasaki, Y., Sigvardsson, M. & Jacobsen, S. E. (2005). Identification of Flt3+ lympho-myeloid stem cells lacking erythro-megakaryocytic potential a revised road map for adult blood lineage commitment. *Cell*, 121,(2): 295-306.

Akashi, K., Traver, D., Miyamoto, T. & Weissman, I. L. (2000). A clonogenic common myeloid progenitor that gives rise to all myeloid lineages. *Nature*, 404,(6774): 193-197.

An, Q., Wright, S. L., Konn, Z. J., Matheson, E., Minto, L., Moorman, A. V., Parker, H., Griffiths, M., Ross, F. M., Davies, T., Hall, A. G., Harrison, C. J., Irving, J. A. & Strefford, J. C. (2008). Variable breakpoints target PAX5 in patients with dicentric chromosomes: a model for the basis of unbalanced translocations in cancer. *Proc Natl Acad Sci U S A*, 105,(44): 17050-17054.

An, Q., Wright, S. L., Moorman, A. V., Parker, H., Griffiths, M., Ross, F. M., Davies, T., Harrison, C. J. & Strefford, J. C. (2009). Heterogeneous breakpoints in patients with acute lymphoblastic leukemia and the dic(9;20)(p11-13;q11) show recurrent involvement of genes at 20q11.21. *Haematologica*, 94,(8): 1164-1169.

Balciunaite, G., Ceredig, R., Massa, S. & Rolink, A. G. (2005). A B220+ CD117+ CD19- hematopoietic progenitor with potent lymphoid and myeloid developmental potential. *Eur. J. Immunol. 2005*, 35,(2019-2030.

Benz, C. & Bleul, C. C. (2005). A multipotent precursor in the thymus maps to the branching point of the T versus B lineage decision. *J Exp Med*, 202,(1): 21-31.

Bohlander, S. K. (2005). ETV6: a versatile player in leukemogenesis. *Semin Cancer Biol*, 15,(3): 162-174.

Bousquet, M., Broccardo, C., Quelen, C., Meggetto, F., Kuhlein, E., Delsol, G., Dastugue, N. & Brousset, P. (2007). A novel PAX5-ELN fusion protein identified in B-cell acute lymphoblastic leukemia acts as a dominant negative on the wild type PAX5. *Blood,* 109,(8): 3417-3423.

Burger, J. A. & Burkle, A. (2007). The CXCR4 chemokine receptor in acute and chronic leukemia: a marrow homing receptor and potential therapeutic target. *British Journal of Haematology,* 137,(288-296.

Busslinger, M., Klix, N., Pfeffer, P., Graninger, P. G. & Kozmik, Z. (1996). Deregulation of PAX-5 by translocation of the Em enhancer of the IgH locus adjacent to two alternative PAX-5 promoters in a diffuse large-cell lymphoma. *Proc. Natl. Acad. Sci. USA,* 93, 6129-6134.

Busslinger, M. (2004). Transcriptional control of early B cell development. *Annu. Rev. Immunol.,* 22, 55-79.

Cazzaniga, G., Daniotti, M., Tosi, S., Giudici, G., Aloisi, A., Pogliani, E., Kearney, L. & Biondi, A. (2001). The paired box domain gene PAX5 is fused to ETV6/TEL in an acute lymphoblastic leukemia case. *Cancer Res,* 61,(12): 4666-4670.

Ceredig, R., Rolink, A. G. & Brown, G. (2009). Models of haematopoiesis: seeing the wood for the trees. *Nat Rev Immunol,* 9,(4): 293-300.

Cobaleda, C., Schebesta, A., Delogu, A. & Busslinger, M. (2007a). Pax5: the guardian of B cell identity and function. *Nature Immunology,* 8,(5): 463-470.

Cobaleda, C., Jochum, W. & M., B. (2007b). Conversion of mature B cells into T cells by dedifferentiation to uncommitted progenitors. *Nature,* 449,(473-479.

Cotta, C. V., Zhang, Z., Kim, H. G. & Klug, C. A. (2003). Pax5 determines B- versus T-cell fate and does not block early myeloid-lineage development. *Blood,* 101,(11): 4342-4346.

Coyaud, E., Struski, S., Prade, N., Familiades, J., Eichner, R., Quelen, C., Bousquet, M., Mugneret, F., Talmant, P., Pages, M. P., Lefebvre, C., Penther, D., Lippert, E., Nadal, N., Taviaux, S., Poppe, B., Luquet, I., Baranger, L., Eclache, V., Radford, I., Barin, C., Mozziconacci, M. J., Lafage-Pochitaloff, M., Antoine-Poirel, H., Charrin, C., Perot, C., Terre, C., Brousset, P., Dastugue, N. & Broccardo, C. (2010a). Wide diversity of PAX5 alterations in B-ALL: a Groupe Francophone de Cytogenetique Hematologique study. *Blood,* 115,(15): 3089-3097.

Coyaud, E., Struski, S., Dastugue, N., Brousset, P., Broccardo, C. & Bradtke, J. (2010b). PAX5-AUTS2 fusion resulting from t(7;9)(q11.2;p13.2) can now be classified as recurrent in B cell acute lymphoblastic leukemia. *Leuk Res,* 34,(12): e323-325.

Czerny, T. B. M. (1995). DNA-Binding and Transactivation Properties of Pax-6: Three Amino Acids in the Paired Domain Are Responsible for the Different Sequence Recognition of Pax-6 and BSAP (Pax-5). *Molecular and Cellular Biology,* 15,(5): 2858-2871.

Delogu, A., Schebesta, A., Sun, Q., Aschenbrenner, K., Perlot, T. & Busslinger, M. (2006). Gene repression by Pax5 in B cells is essential for blood cell homeostasis and is reversed in plasma cells. *Immunity,* 24,(3): 269-281.

Den Boer, M. L., van Slegtenhorst, M., De Menezes, R. X., Cheok, M. H., Buijs-Gladdines, J. G., Peters, S. T., Van Zutven, L. J., Beverloo, H. B., Van der Spek, P. J., Escherich, G., Horstmann, M. A., Janka-Schaub, G. E., Kamps, W. A., Evans, W. E. & Pieters, R.

(2009). A subtype of childhood acute lymphoblastic leukaemia with poor treatment outcome: a genome-wide classification study. *Lancet Oncol*, 10,(2): 125-134.

Dong, M. & Blobe, G. C. (2006). Role of transforming growth factor-beta in hematologic malignancies. *Blood*, 107,(12): 4589-4596.

Familiades, J., Bousquet, M., Lafage-Pochitaloff, M., Bene, M. C., Beldjord, K., De Vos, J., Dastugue, N., Coyaud, E., Struski, S., Quelen, C., Prade-Houdellier, N., Dobbelstein, S., Cayuela, J. M., Soulier, J., Grardel, N., Preudhomme, C., Cave, H., Blanchet, O., Lheritier, V., Delannoy, A., Chalandon, Y., Ifrah, N., Pigneux, A., Brousset, P., Macintyre, E. A., Huguet, F., Dombret, H., Broccardo, C. & Delabesse, E. (2009). PAX5 mutations occur frequently in adult B-cell progenitor acute lymphoblastic leukemia and PAX5 haploinsufficiency is associated with BCR-ABL1 and TCF3-PBX1 fusion genes: a GRAALL study. *Leukemia*, 23,(11): 1989-1998.

Fazio, G., Palmi, C., Rolink, A., Biondi, A. & Cazzaniga, G. (2008). PAX5/TEL acts as a transcriptional repressor causing down-modulation of CD19, enhances migration to CXCL12, and confers survival advantage in pre-BI cells. *Cancer Res*, 68,(1): 181-189.

Fazio, G., Cazzaniga, V., Palmi, C., Galbiati, M., Giordan, M., te Kronnie, G., Rolink, A., Biondi, A. & Cazzaniga, G. (2010). PAX5/TEL has an opposite dominant effect on endogenous PAX5, affecting its transcriptional regulation, B cell adhesion and BCR signalling in murine pre-BI cells. *Proceedings of American Society for Hematology (ASH) – 52nd Congress, Orlando, Florida, USA. Blood,* 116(11))#2482.

Fuxa, M. & Skok, J. A. (2007). Transcriptional regulation in early B cell development. *Current Opinion in Immunology*, 19, 129-136.

Ghia, P., ten Boekel, E., Rolink, A. G. & Melchers, F. (1998). B-cell development: a comparison between mouse and man. *Immunol Today*, 19,(10): 480-485.

Golub, T. R. (2007). Global views of leukaemia. *Nature*, 446, 739-740.

Gregory, J. & Feusner, J. (2009). Acute promyelocytic leukemia in childhood. *Curr Oncol Rep*, 11,(6): 439-445.

Guastadisegni, M. C., Lonoce, A., Impera, L., Di Terlizzi, F., Fugazza, G., Aliano, S., Grasso, R., Cluzeau, T., Raynaud, S., Rocchi, M. & Storlazzi, C. T. (2010). CBFA2T2 and C20orf112: two novel fusion partners of RUNX1 in acute myeloid leukemia. *Leukemia*, 24,(8): 1516-1519.

Hagman, J. & Lukin, K. (2005). Early B-cell factor 'pioneers' the way for B-cell development. *Trends Immunol*, 26,(9): 455-461.

Hagman, J. & Lukin, K. (2006). Transcription factors drive B cell development. *Current Opinion in Immunology*, 18, 127-134.

Harrison, C. J. (2001). Acute lymphoblastic leukaemia. *Best Practice & Research Clinical Haematology*, 14,(3): 593-607.

Holmes, M. L., Carotta, S., Corcoran, L. M. & Nutt, S. L. (2006). Repression of Flt3 by Pax5 is crucial for B-cell lineage commitment. *Genes Dev*, 20,(8): 933-938.

Horcher, M., Souabni, A. & Busslinger, M. (2001). Pax5/BSAP Maintains the Identity of B Cells in Late B Lymphopoiesis. *Immunity*, 14,(779-790.

Iacobucci, I., Lonetti, A., Paoloni, F., Papayannidis, C., Ferrari, A., Storlazzi, C. T., Vignetti, M., Cilloni, D., Messa, F., Guadagnuolo, V., Paolini, S., Elia, L., Messina, M., Vitale, A., Meloni, G., Soverini, S., Pane, F., Baccarani, M., Foa, R. & Martinelli, G. (2010). The PAX5 gene is frequently rearranged in BCR-ABL1-positive acute lymphoblastic leukemia but is not associated with outcome. A report on behalf of the GIMEMA Acute Leukemia Working Party. *Haematologica*, 95,(10): 1683-1690.

Janeway, C. A. J., Travers, P., Walport, M. & Shlomchik, M. J. (2001). Immunobiology. The Immune System in Health and Disease. New York, Garland Science.

Kawamata, N., Ogawa, S., Zimmermann, M., Kato, M., Sanada, M., Hemminki, K., Yamatomo, G., Nannya, Y., Koehler, R., Flohr, T., Miller, C. W., Harbott, J., Ludwig, W. D., Stanulla, M., Schrappe, M., Bartram, C. R. & Koeffler, H. P. (2008). Molecular allelokaryotyping of pediatric acute lymphoblastic leukemias by high-resolution single nucleotide polymorphism oligonucleotide genomic microarray. *Blood*, 111,(2): 776-784.

Koon, H. B., Ippolito, G. C., Banham, A. H. & Tucker, P. W. (2007). FOXP1: a potential therapeutic target in cancer. *Expert Opin Ther Targets*, 11,(7): 955-965.

Kozmik, Z., Wang, S., Dorfler, P., Adams, B. & Busslinger, M. (1992). The Promoter of the CD19 Gene Is a Target for the B-Cell-Specific Transcription Factor BSAP. *Molecular and Cellular Biology*, 12,(6): 2662-2672.

Kurahashi, S., Hayakawa, F., Miyata, Y., Yasuda, T., Minami, Y., Tsuzuki, S., Abe, A. & Naoe, T. (2011). PAX5-PML acts as a dual dominant-negative form of both PAX5 and PML. *Oncogene*, 30,(15): 1822-1830.

Lida, S., Rao, P., Nallasivam, P., Hibshoosh, H., Butler, M., Louie, D., Dyomin, V., Ohno, H., Chaganti, R. & Dalla-Favera, R. (1996). The t(9;14)(p13;q32) Chromosomal Translocation Associated With Lymphoplasmacytoid Lymphoma Involves the PAX-5 Gene. *Blood*, 88,(11): 4110-4117.

Maier, H., Ostraat, R., Parenti, S., Fitzsimmons, D., Abraham, L. J., Garvie, C. W. & Hagman, J. (2003). Requirements for selective recruitment of Ets proteins and activation of mb-1/Ig-a gene transcription by Pax-5 (BSAP). *Nucleic Acids Research*, 31,(19): 5483-5489.

Manz, M. G., Miyamoto, T., Akashi, K. & Weissman, I. L. (2002). Prospective isolation of human clonogenic common myeloid progenitors. *Proc Natl Acad Sci U S A*, 99,(18): 11872-11877.

Matthias, P. & Rolink, A. G. (2005). Transcriptional Networks In Developing And Mature B Cells. *Nature Reviews*, 5, 497-508.

Morrison, A. M., Nutt, S. L., Thevenin, C., Rolink, A. & Busslinger, M. (1998). Loss- and gain-of-function mutations reveal an important role of BSAP (Pax-5) at the start and end of B cell differentiation. *Semin Immunol*, 10,(2): 133-142.

Mullighan, C. G., Goorha, S., Radtke, I., Miller, C. B., Coustan-Smith, E., Dalton, J. D., Girtman, K., Mathew, S., Ma, J., Pounds, S. B., Su, X., Pui, C. H., Relling, M. V., Evans, W. E., Shurtleff, S. A. & Downing, J. R. (2007). Genome-wide analysis of genetic alterations in acute lymphoblastic leukaemia. *Nature*, 446,(7137): 758-764.

Mullighan, C. G., Phillips, L. A., Su, X., Ma, J., Miller, C. B., Shurtleff, S. A. & Downing, J. R. (2008). Genomic analysis of the clonal origins of relapsed acute lymphoblastic leukemia. *Science*, 322,(5906): 1377-1380.

Mullighan, C. G., Su, X., Zhang, J., Radtke, I., Phillips, L. A., Miller, C. B., Ma, J., Liu, W., Cheng, C., Schulman, B. A., Harvey, R. C., Chen, I. M., Clifford, R. J., Carroll, W. L., Reaman, G., Bowman, W. P., Devidas, M., Gerhard, D. S., Yang, W., Relling, M. V., Shurtleff, S. A., Campana, D., Borowitz, M. J., Pui, C. H., Smith, M., Hunger, S. P.,

Willman, C. L. & Downing, J. R. (2009). Deletion of IKZF1 and prognosis in acute lymphoblastic leukemia. *N Engl J Med*, 360,(5): 470-480.

Myatt, S. S. & Lam, E. W. (2007). The emerging roles of forkhead box (Fox) proteins in cancer. *Nat Rev Cancer*, 7,(11): 847-859.

Nebral, K., Konig, M., Harder, L., Siebert, R., Haas, O. A. & Strehl, S. (2007). Identification of PML as novel *PAX5* fusion partner in childhood acute lymphoblastic leukaemia. *British Journal of Haematology*, 139, 269-274.

Nebral, K., Denk, D., Attarbaschi, A., Konig, M., Mann, G., Haas, O. A. & Strehl, S. (2009). Incidence and diversity of *PAX5* fusion genes in childhood acute lymphoblastic leukemia. *Leukemia*, 23,(1): 134-143.

Nutt, S. L., Morrison, A. M., Dorfler, P., Rolink, A. & Busslinger, M. (1998). Indentification of BSAP (Pax-5) target genes in early B-cell development by loss- and gain-of-function experiments. *The EMBO Journal*, 17,(8): 2319-2333.

Nutt, S. L., Heavey, B., Rolink, A. G. & Busslinger, M. (1999). Commitment to the B-lymphoid lineage depends on the transcription factor Pax5. *Nature*, 401,(6753): 556-562.

Nutt, S. L. & Kee, B. L. (2007). The Transcriptional Regulation of B Cell Lineage Commitment. *Immunity Reviews*, 26, 715-725.

O'Neil, J. & Look, A. T. (2007). Mechanisms of transcription factor deregulation in lymphoid cell transformation. *Oncogene*, 26,(47): 6838-6849.

Paulsson, K., Cazier, J. B., Macdougall, F., Stevens, J., Stasevich, I., Vrcelj, N., Chaplin, T., Lillington, D. M., Lister, T. A. & Young, B. D. (2008). Microdeletions are a general feature of adult and adolescent acute lymphoblastic leukemia: Unexpected similarities with pediatric disease. *Proc Natl Acad Sci U S A*, 105,(18): 6708-6713.

Qiu, J. J., Chu, H., Lu, X., Jiang, X. & Dong, S. (2011). The reduced and altered activities of PAX5 are linked to the protein-protein interaction motif (coiled-coil domain) of the PAX5-PML fusion protein in t(9;15)-associated acute lymphocytic leukemia. *Oncogene*, 30,(8): 967-977.

Rolink, A. G., Schaniel, C., Bruno, L. & Melchers, F. (2002a). In vitro and in vivo plasticity of Pax5-deficient pre-B I cells. *Immunol Lett*, 82,(1-2): 35-40.

Rolink, A. G. & Melchers, F. (2002b). BAFF led B cells survive and thrive: roles of BAFF in B-cell development. *Curr Opin Immunol*, 14,(2): 266-275.

Rolink, A. G., Tschopp, J., Schneider, P. & Melchers, F. (2002c). BAFF is a survival and maturation factor for mouse B cells. *Eur J Immunol*, 32,(7): 2004-2010.

Santoro, A., Bica, M. G., Dagnino, L., Agueli, C., Salemi, D., Cannella, S., Veltroni, M., Cetica, V., Giarin, E., Fabbiano, F., Basso, G. & Arico, M. (2009). Altered mRNA expression of PAX5 is a common event in acute lymphoblastic leukaemia. *Br J Haematol*, 146,(6): 686-689.

Schebesta, M., Pfeffer, P. L. & Busslinger, M. (2002). Control of Pre-BCR Signaling by Pax5-Dependent Activation of the BLNK Gene. *Immunity*, 17, 473-485.

Schebesta, A., McManus, S., Salvagiotto, G., Delogu, A., Busslinger, G. A. & M., B. (2007). Transcription Factor Pax5 Activates the Chromatin of Key Genes Involved in B Cell Signaling, Adhesion, Migration, and Immune Function. *Immunity*, 27, 49-63.

Souabni, A., Cobaleda, C., Schebesta, M. & Busslinger, M. (2002). Pax5 Promotes B Lymphopoiesis and Blocks T Cell Development by Repressing Notch1. *Immunity*, 17, 781-793.

Souabni, A., Jochum, W. & Busslinger, M. (2007). Oncogenic role of Pax5 in the T-lymphoid lineage upon ectopic expression from the immunoglobulin heavy-chain locus. *Blood*, 109, 281-289.

Strehl, S., Konig, M., Dworzak, M. N., Kalwak, K. & Haas, O. A. (2003). PAX5/ETV6 fusion defines cytogenetic entity dic(9;12)(p13;p13). *Leukemia*, 17,(6): 1121-1123.

Trageser, D., Iacobucci, I., Nahar, R., Duy, C., von Levetzow, G., Klemm, L., Park, E., Schuh, W., Gruber, T., Herzog, S., Kim, Y. M., Hofmann, W. K., Li, A., Storlazzi, C. T., Jack, H. M., Groffen, J., Martinelli, G., Heisterkamp, N., Jumaa, H. & Muschen, M. (2009). Pre-B cell receptor-mediated cell cycle arrest in Philadelphia chromosome-positive acute lymphoblastic leukemia requires IKAROS function. *J Exp Med*, 206,(8): 1739-1753.

van Zelm, M. C., van der Burg, M., de Ridder, D., Barendregt, B. H., de Haas, E. F., Reinders, M. J., Lankester, A. C., Revesz, T., Staal, F. J. & van Dongen, J. J. (2005). Ig gene rearrangement steps are initiated in early human precursor B cell subsets and correlate with specific transcription factor expression. *J Immunol*, 175,(9): 5912-5922.

Waterhouse, A., Wise, S. G., Ng, M. K. & Weiss, A. S. (2011). Elastin as a nonthrombogenic biomaterial. *Tissue Eng Part B Rev*, 17,(2): 93-99.

11

p53 as a Therapeutic Target in T-ALL

Irene Riz[1], Wenjing Yang[2], Weiqun Peng[2] and Robert G. Hawley[1]
[1]*Department of Anatomy and Regenerative Biology*
[2]*Department of Physics, The George Washington University, Washington, DC*
USA

1. Introduction

TP53 is a central hub integrating stress signals from oncogenic genetic lesions and cytotoxic anti-cancer agents. The function of p53 as a regulator of transcription is well documented. More recently it was shown to directly interact with BCL2 family members and induce mitochondrial cell death. Stress-induced activation of p53 leads to cell cycle arrest that allows metabolic adjustments and repair mechanisms to take place prior to the next cycle; p53 may also induce senescence or apoptosis depending on the strength and nature of stress stimuli and/or cell type.

In 50% of human cancers, the TP53 gene is deleted or mutated with a high proportion of gain of oncogenic function mutations. It is noteworthy therefore that TP53 is rarely mutated in T-ALL. However, its tumor suppressor activity is circumvented by genetic lesions. We will discuss here the most frequent T-ALL genetic abnormalities of INK4A/ARF, NOTCH1 and PTEN genes and how they affect TP53 expression and function. Current understanding of the signaling pathways governed by these oncogenes is advanced enough to find points of intersection with p53 downstream targets and attempt to translate the accumulated knowledge to the clinic.

In addition, we will discuss the results of our analysis of publicly available expression profiling data indicating the existence of a TP53-anchored transcriptional program targeted by T-ALL oncogenes such as NOTCH, MYC and TLX1 in primary leukemic cells and how it can be exploited for cancer intervention.

Overall, the goal of this chapter is to describe how T-ALL pathobiology affects the p53-interacting network, highlighting some new potential therapeutic targets as well as some still unresolved questions.

2. INK4A-ARF inactivation circumvents oncogene-induced p53

Inactivation of INK4A-ARF occurs in 70% of T-ALL cases by mutations, biallelic deletions or hypermethylation (Hebert et al., 1994; Gardie et al., 1998; Sulong et al., 2009; Van Vlierberghe et al., 2008; Ferrando et al., 2002; Omura-Minamisawa et al., 2000). The locus encodes two stress-induced proteins with distinct tumor suppressing functions (Quelle et al., 1995): one, INK4A, targets cell cycle entry and another, ARF, inhibits cell cycle progression and cell survival. The two completely unrelated protein sequences derive from the same locus via expression of two alterative reading frames. This unusual feature was suggested to be important for coordinate regulation of these gene products in response to stress signals (Gil & Peters, 2006; Popov & Gil, 2010). The tumor suppressor functions of INK4A and ARF are not redundant since animals with individually inactivated products of the locus showed less spontaneous tumors than the double knockouts (Sharpless et al., 2004). It is well established that the function of INK4A is to inhibit cyclin D-dependent protein kinases and thus suppress proliferation, loss of function contributing to signal-independent cell cycle entry (Serrano et al., 1993). Recently, INK4A was also implicated in regulation of thymocyte apoptosis in response to oxidative stress or gamma irradiation (Bianchi et al., 2006). An excellent review summarizing the biological functions of the INK4 family of proteins has been published (Canepa et al., 2007). Our focus will be on the ARF protein since, as shown in Figure 1, the best characterized activity of ARF is activation of p53. The mechanisms include direct inhibition of the enzymatic activity of the MDM2 E3 ubiquitin ligase and sequestering of the protein in nucleoli (Llanos et al., 2001; Honda & Yasuda, 1999): MDM2 binding is one of the major mechanisms keeping the apoptotic and growth-arresting function of p53 in check. MDM2 blocks p53 transactivation function and enforces its nuclear export and proteasomal degradation (Honda et al., 1997; Zhang & Xiong, 2001; Weber et al., 1999) (See Figure 1 for more details). In addition ARF was suggested to have p53-independent functions; for example, modulation of activity of transcription factors such as MYC, E2F and NFκB family members leads to their enhanced apoptotic activity or stress-induced inhibition of protein synthesis (Sherr, 2006; Qi et al., 2004).

ARF is regulated at multiple levels. Its protein stability and subcellular localization is controlled by the nucleolar phosphoprotein NPM1. ARF-NPM1 complexes are predominantly localized in nucleoli where ARF is more stable (Bertwistle et al., 2004; Brady et al., 2004). Its half life significantly decreases in the nucleoplasm via ubiquitination and proteasome-mediated degradation (Rodway et al., 2004; Kuo et al., 2004). Perhaps the most important aspect of ARF regulation is at the level of transcription. ARF is not expressed in most normal tissues; however, it can be activated in response to stress or aberrant hyperproliferative signals (e.g. RAS mutations, MYC overexpression, BCR-ABL translocation).

In adult hematopoietic stem cells and in immature thymocytes, the INK4A-ARF locus is silenced by the Polycomb-group gene BMI1 (Jacobs et al., 1999; Bracken et al., 2007). This epigenetic regulation is required for survival of normal T cell precursors (Miyazaki et al., 2008). However, ARF expression can be induced at this stage and activates apoptosis in cells with aberrant T cell receptor gene rearrangements or other genetic lesions leading to ectopic activation of protooncogenes. The most frequent T-ALL-associated oncogenic events, involving NOTCH1 (50%) and TAL1 (60%), as well as other less frequent genetic abnormalities, such as activation of LMO2 (9%), were directly demonstrated to cooperate with the loss of INK4A-ARF function (Shank-Calvo et al., 2006; Treanor et al., 2011). The response of the locus may be developmentally specific. For example, the responsiveness of the INK4A-ARF locus to the constitutively-active truncated form of NOTCH1 depends on the stage of development, with the locus being silent in hematopoietic stem cells but inducible in thymocytes (Volanakis et al., 2009). From that perspective, it is noteworthy that in immature T-ALL cases, the INK4A-ARF locus is predominantly found intact but kept inactive by epigenetic mechanisms (Ferrando et al., 2002). Thus these silencing mechanisms may serve as potential therapeutic targets in immature T-ALLs.

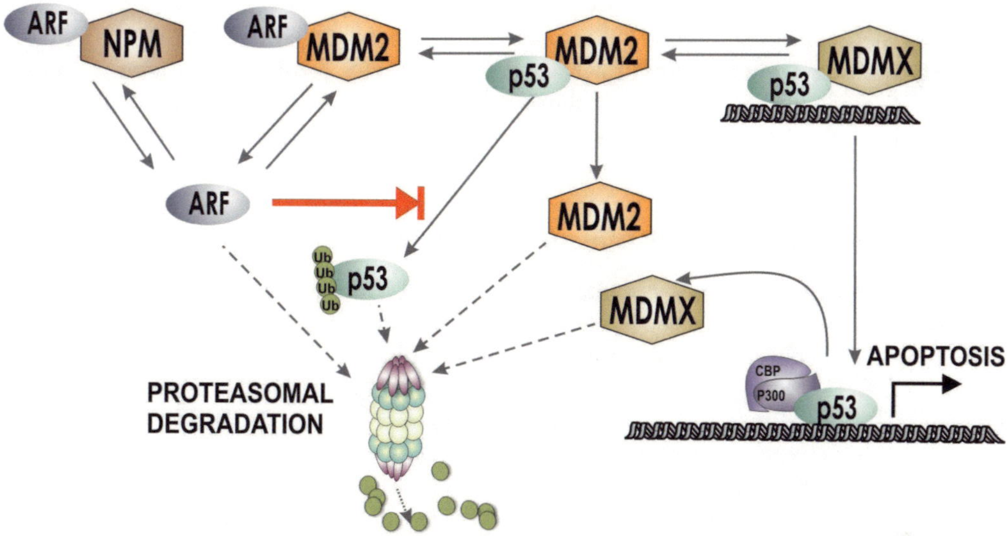

Fig. 1. Regulation of p53 protein stability via ARF and MDM2/MDMX. From left to right: nucleolar phosphoprotein NPM1 controls ARF protein stability and subcellular localization. ARF-NPM1 complexes are predominantly localized in nucleoli where ARF is more stable. Liberated ARF may be degraded by proteasomes or may associate with MDM2 and prevent degradation of p53 via direct binding to MDM2 and inhibition of its ubiquitin ligase activity. p53 is stabilized in MDMX complexes, but for full activation of p53-dependent transcription MDMX is replaced by transcriptional cofactors. MDM2 and MDMX are subjected to stress-induced proteasomal degradation.

Because the immature T-ALL subset represents the highest risk among T-ALL, we will describe in more detail BMI1 function and regulation to highlight potential therapeutic strategies aiming to reactivate the INK4A-ARF locus. In thymocytes, BMI1 binds directly to the locus and specifically maintains trimethylation of histone H3 at lysine 27 (3mH3K27 modification) (Miyazaki et al., 2008). For maintenance of the repressed state through multiple rounds of cell divisions, DNA methylation markers are necessary. Polycomb proteins interpret DNA methylation marks and translate them into histone modifications to initiate/maintain repression (Spivakov & Fisher, 2007). Thus it is not surprising, but may be very important for potential clinical translation, that inhibition of DNA methyltransferase (DNMT) was shown to derepress the INK4A-ARF locus by affecting this mechanism in human cord blood-derived multipotent stem cells. The authors used 5-azacytidine, an inhibitor of DNMT analogous to cytidine; they showed that loss of DNA methylation marks caused diminished recruitment of EZH2, a key histone methyltransferase, and decreased 3mH3K27 modification of the INK4A-ARF locus (So et al., 2011). Another attractive candidate for therapeutic intervention is Hedgehog signaling, required for survival and proliferation of early thymocyte precursors (El Andaloussi et al., 2006). Moreover, it was recently shown that Sonic hedgehog activates BMI1 expression during cerebellar development (Leung et al., 2004). Thus testing Hedgehog inhibitors such as cyclopamine or vismodegib on immature T-ALL samples might be a promising approach. The strategy of reactivating the INK4A-ARF locus is complicated, however, by the fact that the locus responds to the same oncogenic signals that support the survival and proliferation of malignant cells. For example, a powerful pro-survival kinase AKT1 targets EZH2 and suppresses methylation of histone H3 at lysine 27 (Cha et al., 2005) while MAPKAP kinase 3, a convergence point downstream of activated ERK and p38, inhibits BMI1 association with chromatin (Voncken et al., 2005). For these reasons and because the INK4A-ARF locus is deleted in the majority of T-ALL cases, current therapeutic strategies are based on activation of p53 in an ARF-independent manner.

3. NOTCH-governed network affects ARF and p53

Mutations activating the developmental regulator NOTCH1 occur in more than 50% of T-ALL cases (Weng et al., 2004). NOTCH1 was initially implicated in T-cell leukemogenesis by the finding of rare chromosomal translocations that place a constitutively-active truncated form of NOTCH1 (NIC) under the T cell receptor (TCR) beta chain promoter (Ellisen et al., 1991). NOTCH1 is a transmembrane receptor (Kopan & Ilagan, 2009). The Delta-like and Jagged ligands activate proteolytic processing of NOTCH1 that releases its cytoplasmic portion allowing it to translocate to the nucleus. In the nucleus, NOTCH1 activates transcription via a DNA-bound protein CSL (Aster et al., 2008). Subsequently, a high frequency of NOTCH1-activating mutations were characterized that enhance its proteolytic processing and/or stabilize its intracellular portion (Weng et al., 2004). Thus in T-ALL, NOTCH signaling is represented by a broad spectrum of levels of activation that may still be ligand dependent and also inhibited by drugs targeting the NOTCH1 processing machinery (Lewis et al., 2007; Sulis et al., 2011).

NOTCH signaling is required for several consecutive stages of normal thymocyte development, from the earliest stage of T-cell fate commitment until the late cortical thymocyte stage with fully rearranged TCR genes (Tanigaki & Honjo, 2007). NOTCH1 provides survival and stimulates growth of normal thymocytes and leukemic T cells (Grabher et al., 2006; Ciofani & Zuniga-Pflucker, 2005). That said, the functional role of NOTCH1 in T-ALL cells undergoing chemotherapeutic treatment is less clear. As NOTCH1 promotes their survival, NOTCH1 mutations would be expected to confer enhanced drug resistance. Interestingly, however, mutations activating NOTCH1 were found to associate with good initial response to treatment (Kox et al., 2010; Asnafi et al., 2009). In this context, and consistent with these observations, it is worth mentioning that we and others observed that NOTCH1 inhibition decreases sensitivity of T-ALL cell lines to selected chemotherapeutic agents while NOTCH1 activation enhances the response (De Keersmaecker et al., 2008; Liu et al., 2009; Riz et al., 2011).

The function of NOTCH1 is mediated by several signaling hubs that in turn impact ARF and p53 function: among them, mTOR kinase, a key growth regulator constitutively activated in many cancers; eIF4E, a selective regulator of translation initiation; SKP2, an E3 ubiqutin ligase; and transcription factors such as MYC and NFκB (Chan et al., 2007; Mungamuri et al., 2006; Hsieh & Ruggero, 2010; Kao et al., 2009; Dohda et al., 2007; Murphy et al., 2008).

The accumulated evidence indicates that ectopic activation of NOTCH1 in premalignant thymocytes may lead to ARF induction. First, in T-ALL, NOTCH1 mutations frequently coincide with INK4A-ARF inactivation (Ferrando et al., 2002; Treanor et al., 2011). Second, in mice, progression to full malignancy in NIC-expressing thymocytes is associated with decreased ARF expression (Li et al., 2008). And finally, oncogenic cooperation of these two genetic aberrations was directly demonstrated in a murine T-ALL model (Volanakis et al., 2009). Moreover, the authors showed indirect activation of the ARF promoter by expression of NIC. Thus these data demonstrated that NOTCH1 mutations may activate ectopic signaling that triggers the oncogene-induced stress response exemplified by ARF induction. However, there is also evidence suggesting that NOTCH1 may downregulate the tumor suppressor function of p53. In an elegant system allowing regulatable NIC expression, it was shown that downregulation of NIC levels in mouse lymphomas *in vivo* is associated with activation of p53 (Beverly et al., 2005). Other work also demonstrated that ectopic expression of NIC partially downregulates the p53-mediated apoptotic response to DNA-damaging drugs in human leukemic cell lines (Mungamuri et al., 2006). The effect was mediated by the mTOR kinase. The authors showed that mTOR inhibition by rapamycin prevented (and eIF4E overexpression restored) the NOTCH1 pro-survival effect. Subsequently, in experiments with loss or gain of NOTCH1 function, MYC was placed upstream of the mTOR-eIF4E pathway (Chan et al., 2007). In agreement with these findings, eIF4E-driven CAP-mediated translation was shown to be required for MYC transforming function (Ruggero et al., 2004; Lin et al., 2008; Barna et al., 2008). Other work indicated that the oncogenic function of the mTOR-eIF4E pathway is mediated at least in part by inhibition of p53 via enhanced translation of MDM2 (Kao et al., 2009). The authors reported that rapamycin increases the p53/MDM2 protein ratio by inhibition of MDM2 translation without affecting its mRNA expression or protein stability. Ectopic expression of eIF4E abrogated the effect. With some gaps yet to be filled, the accumulated data indicate the existence of a signaling axis in T-ALL cells connecting the following components NOTCH1-MYC-mTOR-eIF4E-MDM2-p53 (see Figure 2 for a complete representation of the pathway).

NOTCH1 was shown to positively regulate the ubiqutin ligase SKP2 and, as a result, downregulate the p27 Kip1 and p21 Cip1 cell cycle inhibitors in T-ALL cell lines (Dohda et al., 2007; Sarmento et al., 2005). Moreover, SKP2 was shown to inhibit p53 function by targeting the acetyltransferase p300 (Kitagawa et al., 2008). Notably, MYC protein is targeted for degradation by SKP2 (Kim et al., 2003; von der Lehr et al., 2003) and SKP2 is not required for the transforming function of MYC (Old et al., 2010). However, as mentioned earlier, MYC gene expression is directly activated by NOTCH1 (Weng et al., 2006; Sharma et al., 2007). It is possible therefore that NOTCH1-induced SKP2 counteracts the NOTCH1-mediated transcriptional activation of MYC to keep MYC protein levels within a pro-survival range. Recently published data suggest that this is indeed the case. It was reported (although not discussed by the authors) that downregulation of NIC in murine T-cell lymphomas expressing MYC under a NOTCH1-independent constitutive promoter showed very strong activation of MYC protein levels without affecting mRNA levels [see Figure 4A and C in (Demarest et al., 2011)]; of note, the process coincided with strong upregulation of p53 protein and tumor regression. Because overexpression of MYC was documented to activate oncogene-induced stress via p53 in ARF-dependent and -independent manners (Murphy et al., 2008), it is tempting to propose that another potential NOTCH1 survival function is mediated by SKP2 control of MYC protein levels. This mechanism may play a particularly prominent role in those cases when, as a result of chromosomal rearrangements, MYC transcription is constitutive and no longer dependent on NOTCH1.

Finally, it is important to note that NOTCH was shown to activate NFκB transcriptional function on multiple levels that includes upregulation of expression of NFκB subunits,

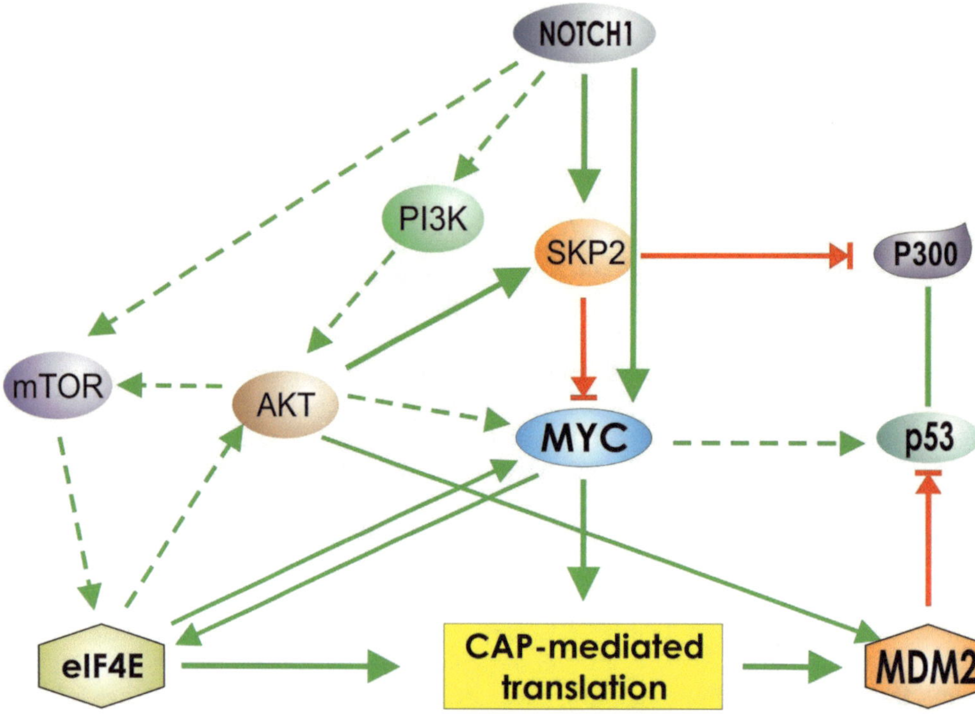

Fig. 2. NOTCH and p53 network. The function of NOTCH1 is mediated by several signaling hubs that in turn impact ARF and p53 function: NOTCH1 activates AKT, AKT directly activates MDM2. NOTCH activates SKP2 and Skp2 suppresses p300-mediated acetylation of p53 and the transactivation ability of p53. MYC gene expression is directly activated by NOTCH; MYC protein levels are controlled by SKP2 and AKT; ectopic MYC activation may cause activation of p53. NOTCH and/or MYC activate mTOR and eIF4E; eIF4E mediates protein synthesis of MYC and activators of AKT kinase; MYC and eIF4E promote CAP-mediated translation of MDM2. Solid arrows indicate direct interaction, dashed arrows indicate functional interaction via one or more intermediaries.

direct interaction with its upstream regulatory components such as IKK kinase, and inhibition of a negative loop of regulation (Osipo et al., 2008; Shin et al., 2006; Espinosa et al., 2010). NFκB and p53 exhibit a well documented history of cross-talk as well as synergistic interactions. For example, p53 and the p52 NFκB subunit coordinately regulate SKP2 gene expression (Barre & Perkins, 2010). NFκB is not only a pro-survival factor, it was shown to activate apoptosis in response to chemotherapeutic drug treatments (Radhakrishnan & Kamalakaran, 2006). Moreover, NFκB can induce p53 function, while p53 was shown to selectively inhibit the survival function of NFκB but to cooperate with the NFκB-mediated transcriptional activation of apoptotic genes (Meley et al., 2010; Ryan et al., 2000). Thus the functional outcome of NOTCH1-NFκB-p53 pathway interaction is not easy to predict; and, depending on the conditions (e.g., chemotherapy-induced stress levels), the NOTCH1-NFκB-p53 pathways may cooperate in promoting apoptosis. In addition, our data indicate that NOTCH1 may positively contribute to NFκB apoptotic function in a p53-independent manner.

We believe therefore that additional studies should be carried out to address the conflicting laboratory and clinical findings about the role of NOTCH1 activation in the regulation of T-

ALL cell survival in response to therapy. Briefly, as mentioned above, a number of preclinical studies have demonstrated a pro-survival role of NOTCH signaling in T-ALL; based on these studies, T-ALL clinical trials investigating the therapeutic potential of γ-secretase inhibitors have been initiated (ClinicalTrials.gov, NCT01088763; NCT00878189); so far, the drugs tested have demonstrated low anti-leukemic efficacy. A novel approach targeting NOTCH1 processing via inhibition of ADAM10 (a disintegrin and metalloprotease 10) was also suggested (Sulis et al., 2011). Moreover, on the basis of results obtained with T-ALL cell lines, in which inhibition of NOTCH signaling was reported to enhance glucocorticoid sensitivity, combination therapies of γ-secretase inhibitors and glucocorticoids were proposed (Real & Ferrando, 2009; Real et al., 2009). Clearly, the inclusion of γ-secretase inhibitors in T-ALL protocols needs to be reevaluated in light of the new clinical data showing that activated NOTCH1 is associated with a better initial response regardless of the type of treatment and particularly to prednisone (Kox et al., 2010). On the other hand, perhaps if it is not combined with conventional therapy, NOTCH1 inhibition may prove to be a successful approach; for example, in combination with Sonic hedgehog inhibition (Okuhashi et al., 2011) or mTOR and PTEN-PI3K/AKT modulation (see below).

4. PTEN: AKT-dependent and -independent activation of p53

Recurring oncogenic events in T-ALL involve inactivation of the PTEN tumor suppressor gene (Zhang et al., 2006; Palomero et al., 2008). The frequency of PTEN mutations was estimated to be about 20%; however, its functional downregulation is more common (Jotta et al., 2010; Silva et al., 2008). PTEN is a lipid phosphatase hydrolyzing phosphate in position 3 from phosphoinositides. In primary T-ALL, PTEN was suggested to be a major factor contributing to elevated levels of phosphoinositides and thus indirectly contributing to MYC protein stability (Silva et al., 2010; Bonnet et al., 2011).

Phosphoinositides, such as phosphatidylinositol-(3,4,5)-trisphosphate (PIP3), are membrane second messengers connecting cytokine and growth factor signaling with intracellular components such as the serine threonine protein kinase AKT (Carracedo & Pandolfi, 2008). PTEN dephosphorylates PIP3 while phosphoinositide-3 kinase (PI3K) reverses the reaction such that the levels of PIP3 are controlled by the balance of these two enzymes (Figure 3). PI3K is activated by various genetic lesions, the most common of which activate NOTCH1 (Sade et al., 2004). In addition, about 20% of mutations are in genes encoding upstream activators of the PI3K pathway; among them, IGF signaling components are the most prominent (Remke et al., 2009) while mutations directly affecting PI3K subunits are more rare (Gutierrez et al., 2009). Thus, as a result of PTEN inhibition and/or PI3K activation, close to 90% of T-ALL show elevated PIP3 levels (Silva et al., 2008). The signal from PIP3 is transmitted via membrane recruitment and activation of a member of the pleckstrin homology domain protein family, one of the best characterized being AKT kinase. Indeed in T-ALL, AKT levels were shown to be activated very frequently (close to 90%) (Silva et al., 2008). AKT phosphorylates about 100 different proteins and mainly promotes survival (by inactivating BAD, MDM2 and forkhead transcription factors) and growth (by inhibition of p27, GSK3 kinase), and regulates glucose homeostasis (by enhancing the glucose transporter GLUT4). Importantly, AKT regulates protein translation and ribosome biogenesis via activation of the mTOR pathway (Carracedo & Pandolfi, 2008). Therefore, the contribution of the PTEN/PI3K-AKT pathway is of central importance to the pathobiology of T-ALL, and especially with regard to p53 regulation.

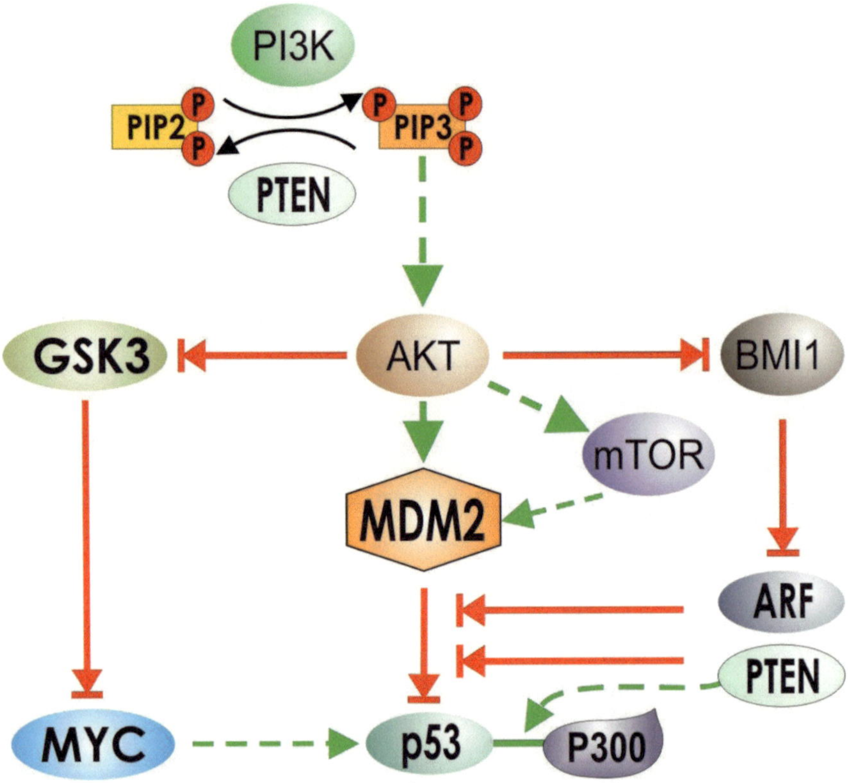

Fig. 3. Role of PTEN in p53 regulation. PTEN hydrolyses the phosphate group in the 3′ position from phosphatidylinositol 3,4,5-triphosphate (PIP3) to form phosphatidylinositol 4,5-biphosphate that counteracts PI3K function. PIP3 activates AKT. AKT phosphorylates and activates MDM2 directly and via mTOR pathways contributes to its protein synthesis. PTEN directly binds p53, enhancing its stability by antagonizing the p53-MDM2 interaction and promoting p300/CBP-mediated acetylation of p53. On the other hand, ectopic AKT activation may induce ARF function, and ectopic MYC activation may induce p53 in ARF -dependent and -independent ways. Solid arrows indicate direct interaction, dashed arrows indicate functional interaction via one or more intermediaries.

Most of the characterized downstream effectors of PTEN are AKT dependent; in T-ALL, they include p53, mTOR and MYC. p53 is regulated by AKT phosphorylation of MDM2 that leads to its nuclear translocation (Mayo & Donner, 2001). In addition, PTEN may directly bind p53 protein, enhance its stability by antagonizing p53-MDM2 interaction, and promote p300/CBP-mediated acetylation of p53 (Zhou et al., 2003; Freeman et al., 2003). Gain or loss of function experiments in T-ALL demonstrated that the PTEN-mTOR axis is important for the growth of the leukemogenic cells (Yilmaz et al., 2006). As previously mentioned, mTOR was also shown to enhance translation of MDM2. A recent publication addressing the frequency of MYC deregulation in T-ALL demonstrated that downregulation of PTEN function is one of the predominant features associated with enhanced MYC protein levels (Bonnet et al., 2011). MYC is regulated via AKT-dependent inhibition of GSK3 kinase. If it is not inhibited by AKT, this constitutively active kinase directly targets MYC protein for degradation (Gregory et al., 2003).

PTEN is a haploinsufficient tumor suppressor since the presence of a single copy does not prevent cancers (Salmena et al., 2008). On the other hand, biallelic loss of PTEN in primary thymocytes causes a cellular stress response resulting in the AKT-dependent induction of cell cycle arrest (Xue et al., 2008) via elevated expression of ARF and p53 proteins (Lee et al., 2010). The data are consistent with earlier work observing that loss of PTEN induces p53 function in other cell types (Chen et al., 2005b; Kim et al., 2007a). Together, the data strongly demonstrate that complete loss of PTEN may activate an oncogene-induced stress response and explains why it usually occurs in advanced cancers with inactivated p53 genes and poor prognosis (Jotta et al., 2010; Gutierrez et al., 2009).

Thus cancer intervention via modulation of PTEN function requires a precise knowledge of PTEN and p53 statuses. For p53 positive cases, PTEN inhibition was proposed as a therapeutic strategy (Mak et al., 2010). A more widely applicable approach is therapeutic restoration/activation of PTEN function. The activity of PTEN is directly inhibited by reactive oxygen species (ROS) oxidation of its catalytic center. Since leukemic cells frequently show increased levels of ROS, antioxidants may contribute to the restoration of PTEN function (Silva et al., 2008). For example, ascorbic acid or resveratrol treatment of T-ALL cell lines was associated with activation of p53; however, PTEN function was not addressed (Harakeh et al., 2007; Cecchinato et al., 2007). The levels of PTEN protein expression are tightly regulated. In T-ALL cells, CK2 was shown to control its protein levels and thus CK2 inhibition was suggested as a therapeutic strategy (Silva et al., 2010). Inhibition of PI3K, AKT and mTOR kinases was also suggested (Chiarini et al., 2010; Chiarini et al., 2009; Evangelisti et al., 2011a; Evangelisti et al., 2011b). However, despite a significant overlap in downstream targets, PTEN loss cannot compensate for NOTCH1 oncogenic function (Medyouf et al., 2010). Thus inhibition of both pathways was shown to cooperate in primary leukemic T cells and in mouse tumor models (Guo et al., 2011; Cullion et al., 2009). Finally, dual inhibition of PI3K and mTOR has been suggested as a therapeutic option for T-ALL (Chiarini et al., 2009).

5. TP53 coexpressed genes — potential chemotherapeutic targets

As discussed above, genetic aberrations may cause activation of a stress response. For example, deregulation of the NOTCH, PTEN, TAL1 or LYL1 loci causes activation of ARF in normal thymocytes. TP53 gene expression can also be induced in response to stress (Vilborg et al., 2010). Despite the secondary adaptive mutations preventing oncogene-induced apoptosis or senescence, cancer cells still frequently show elevated stress levels. The elevated stress together with enhanced growth is exploited in cancer therapies, which aim to selectively kill tumor cells while sparing normal cells. Knowing the transcription programs mediating the stress phenotype of cancer cells is important for the rational design of new "targeted" treatment strategies (Luo et al., 2009).

While analyzing publicly available expression profiles of primary T-ALL cells, we noticed that expression levels of TP53 varied greatly between patient samples. Moreover, in the majority of cases, TP53 was expressed at higher levels than in normal thymocytes, indicating that the complexity of aberrations in T-ALL manifests in various levels of oncogene-induced stress. We asked what transcripts are coregulated with TP53 with the expectation of identifying genes that functionally interact with it. We analyzed expression profiles of primary T-ALL samples and normal thymocytes (Soulier et al., 2005). Genes were selected for analysis that were coexpressed with TP53 (Affymetrix probe set 211300_s_at U133A) based on similarity of their expression patterns (r>0.65) within about 100 T-ALL patient samples. As expected, the set of TP53-profile neighbors contained a number of genes encoding proteins that interact with TP53 at the mRNA or protein levels, regulating its stability and function (Figure 4). Interestingly, among them were genes that counteract p53 function, possibly reflecting neoplastic adaptation to high levels of TP53 gene expression. For example, inactivation of p53 at the level of protein stability is illustrated by PA2G4, PSME3 and HUWE1. Briefly, PA2G4 promotes p53 polyubiquitination and degradation; PSME3, encoding the 26S proteasome subunit, was shown to be required for p53 degradation (Zhang & Zhang, 2008); and HUWE1 (or ARF-BP1) E3 ubiqutin ligase directly binds to p53 and targets it for degradation in an MDM2-independent manner (Chen et al., 2005a). Other examples include G3BP1, which facilitates redistribution of p53 from the nucleus to the cytoplasm (Kim et al., 2007b); UBE2N (or UBC13), which inhibits formation of transcriptionally active p53 tetramers (Topisirovic et al., 2009); and CHD4, which deacetylates p53 and blocks p21 induction (Polo et al., 2010). Finally, inhibition of p53 transcriptional outcome is exemplified by YBX1, which is a component of the repressor complex blocking expression of p53 target genes (Shiota et al., 2008; Kim et al., 2008). Proteins cooperating with p53 function were also found among the set of p53-profile neighbors; for example, HNRNPF promotes p53 mRNA 3′-end formation (Decorsiere et al., 2011); DKC1 facilitates p53 translation; heat shock-induced stabilization of p53 occurs via direct binding to HSP90AA1; the purine biosynthesis enzyme GART is involved in p53- activating posttranslational modifications (Bronder & Moran, 2003); and SSRP1 is a component of the p53 transcriptional complex (Keller & Lu, 2002; Keller et al., 2001). There were also examples of genetic cooperation such as NOLC1 and SMARCC1. TP53 and NOLC1 cooperate in snoRNA-mediated ribosomal RNA editing, an important process for stress-induced stabilization of ribosomes (Krastev et al., 2011). Haploinsufficiency of both SMARCC1 and p53 cooperate to induce tumorigenesis in a mouse model (Ahn et al., 2011).

Because p53 is known to interact in some manner with a large portion of the genome, we asked if the enrichment of the p53-interacting genes in the set of TP53-profile neighbors is statistically significant. An empirical approach was used to determine the p-value. We generated 100 sets of 100 genes randomly selected from all annotated genes. For each set of 100 genes, TP53 was added to the set. The resulting simulated gene sets were subjected to Ingenuity Pathway Analysis and treated the same way as the list of T-ALL TP53-profile neighbors. The tabulated results of the number of p53 connections identified were used to estimate the p-value: this statistical approach indicated that the number of p53 connections within the set of T-ALL TP53-profile neighbors significantly exceeded the number of those within the simulated randomly-selected gene sets (p-value < 0.01). Importantly, our statistical analysis suggests that other less-studied genes among the T-ALL TP53-profile neighbors may also be important regulators of p53. This idea warrants further investigation because novel regulators of p53 might be found that may serve as potential therapeutic targets (Cheok et al., 2011). In support of this notion, certain of the known p53-interacting proteins, such as HUWE1, have already been suggested as possibilities for therapeutic intervention to restore p53 function in cancer cells (Chen et al., 2006).

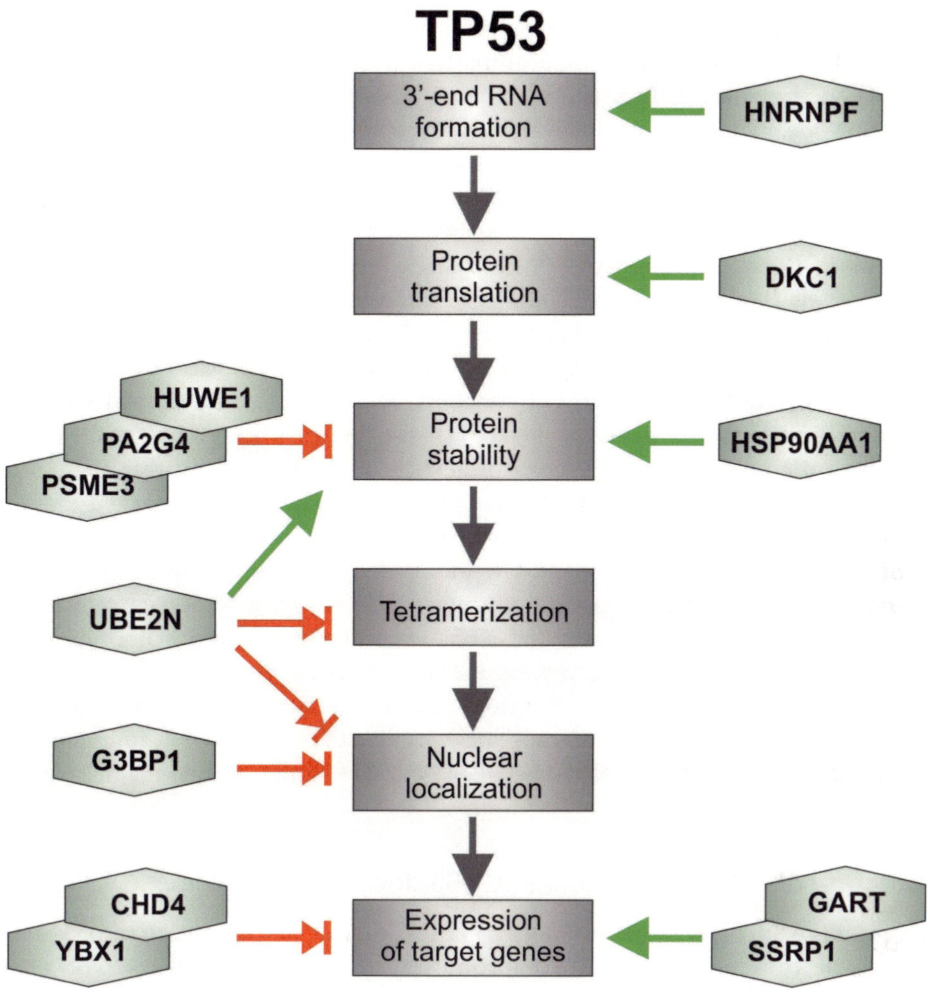

Fig. 4. TP53 profile neighbors in T-ALL regulate its function. Shown are examples of the TP53 profile neighbors known to target sequential steps of p53 activation.

The enrichment of p53-interacting genes and common expression signature also indicated that the set of TP53-profile neighbors is deregulated as a result of leukemogenesis and may be targeted by common T-ALL oncogenes. To ask which oncogenes may be involved in regulation of the set of TP53-coexpressed genes in T-ALL, we used genome-wide chromatin immunoprecipitation data previously published by others (Margolin et al., 2009; De Keersmaecker et al., 2010) to identify direct MYC or TLX1 targets. We found that the set of T-ALL TP53-coexpressed genes is significantly enriched for direct MYC and/or TLX1 targets, accounting for 70% of the set. Specifically, out of 16,697 genes represented on the array, 8,404 of them were bound by either MYC or TLX1. On the other hand, out of the 99 genes found to be coexpressed with TP53 in T-ALL, 69 of them were bound by either MYC or TLX1. Using the hypergeometric distribution, we determined that the p-value for the frequency of MYC or TLX1 target genes within the set of T-ALL p53-profile neighbors is 7×10^{-5}. Notably, NOTCH1 targets were within the subsets of MYC and/or

TLX1 targets. Moreover, the remaining 30% of the genes showed similar expression profiles and functional classification, arguing that they are regulated by one of NOTCH1, MYC or TLX1, but indirectly via downstream transcription factors. Promoter analysis revealed that the incidence of glucocorticoid receptor (GR) binding sites was 10 times more frequent in this set versus the genes directly targeted by MYC and TLX1, suggesting that these genes are potential targets of GR, and that GR may be the transcription factor contributing to the oncogene-induced stress response. A number of observations support this hypothesis. First, TLX1-positive T-ALL cases are characterized by high GR mRNA expression levels (Ferrando et al., 2002). In this regard, we found that shRNA-mediated knockdown of TLX1 in the T-ALL-derived ALL-SIL cell line was associated with increased resistance to glucocorticoid-induced cell death (manuscript in preparation) indicating that TLX1 may contribute positively to GR function. Moreover, recent clinical studies have demonstrated that activation of the NOTCH1 oncogene is associated with a superior initial therapeutic response to glucocorticoids (Kox et al., 2010) indicating that NOTCH1 may also cooperate with GR-induced killing. Finally, we and others observed that ectopic activation of MYC may cause transcriptional induction of pro-apoptotic BIM (Riz et al., 2011), which is a known mediator of GR induced apoptosis in T-ALL cells. Thus we hypothesize based on our analysis that an interacting network of transcription factors—NOTCH1-MYC-TLX1—may activate the TP53-anchored transcriptional program of an oncogene-induced stress response, predominantly via direct binding to promoters and in part via activation of GR function. We hope that our hypothesis will help to stimulate further studies seeking novel therapeutic targets to restore p53 function and to understand the intricate relationships between NOTCH1 and GR, two major targets of T-ALL therapeutic intervention.

6. Interaction of T-ALL mutations and p53 downstream targets

It is important to appreciate that not only p53 function but also execution of p53-governed transcriptional programs is often compromised by T-ALL mutations. For example, NOTCH1 via activation of SKP2 decreases the levels of p21 and thus counteracts one of the best characterized activities of p53 (Sarmento et al., 2005). As discussed above, the pathways downstream of NOTCH and PTEN intersect at the level of PI3K-mTOR. A set of p53 target genes controls this pathway as well (Feng et al., 2005). PTEN itself was shown to be a p53 target gene about 10 years ago (Stambolic et al., 2001). Since then, it has become appreciated that PTEN is activated by p53 in response to high-dose chemotherapy as part of a p53-governed transcriptional program committing cells to apoptosis. NOTCH1 was shown to inhibit PTEN via upregulation of the transcription factor HES1, which directly represses the PTEN promoter (Palomero et al., 2007). Among upstream modulators of PI3K, p53 induces IGF-BP3 (Buckbinder et al., 1995). IGF-BP3 binds to IGF1 or IGF2 and prevents their interaction with the receptor. Mutations involving components of IGF signaling are frequent contributors to PI3K activation in T-ALL (Remke et al., 2009). Other p53 targets affecting the mTOR pathway include TSC2, AMPK beta1, sestrins 1 and 2 and REDD1, all of which contribute to negative regulation of mTOR by targeting the TORC1 complex (which counteracts AKT function) (Feng et al., 2007) (Figure 5).

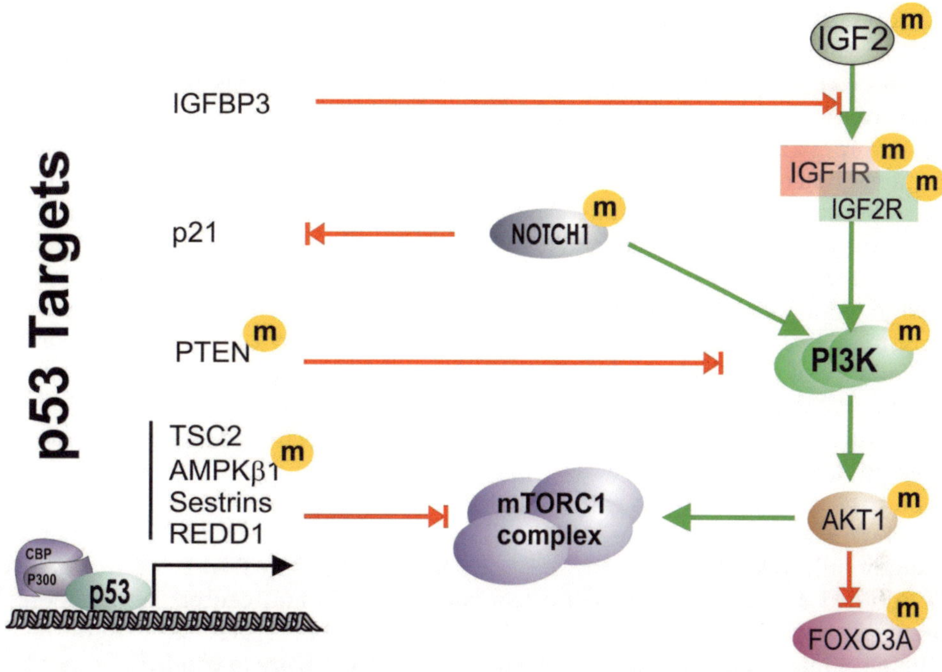

Fig. 5. T-ALL-associated genetic lesions compromise the function of p53 downstream targets. Alterations of NOTCH1 and PTEN loci are complemented by less frequent mutations in the growth-promoting IGF-PI3K/AKT/mTOR network; mutant proteins are indicated by 'm'. By inhibiting this network, the p53 target genes shown adjust metabolic rates in response to stress conditions and stall cell cycle progression.

7. Conclusion

A plethora of inactivating mutations notwithstanding there is still a possibility for therapeutic restoration of p53 apoptotic function because of two major features typical to this cellular regulator: multiplicity of activating stimuli and redundancy of the activating modifications. p53 is activated in response to a variety of stresses such as lack of nutrients, energy deprivation, DNA damage, heat shock, hypoxia or enhanced oxidation, and ER protein overload. Importantly, the apoptotic function of p53 may be activated only in the presence of persistent irreparable stress. For example, while reparable DNA damage activates p53 only partially via Ser-15/20 phosphorylation (which is sufficient for cell cycle arrest), PTEN induction by p53 is triggered by persistent DNA damage and has an additional checkpoint that requires phosphorylation of Ser46 in p53 (Mayo et al., 2005; Zhang et al., 2011). Thus chemotherapeutic agents activating p53 beyond its growth-arresting function should be considered as an aid to p53 protein stabilizers such as blockers of MDM2 function (Hasegawa et al., 2009). Among these regulators, WIP1 phosphatase (PPM1D), a p53 target and negative loop of autoregulation of p53 was suggested as a possibility, however, not tested in T-ALL (Lu et al., 2008; Yoda et al., 2008). Even though the Ser46 phosphorylated form of p53 was shown to associate with apoptotic activity, point mutation substituting this amino acid to alanine did not prevent activation of p53 apoptotic function (Kurihara et al., 2007). This illustration, together with studies showing that the p53-

MDM2 interaction is not affected by single point mutations, supports the idea of p53 regulatory redundancy (Kruse & Gu, 2009).

At the onset of neoplastic development, p53 is often activated as part of an oncogene-induced stress response. It is noteworthy that TP53 is rarely mutated in T-ALL (De Keersmaecker et al., 2005). Despite adaptive genetic and epigenetic mechanisms disrupting its functional outcome [discussed herein and (Vilas-Zornoza et al., 2011)], the p53 pathway still stays partially activated in fully developed T-ALL. Thus selective reactivation of p53 tumor suppressor function in the malignant cells is possible in principle by overcoming the disrupted links of the pathway. The development of personalized medicine providing knowledge of the patient's cancer genome should facilitate efforts to devise the appropriate strategy to activate wild-type p53 function in T-ALL. We believe that combining conventional cytotoxic therapy with molecular targeted approaches restoring p53 activity to its full potential will improve current protocols and prevent relapse. In this regard, there are several small molecule inhibitors of the p53-MDM2 interaction that are currently being investigated (Cheok et al., 2011), at least one of which (RG7112) is undergoing clinical trials in T-ALL patients (ClinicalTrials.gov, NCT00623870).

In spite of over 30 years of p53 research and investigation into the molecular basis of T-ALL, surprisingly little is known about the role and function of p53 in T-ALL. At time of writing, 43,847 PubMed articles were found by searching for "p53 and cancer" whereas only 146 articles could be retrieved for "p53 and T-ALL". T-ALL represents 15% of pediatric hematological malignancies which are the most common cancers in children. So, we believe that the subject is significantly underrepresented. We hope that by summarizing the current state of the art, this chapter will bring more attention to this issue and pave the way for new therapeutic strategies for patients with this disease.

8. Acknowledgments

We thank Sana Ahmad for assistance determining the statistical significance of p53 connections within the set of TP53-profile neighbors and Ian Toma for help preparing the figures. This work was supported in part by an American Cancer Society Pilot Grant for Junior Faculty from The George Washington University Cancer Institute (IRG-08-091-01) and a Pilot Project Award from the Clinical and Translational Science Institute at Children's National Medical Center (NIH UL1RR031988) (I.R.); and by NIH Grants R01HL65519 and R01HL66305, an Elaine H. Snyder Cancer Research Award and a King Fahd Endowment from The George Washington University School of Medicine (R.G.H.). Its contents are solely the responsibility of the authors and do not necessarily represent the official views of the National Center for Research Resources or the National Institutes of Health.
Correspondence: I.R. (anaixr@gwumc.edu) or R.G.H. (rghawley@gwu.edu)

9. References

Ahn, J., Ko, M., Lee, C., Kim, J., Yoon, H., & Seong, R.H. (2011). Srg3, a mouse homolog of BAF155, is a novel p53 target and acts as a tumor suppressor by modulating p21(WAF1/CIP1) expression. *Oncogene* 30, 445-456.

Asnafi, V., Buzyn, A., Le, N.S., Baleydier, F., Simon, A., Beldjord, K., Reman, O., Witz, F., Fagot, T., Tavernier, E., et al. (2009). NOTCH1/FBXW7 mutation identifies a large subgroup with favorable outcome in adult T-cell acute lymphoblastic leukemia (T-

ALL): a Group for Research on Adult Acute Lymphoblastic Leukemia (GRAALL) study. *Blood* 113, 3918-3924.

Aster, J.C., Pear, W.S., & Blacklow, S.C. (2008). Notch signaling in leukemia. *Annu. Rev. Pathol.* 3, 587-613.

Barna, M., Pusic, A., Zollo, O., Costa, M., Kondrashov, N., Rego, E., Rao, P.H., & Ruggero, D. (2008). Suppression of Myc oncogenic activity by ribosomal protein haploinsufficiency. *Nature* 456, 971-975.

Barre, B. & Perkins, N.D. (2010). The Skp2 promoter integrates signaling through the NF-kappaB, p53, and Akt/GSK3beta pathways to regulate autophagy and apoptosis. *Mol. Cell* 38, 524-538.

Bertwistle, D., Sugimoto, M., & Sherr, C.J. (2004). Physical and functional interactions of the Arf tumor suppressor protein with nucleophosmin/B23. *Mol. Cell Biol.* 24, 985-996.

Beverly, L.J., Felsher, D.W., & Capobianco, A.J. (2005). Suppression of p53 by Notch in lymphomagenesis: implications for initiation and regression. *Cancer Res.* 65, 7159-7168.

Bianchi, T., Rufer, N., MacDonald, H.R., & Migliaccio, M. (2006). The tumor suppressor p16Ink4a regulates T lymphocyte survival. *Oncogene* 25, 4110-4115.

Bonnet, M., Loosveld, M., Montpellier, B., Navarro, J.M., Quilichini, B., Picard, C., Di Cristofaro, J., Bagnis, C., Fossat, C., Hernandez, L., et al. (2011). Posttranscriptional deregulation of MYC via PTEN constitutes a major alternative pathway of MYC activation in T-cell acute lymphoblastic leukemia. *Blood* 117, 6650-6659.

Bracken, A.P., Kleine-Kohlbrecher, D., Dietrich, N., Pasini, D., Gargiulo, G., Beekman, C., Theilgaard-Monch, K., Minucci, S., Porse, B.T., Marine, J.C., et al. (2007). The Polycomb group proteins bind throughout the INK4A-ARF locus and are disassociated in senescent cells. *Genes Dev.* 21, 525-530.

Brady, S.N., Yu, Y., Maggi, L.B., Jr., & Weber, J.D. (2004). ARF impedes NPM/B23 shuttling in an Mdm2-sensitive tumor suppressor pathway. *Mol. Cell Biol.* 24, 9327-9338.

Bronder, J.L. & Moran, R.G. (2003). A defect in the p53 response pathway induced by de novo purine synthesis inhibition. *J. Biol .Chem.* 278, 48861-48871.

Buckbinder, L., Talbott, R., Velasco-Miguel, S., Takenaka, I., Faha, B., Seizinger, B.R., & Kley, N. (1995). Induction of the growth inhibitor IGF-binding protein 3 by p53. *Nature* 377, 646-649.

Canepa, E.T., Scassa, M.E., Ceruti, J.M., Marazita, M.C., Carcagno, A.L., Sirkin, P.F., & Ogara, M.F. (2007). INK4 proteins, a family of mammalian CDK inhibitors with novel biological functions. *IUBMB. Life* 59, 419-426.

Carracedo, A. & Pandolfi, P.P. (2008). The PTEN-PI3K pathway: of feedbacks and cross-talks. *Oncogene* 27, 5527-5541.

Cecchinato, V., Chiaramonte, R., Nizzardo, M., Cristofaro, B., Basile, A., Sherbet, G.V., & Comi, P. (2007). Resveratrol-induced apoptosis in human T-cell acute lymphoblastic leukaemia MOLT-4 cells. *Biochem. Pharmacol.* 74, 1568-1574.

Cha, T.L., Zhou, B.P., Xia, W., Wu, Y., Yang, C.C., Chen, C.T., Ping, B., Otte, A.P., & Hung, M.C. (2005). Akt-mediated phosphorylation of EZH2 suppresses methylation of lysine 27 in histone H3. *Science* 310, 306-310.

Chan, S.M., Weng, A.P., Tibshirani, R., Aster, J.C., & Utz, P.J. (2007). Notch signals positively regulate activity of the mTOR pathway in T-cell acute lymphoblastic leukemia. *Blood* 110, 278-286.

Chen, D., Brooks, C.L., & Gu, W. (2006). ARF-BP1 as a potential therapeutic target. *Br. J. Cancer* 94, 1555-1558.

Chen, D., Kon, N., Li, M., Zhang, W., Qin, J., & Gu, W. (2005a). ARF-BP1/Mule is a critical mediator of the ARF tumor suppressor. *Cell* 121, 1071-1083.

Chen, Z., Trotman, L.C., Shaffer, D., Lin, H.K., Dotan, Z.A., Niki, M., Koutcher, J.A., Scher, H.I., Ludwig, T., Gerald, W., et al. (2005b). Crucial role of p53-dependent cellular senescence in suppression of Pten-deficient tumorigenesis. *Nature* 436, 725-730.

Cheok, C.F., Verma, C.S., Baselga, J., & Lane, D.P. (2011). Translating p53 into the clinic. *Nat. Rev. Clin. Oncol.* 8, 25-37.

Chiarini, F., Fala, F., Tazzari, P.L., Ricci, F., Astolfi, A., Pession, A., Pagliaro, P., McCubrey, J.A., & Martelli, A.M. (2009). Dual inhibition of class IA phosphatidylinositol 3-kinase and mammalian target of rapamycin as a new therapeutic option for T-cell acute lymphoblastic leukemia. *Cancer Res.* 69, 3520-3528.

Chiarini, F., Grimaldi, C., Ricci, F., Tazzari, P.L., Evangelisti, C., Ognibene, A., Battistelli, M., Falcieri, E., Melchionda, F., Pession, A., et al. (2010). Activity of the novel dual phosphatidylinositol 3-kinase/mammalian target of rapamycin inhibitor NVP-BEZ235 against T-cell acute lymphoblastic leukemia. *Cancer Res.* 70, 8097-8107.

Ciofani, M. & Zuniga-Pflucker, J.C. (2005). Notch promotes survival of pre-T cells at the beta-selection checkpoint by regulating cellular metabolism. *Nat. Immunol.* 6, 881-888.

Cullion, K., Draheim, K.M., Hermance, N., Tammam, J., Sharma, V.M., Ware, C., Nikov, G., Krishnamoorthy, V., Majumder, P.K., & Kelliher, M.A. (2009). Targeting the Notch1 and mTOR pathways in a mouse T-ALL model. *Blood* 113, 6172-6181.

De Keersmaecker, K., Lahortiga, I., Mentens, N., Folens, C., Van Neste, L., Bekaert, S., Vandenberghe, P., Odero, M.D., Marynen, P., & Cools, J. (2008). *In vitro* validation of gamma-secretase inhibitors alone or in combination with other anti-cancer drugs for the treatment of T-cell acute lymphoblastic leukemia. *Haematologica* 93, 533-542.

De Keersmaecker, K., Marynen, P., & Cools, J. (2005). Genetic insights in the pathogenesis of T-cell acute lymphoblastic leukemia. *Haematologica* 90, 1116-1127.

De Keersmaecker, K., Real, P.J., Gatta, G.D., Palomero, T., Sulis, M.L., Tosello, V., Van Vlierberghe, P., Barnes, K., Castillo, M., Sole, X., et al. (2010). The TLX1 oncogene drives aneuploidy in T cell transformation. *Nat. Med.* 16, 1321-1327.

Decorsiere, A., Cayrel, A., Vagner, S., & Millevoi, S. (2011). Essential role for the interaction between hnRNP H/F and a G quadruplex in maintaining p53 pre-mRNA 3'-end processing and function during DNA damage. *Genes Dev.* 25, 220-225.

Demarest, R.M., Dahmane, N., & Capobianco, A.J. (2011). Notch is oncogenic dominant in T-cell acute lymphoblastic leukemia. *Blood* 117, 2901-2909.

Dohda, T., Maljukova, A., Liu, L., Heyman, M., Grander, D., Brodin, D., Sangfelt, O., & Lendahl, U. (2007). Notch signaling induces SKP2 expression and promotes reduction of p27Kip1 in T-cell acute lymphoblastic leukemia cell lines. *Exp. Cell Res.* 313, 3141-3152.

El Andaloussi, A., Graves, S., Meng, F., Mandal, M., Mashayekhi, M., & Aifantis, I. (2006). Hedgehog signaling controls thymocyte progenitor homeostasis and differentiation in the thymus. *Nat. Immunol.* 7, 418-426.

Ellisen, L.W., Bird, J., West, D.C., Soreng, A.L., Reynolds, T.C., Smith, S.D., & Sklar, J. (1991). TAN-1, the human homolog of the Drosophila notch gene, is broken by chromosomal translocations in T lymphoblastic neoplasms. *Cell* 66, 649-661.

Espinosa, L., Cathelin, S., D'Altri, T., Trimarchi, T., Statnikov, A., Guiu, J., Rodilla, V., Ingles-Esteve, J., Nomdedeu, J., Bellosillo, B., et al. (2010). The Notch/Hes1 pathway sustains NF-kappaB activation through CYLD repression in T cell leukemia. *Cancer Cell* 18, 268-281.

Evangelisti, C., Ricci, F., Tazzari, P., Chiarini, F., Battistelli, M., Falcieri, E., Ognibene, A., Pagliaro, P., Cocco, L., McCubrey, J.A., et al. (2011a). Preclinical testing of the Akt inhibitor triciribine in T-cell acute lymphoblastic leukemia. *J. Cell Physiol* 226, 822-831.

Evangelisti, C., Ricci, F., Tazzari, P., Tabellini, G., Battistelli, M., Falcieri, E., Chiarini, F., Bortul, R., Melchionda, F., Pagliaro, P., et al. (2011b). Targeted inhibition of mTORC1 and mTORC2 by active-site mTOR inhibitors has cytotoxic effects in T-cell acute lymphoblastic leukemia. *Leukemia* 25, 781-791.

Feng, Z., Hu, W., de Stanchina, E., Teresky, A.K., Jin, S., Lowe, S., & Levine, A.J. (2007). The regulation of AMPK beta1, TSC2, and PTEN expression by p53: stress, cell and tissue specificity, and the role of these gene products in modulating the IGF-1-AKT-mTOR pathways. *Cancer Res.* 67, 3043-3053.

Feng, Z., Zhang, H., Levine, A.J., & Jin, S. (2005). The coordinate regulation of the p53 and mTOR pathways in cells. *Proc. Natl. Acad. Sci. USA* 102, 8204-8209.

Ferrando, A.A., Neuberg, D.S., Staunton, J., Loh, M.L., Huard, C., Raimondi, S.C., Behm, F.G., Pui, C.H., Downing, J.R., Gilliland, D.G., et al. (2002). Gene expression signatures define novel oncogenic pathways in T cell acute lymphoblastic leukemia. *Cancer Cell* 1, 75-87.

Freeman, D.J., Li, A.G., Wei, G., Li, H.H., Kertesz, N., Lesche, R., Whale, A.D., Martinez-Diaz, H., Rozengurt, N., Cardiff, R.D., et al. (2003). PTEN tumor suppressor regulates p53 protein levels and activity through phosphatase-dependent and -independent mechanisms. *Cancer Cell* 3, 117-130.

Gardie, B., Cayuela, J.M., Martini, S., & Sigaux, F. (1998). Genomic alterations of the p19ARF encoding exons in T-cell acute lymphoblastic leukemia. *Blood* 91, 1016-1020.

Gil, J. & Peters, G. (2006). Regulation of the INK4b-ARF-INK4a tumour suppressor locus: all for one or one for all. *Nat. Rev. Mol. Cell Biol.* 7, 667-677.

Grabher, C., von Boehmer, H., & Look, A.T. (2006). Notch 1 activation in the molecular pathogenesis of T-cell acute lymphoblastic leukaemia. *Nat. Rev. Cancer* 6, 347-359.

Gregory, M.A., Qi, Y., & Hann, S.R. (2003). Phosphorylation by glycogen synthase kinase-3 controls c-myc proteolysis and subnuclear localization. *J. Biol. Chem.* 278, 51606-51612.

Guo, D., Teng, Q., & Ji, C. (2011). NOTCH and phosphatidylinositide 3-kinase/phosphatase and tensin homolog deleted on chromosome ten/AKT/mammalian target of rapamycin (mTOR) signaling in T-cell development and T-cell acute lymphoblastic leukemia. *Leuk. Lymphoma.*

Gutierrez, A., Sanda, T., Grebliunaite, R., Carracedo, A., Salmena, L., Ahn, Y., Dahlberg, S., Neuberg, D., Moreau, L.A., Winter, S.S., et al. (2009). High frequency of PTEN, PI3K, and AKT abnormalities in T-cell acute lymphoblastic leukemia. *Blood* 114, 647-650.

Harakeh, S., Diab-Assaf, M., Khalife, J.C., Abu-el-Ardat, K.A., Baydoun, E., Niedzwiecki, A., El-Sabban, M.E., & Rath, M. (2007). Ascorbic acid induces apoptosis in adult T-cell leukemia. *Anticancer Res.* 27, 289-298.

Hasegawa, H., Yamada, Y., Iha, H., Tsukasaki, K., Nagai, K., Atogami, S., Sugahara, K., Tsuruda, K., Ishizaki, A., & Kamihira, S. (2009). Activation of p53 by Nutlin-3a, an antagonist of MDM2, induces apoptosis and cellular senescence in adult T-cell leukemia cells. *Leukemia* 23, 2090-2101.

Hebert, J., Cayuela, J.M., Berkeley, J., & Sigaux, F. (1994). Candidate tumor-suppressor genes MTS1 (p16INK4A) and MTS2 (p15INK4B) display frequent homozygous deletions in primary cells from T- but not from B-cell lineage acute lymphoblastic leukemias. *Blood* 84, 4038-4044.

Honda, R., Tanaka, H., & Yasuda, H. (1997). Oncoprotein MDM2 is a ubiquitin ligase E3 for tumor suppressor p53. *FEBS Lett.* 420, 25-27.

Honda, R. & Yasuda, H. (1999). Association of p19(ARF) with Mdm2 inhibits ubiquitin ligase activity of Mdm2 for tumor suppressor p53. *EMBO J.* 18, 22-27.

Hsieh, A.C. & Ruggero, D. (2010). Targeting eukaryotic translation initiation factor 4E (eIF4E) in cancer. *Clin. Cancer Res.* 16, 4914-4920.

Jacobs, J.J., Kieboom, K., Marino, S., DePinho, R.A., & van Lohuizen, M. (1999). The oncogene and Polycomb-group gene bmi-1 regulates cell proliferation and senescence through the ink4a locus. *Nature* 397, 164-168.

Jotta, P.Y., Ganazza, M.A., Silva, A., Viana, M.B., da Silva, M.J., Zambaldi, L.J., Barata, J.T., Brandalise, S.R., & Yunes, J.A. (2010). Negative prognostic impact of PTEN mutation in pediatric T-cell acute lymphoblastic leukemia. *Leukemia* 24, 239-242.

Kao, C.L., Hsu, H.S., Chen, H.W., & Cheng, T.H. (2009). Rapamycin increases the p53/MDM2 protein ratio and p53-dependent apoptosis by translational inhibition of mdm2 in cancer cells. *Cancer Lett.* 286, 250-259.

Keller, D.M. & Lu, H. (2002). p53 serine 392 phosphorylation increases after UV through induction of the assembly of the CK2.hSPT16.SSRP1 complex. *J. Biol. Chem.* 277, 50206-50213.

Keller, D.M., Zeng, X., Wang, Y., Zhang, Q.H., Kapoor, M., Shu, H., Goodman, R., Lozano, G., Zhao, Y., & Lu, H. (2001). A DNA damage-induced p53 serine 392 kinase complex contains CK2, hSpt16, and SSRP1. *Mol. Cell* 7, 283-292.

Kim, J.S., Lee, C., Bonifant, C.L., Ressom, H., & Waldman, T. (2007a). Activation of p53-dependent growth suppression in human cells by mutations in PTEN or PIK3CA. *Mol. Cell Biol.* 27, 662-677.

Kim, K., Choi, J., Heo, K., Kim, H., Levens, D., Kohno, K., Johnson, E.M., Brock, H.W., & An, W. (2008). Isolation and characterization of a novel H1.2 complex that acts as a repressor of p53-mediated transcription. *J. Biol. Chem.* 283, 9113-9126.

Kim, M.M., Wiederschain, D., Kennedy, D., Hansen, E., & Yuan, Z.M. (2007b). Modulation of p53 and MDM2 activity by novel interaction with Ras-GAP binding proteins (G3BP). *Oncogene* 26, 4209-4215.

Kim, S.Y., Herbst, A., Tworkowski, K.A., Salghetti, S.E., & Tansey, W.P. (2003). Skp2 regulates Myc protein stability and activity. *Mol. Cell* 11, 1177-1188.

Kitagawa, M., Lee, S.H., & McCormick, F. (2008). Skp2 suppresses p53-dependent apoptosis by inhibiting p300. *Mol. Cell* 29, 217-231.

Kopan, R. & Ilagan, M.X. (2009). The canonical Notch signaling pathway: unfolding the activation mechanism. *Cell* 137, 216-233.

Kox, C., Zimmermann, M., Stanulla, M., Leible, S., Schrappe, M., Ludwig, W.D., Koehler, R., Tolle, G., Bandapalli, O.R., Breit, S., et al. (2010). The favorable effect of activating NOTCH1 receptor mutations on long-term outcome in T-ALL patients treated on the ALL-BFM 2000 protocol can be separated from FBXW7 loss of function. *Leukemia* 24, 2005-2013.

Krastev, D.B., Slabicki, M., Paszkowski-Rogacz, M., Hubner, N.C., Junqueira, M., Shevchenko, A., Mann, M., Neugebauer, K.M., & Buchholz, F. (2011). A systematic RNAi synthetic interaction screen reveals a link between p53 and snoRNP assembly. *Nat. Cell Biol.* 13, 809-818.

Kruse, J.P. & Gu, W. (2009). Modes of p53 regulation. *Cell* 137, 609-622.

Kuo, M.L., den Besten, W., Bertwistle, D., Roussel, M.F., & Sherr, C.J. (2004). N-terminal polyubiquitination and degradation of the Arf tumor suppressor. *Genes Dev.* 18, 1862-1874.

Kurihara, A., Nagoshi, H., Yabuki, M., Okuyama, R., Obinata, M., & Ikawa, S. (2007). Ser46 phosphorylation of p53 is not always sufficient to induce apoptosis: multiple mechanisms of regulation of p53-dependent apoptosis. *Genes Cells* 12, 853-861.

Lee, J.Y., Nakada, D., Yilmaz, O.H., Tothova, Z., Joseph, N.M., Lim, M.S., Gilliland, D.G., & Morrison, S.J. (2010). mTOR activation induces tumor suppressors that inhibit leukemogenesis and deplete hematopoietic stem cells after Pten deletion. *Cell Stem Cell* 7, 593-605.

Leung, C., Lingbeek, M., Shakhova, O., Liu, J., Tanger, E., Saremaslani, P., van Lohuizen, M., & Marino, S. (2004). Bmi1 is essential for cerebellar development and is overexpressed in human medulloblastomas. *Nature* 428, 337-341.

Lewis, H.D., Leveridge, M., Strack, P.R., Haldon, C.D., O'Neil, J., Kim, H., Madin, A., Hannam, J.C., Look, A.T., Kohl, N., et al. (2007). Apoptosis in T cell acute lymphoblastic leukemia cells after cell cycle arrest induced by pharmacological inhibition of notch signaling. *Chem. Biol.* 14, 209-219.

Li, X., Gounari, F., Protopopov, A., Khazaie, K., & von Boehmer, H. (2008). Oncogenesis of T-ALL and nonmalignant consequences of overexpressing intracellular NOTCH1. *J. Exp. Med.* 205, 2851-2861.

Lin, C.J., Cencic, R., Mills, J.R., Robert, F., & Pelletier, J. (2008). c-Myc and eIF4F are components of a feedforward loop that links transcription and translation. *Cancer Res.* 68, 5326-5334.

Liu, S., Breit, S., Danckwardt, S., Muckenthaler, M.U., & Kulozik, A.E. (2009). Downregulation of Notch signaling by gamma-secretase inhibition can abrogate chemotherapy-induced apoptosis in T-ALL cell lines. *Ann. Hematol.* 88, 613-621.

Llanos, S., Clark, P.A., Rowe, J., & Peters, G. (2001). Stabilization of p53 by p14ARF without relocation of MDM2 to the nucleolus. *Nat. Cell Biol.* 3, 445-452.

Lu, X., Nguyen, T.A., Moon, S.H., Darlington, Y., Sommer, M., & Donehower, L.A. (2008). The type 2C phosphatase Wip1: an oncogenic regulator of tumor suppressor and DNA damage response pathways. *Cancer Metastasis Rev.* 27, 123-135.

Luo, J., Solimini, N.L., & Elledge, S.J. (2009). Principles of cancer therapy: oncogene and non-oncogene addiction. *Cell* 136, 823-837.

Mak, L.H., Vilar, R., & Woscholski, R. (2010). Characterisation of the PTEN inhibitor VO-OHpic. *J.Chem.Biol.* 3, 157-163.

Margolin, A.A., Palomero, T., Sumazin, P., Califano, A., Ferrando, A.A., & Stolovitzky, G. (2009). ChIP-on-chip significance analysis reveals large-scale binding and regulation by human transcription factor oncogenes. *Proc. Natl. Acad. Sci. USA* 106, 244-249.

Mayo, L.D. & Donner, D.B. (2001). A phosphatidylinositol 3-kinase/Akt pathway promotes translocation of Mdm2 from the cytoplasm to the nucleus. *Proc. Natl. Acad. Sci. USA* 98, 11598-11603.

Mayo, L.D., Seo, Y.R., Jackson, M.W., Smith, M.L., Guzman, J.R., Korgaonkar, C.K., & Donner, D.B. (2005). Phosphorylation of human p53 at serine 46 determines promoter selection and whether apoptosis is attenuated or amplified. *J. Biol. Chem.* 280, 25953-25959.

Medyouf, H., Gao, X., Armstrong, F., Gusscott, S., Liu, Q., Gedman, A.L., Matherly, L.H., Schultz, K.R., Pflumio, F., You, M.J., et al. (2010). Acute T-cell leukemias remain dependent on Notch signaling despite PTEN and INK4A/ARF loss. *Blood* 115, 1175-1184.

Meley, D., Spiller, D.G., White, M.R., McDowell, H., Pizer, B., & See, V. (2010). p53-mediated delayed NF-kappaB activity enhances etoposide-induced cell death in medulloblastoma. *Cell Death. Dis.* 1, e41.

Miyazaki, M., Miyazaki, K., Itoi, M., Katoh, Y., Guo, Y., Kanno, R., Katoh-Fukui, Y., Honda, H., Amagai, T., van Lohuizen, M., et al. (2008). Thymocyte proliferation induced by pre-T cell receptor signaling is maintained through polycomb gene product Bmi-1-mediated Cdkn2a repression. *Immunity.* 28, 231-245.

Mungamuri, S.K., Yang, X., Thor, A.D., & Somasundaram, K. (2006). Survival signaling by Notch1: mammalian target of rapamycin (mTOR)-dependent inhibition of p53. *Cancer Res.* 66, 4715-4724.

Murphy, D.J., Junttila, M.R., Pouyet, L., Karnezis, A., Shchors, K., Bui, D.A., Brown-Swigart, L., Johnson, L., & Evan, G.I. (2008). Distinct thresholds govern Myc's biological output *in vivo*. *Cancer Cell* 14, 447-457.

Okuhashi, Y., Itoh, M., Nara, N., & Tohda, S. (2011). Effects of combination of notch inhibitor plus hedgehog inhibitor or Wnt inhibitor on growth of leukemia cells. *Anticancer Res.* 31, 893-896.

Old, J.B., Kratzat, S., Hoellein, A., Graf, S., Nilsson, J.A., Nilsson, L., Nakayama, K.I., Peschel, C., Cleveland, J.L., & Keller, U.B. (2010). Skp2 directs Myc-mediated suppression of p27Kip1 yet has modest effects on Myc-driven lymphomagenesis. *Mol. Cancer Res.* 8, 353-362.

Omura-Minamisawa, M., Diccianni, M.B., Batova, A., Chang, R.C., Bridgeman, L.J., Yu, J., Pullen, J., Bowman, W.P., & Yu, A.L. (2000). Universal inactivation of both p16 and p15 but not downstream components is an essential event in the pathogenesis of T-cell acute lymphoblastic leukemia. *Clin. Cancer Res.* 6, 1219-1228.

Osipo, C., Golde, T.E., Osborne, B.A., & Miele, L.A. (2008). Off the beaten pathway: the complex cross talk between Notch and NF-kappaB. *Lab Invest.* 88, 11-17.

Palomero, T., Dominguez, M., & Ferrando, A.A. (2008). The role of the PTEN/AKT pathway in NOTCH1-induced leukemia. *Cell Cycle* 7, 965-970.

Palomero, T., Sulis, M.L., Cortina, M., Real, P.J., Barnes, K., Ciofani, M., Caparros, E., Buteau, J., Brown, K., Perkins, S.L., et al. (2007). Mutational loss of PTEN induces resistance to NOTCH1 inhibition in T-cell leukemia. *Nat. Med.* 13, 1203-1210.

Polo, S.E., Kaidi, A., Baskcomb, L., Galanty, Y., & Jackson, S.P. (2010). Regulation of DNA-damage responses and cell-cycle progression by the chromatin remodelling factor CHD4. *EMBO J.* 29, 3130-3139.

Popov, N. & Gil, J. (2010). Epigenetic regulation of the INK4b-ARF-INK4a locus: in sickness and in health. *Epigenetics* 5, 685-690.

Qi, Y., Gregory, M.A., Li, Z., Brousal, J.P., West, K., & Hann, S.R. (2004). p19ARF directly and differentially controls the functions of c-Myc independently of p53. *Nature* 431, 712-717.

Quelle, D.E., Zindy, F., Ashmun, R.A., & Sherr, C.J. (1995). Alternative reading frames of the INK4a tumor suppressor gene encode two unrelated proteins capable of inducing cell cycle arrest. *Cell* 83, 993-1000.

Radhakrishnan, S.K. & Kamalakaran, S. (2006). Pro-apoptotic role of NF-kappaB: implications for cancer therapy. *Biochim. Biophys. Acta* 1766, 53-62.

Real, P.J. & Ferrando, A.A. (2009). NOTCH inhibition and glucocorticoid therapy in T-cell acute lymphoblastic leukemia. *Leukemia* 23, 1374-1377.

Real, P.J., Tosello, V., Palomero, T., Castillo, M., Hernando, E., de Stanchina, E., Sulis, M.L., Barnes, K., Sawai, C., Homminga, I., et al. (2009). Gamma-secretase inhibitors reverse glucocorticoid resistance in T cell acute lymphoblastic leukemia. *Nat. Med.* 15, 50-58.

Remke, M., Pfister, S., Kox, C., Toedt, G., Becker, N., Benner, A., Werft, W., Breit, S., Liu, S., Engel, F., et al. (2009). High-resolution genomic profiling of childhood T-ALL reveals frequent copy-number alterations affecting the TGF-beta and PI3K-AKT pathways and deletions at 6q15-16.1 as a genomic marker for unfavorable early treatment response. *Blood* 114, 1053-1062.

Riz, I., Zweier-Renn, L.A., Toma, I., Hawley, T.S., & Hawley, R.G. (2011). Apoptotic role of IKK in T-ALL therapeutic response. *Mol. Cancer Res.* 9, 979-984.

Rodway, H., Llanos, S., Rowe, J., & Peters, G. (2004). Stability of nucleolar versus non-nucleolar forms of human p14(ARF). *Oncogene* 23, 6186-6192.

Ruggero, D., Montanaro, L., Ma, L., Xu, W., Londei, P., Cordon-Cardo, C., & Pandolfi, P.P. (2004). The translation factor eIF-4E promotes tumor formation and cooperates with c-Myc in lymphomagenesis. *Nat. Med.* 10, 484-486.

Ryan, K.M., Ernst, M.K., Rice, N.R., & Vousden, K.H. (2000). Role of NF-kappaB in p53-mediated programmed cell death. *Nature* 404, 892-897.

Sade, H., Krishna, S., & Sarin, A. (2004). The anti-apoptotic effect of Notch-1 requires p56lck-dependent, Akt/PKB-mediated signaling in T cells. *J. Biol. Chem.* 279, 2937-2944.

Salmena, L., Carracedo, A., & Pandolfi, P.P. (2008). Tenets of PTEN tumor suppression. *Cell* 133, 403-414.

Sarmento, L.M., Huang, H., Limon, A., Gordon, W., Fernandes, J., Tavares, M.J., Miele, L., Cardoso, A.A., Classon, M., & Carlesso, N. (2005). Notch1 modulates timing of G1-S progression by inducing SKP2 transcription and p27 Kip1 degradation. *J. Exp. Med.* 202, 157-168.

Serrano, M., Hannon, G.J., & Beach, D. (1993). A new regulatory motif in cell-cycle control causing specific inhibition of cyclin D/CDK4. *Nature* 366, 704-707.

Shank-Calvo, J.A., Draheim, K., Bhasin, M., & Kelliher, M.A. (2006). p16Ink4a or p19Arf loss contributes to Tal1-induced leukemogenesis in mice. *Oncogene* 25, 3023-3031.

Sharma, V.M., Draheim, K.M., & Kelliher, M.A. (2007). The Notch1/c-Myc pathway in T cell leukemia. *Cell Cycle* 6, 927-930.

Sharpless, N.E., Ramsey, M.R., Balasubramanian, P., Castrillon, D.H., & DePinho, R.A. (2004). The differential impact of p16(INK4a) or p19(ARF) deficiency on cell growth and tumorigenesis. *Oncogene* 23, 379-385.

Sherr, C.J. (2006). Divorcing ARF and p53: an unsettled case. *Nat. Rev. Cancer* 6, 663-673.

Shin, H.M., Minter, L.M., Cho, O.H., Gottipati, S., Fauq, A.H., Golde, T.E., Sonenshein, G.E., & Osborne, B.A. (2006). Notch1 augments NF-kappaB activity by facilitating its nuclear retention. *EMBO J.* 25, 129-138.

Shiota, M., Izumi, H., Onitsuka, T., Miyamoto, N., Kashiwagi, E., Kidani, A., Hirano, G., Takahashi, M., Naito, S., & Kohno, K. (2008). Twist and p53 reciprocally regulate target genes via direct interaction. *Oncogene* 27, 5543-5553.

Silva, A., Jotta, P.Y., Silveira, A.B., Ribeiro, D., Brandalise, S.R., Yunes, J.A., & Barata, J.T. (2010). Regulation of PTEN by CK2 and Notch1 in primary T-cell acute lymphoblastic leukemia: rationale for combined use of CK2- and gamma-secretase inhibitors. *Haematologica* 95, 674-678.

Silva, A., Yunes, J.A., Cardoso, B.A., Martins, L.R., Jotta, P.Y., Abecasis, M., Nowill, A.E., Leslie, N.R., Cardoso, A.A., & Barata, J.T. (2008). PTEN posttranslational inactivation and hyperactivation of the PI3K/Akt pathway sustain primary T cell leukemia viability. *J. Clin. Invest* 118, 3762-3774.

So, A.Y., Jung, J.W., Lee, S., Kim, H.S., & Kang, K.S. (2011). DNA methyltransferase controls stem cell aging by regulating BMI1 and EZH2 through microRNAs. *PLoS One* 6, e19503.

Soulier, J., Clappier, E., Cayuela, J.M., Regnault, A., Garcia-Peydro, M., Dombret, H., Baruchel, A., Toribio, M.L., & Sigaux, F. (2005). HOXA genes are included in genetic and biologic networks defining human acute T-cell leukemia (T-ALL). *Blood* 106, 274-286.

Spivakov, M. & Fisher, A.G. (2007). Epigenetic signatures of stem-cell identity. *Nat. Rev. Genet.* 8, 263-271.

Stambolic, V., MacPherson, D., Sas, D., Lin, Y., Snow, B., Jang, Y., Benchimol, S., & Mak, T.W. (2001). Regulation of PTEN transcription by p53. *Mol. Cell* 8, 317-325.

Sulis, M.L., Saftig, P., & Ferrando, A.A. (2011). Redundancy and specificity of the metalloprotease system mediating oncogenic NOTCH1 activation in T-ALL. *Leukemia* doi:10.1038/leu.2011.130 [Epub ahead of print].

Sulong, S., Moorman, A.V., Irving, J.A., Strefford, J.C., Konn, Z.J., Case, M.C., Minto, L., Barber, K.E., Parker, H., Wright, S.L., et al. (2009). A comprehensive analysis of the CDKN2A gene in childhood acute lymphoblastic leukemia reveals genomic deletion, copy number neutral loss of heterozygosity, and association with specific cytogenetic subgroups. *Blood* 113, 100-107.

Tanigaki, K. & Honjo, T. (2007). Regulation of lymphocyte development by Notch signaling. *Nat. Immunol.* 8, 451-456.

Topisirovic, I., Gutierrez, G.J., Chen, M., Appella, E., Borden, K.L., & Ronai, Z.A. (2009). Control of p53 multimerization by Ubc13 is JNK-regulated. *Proc. Natl. Acad. Sci. USA* 106, 12676-12681.

Treanor, L.M., Volanakis, E.J., Zhou, S., Lu, T., Sherr, C.J., & Sorrentino, B.P. (2011). Functional interactions between Lmo2, the Arf tumor suppressor, and Notch1 in murine T-cell malignancies. *Blood* 117, 5453-5462.

Van Vlierberghe, P., Homminga, I., Zuurbier, L., Gladdines-Buijs, J., van Wering, E.R., Horstmann, M., Beverloo, H.B., Pieters, R., & Meijerink, J.P. (2008). Cooperative genetic defects in TLX3 rearranged pediatric T-ALL. *Leukemia* 22, 762-770.

Vilas-Zornoza, A., Agirre, X., Martin-Palanco, V., Martin-Subero, J.I., San Jose-Eneriz, E., Garate, L., Alvarez, S., Miranda, E., Rodriguez-Otero, P., Rifon, J., et al. (2011). Frequent and simultaneous epigenetic inactivation of TP53 pathway genes in acute lymphoblastic leukemia. *PLoS One* 6, e17012.

Vilborg, A., Wilhelm, M.T., & Wiman, K.G. (2010). Regulation of tumor suppressor p53 at the RNA level. *J. Mol. Med. (Berl)* 88, 645-652.

Volanakis, E.J., Williams, R.T., & Sherr, C.J. (2009). Stage-specific Arf tumor suppression in Notch1-induced T-cell acute lymphoblastic leukemia. *Blood* 114, 4451-4459.

von der Lehr, N., Johansson, S., Wu, S., Bahram, F., Castell, A., Cetinkaya, C., Hydbring, P., Weidung, I., Nakayama, K., Nakayama, K.I., et al. (2003). The F-box protein Skp2 participates in c-Myc proteasomal degradation and acts as a cofactor for c-Myc-regulated transcription. *Mol. Cell* 11, 1189-1200.

Voncken, J.W., Niessen, H., Neufeld, B., Rennefahrt, U., Dahlmans, V., Kubben, N., Holzer, B., Ludwig, S., & Rapp, U.R. (2005). MAPKAP kinase 3pK phosphorylates and regulates chromatin association of the polycomb group protein Bmi1. *J. Biol. Chem.* 280, 5178-5187.

Weber, J.D., Taylor, L.J., Roussel, M.F., Sherr, C.J., & Bar-Sagi, D. (1999). Nucleolar Arf sequesters Mdm2 and activates p53. *Nat. Cell Biol.* 1, 20-26.

Weng, A.P., Ferrando, A.A., Lee, W., Morris, J.P., Silverman, L.B., Sanchez-Irizarry, C., Blacklow, S.C., Look, A.T., & Aster, J.C. (2004). Activating mutations of NOTCH1 in human T cell acute lymphoblastic leukemia. *Science* 306, 269-271.

Weng, A.P., Millholland, J.M., Yashiro-Ohtani, Y., Arcangeli, M.L., Lau, A., Wai, C., Del, B.C., Rodriguez, C.G., Sai, H., Tobias, J., et al. (2006). c-Myc is an important direct target of Notch1 in T-cell acute lymphoblastic leukemia/lymphoma. *Genes Dev.* 20, 2096-2109.

Xue, L., Nolla, H., Suzuki, A., Mak, T.W., & Winoto, A. (2008). Normal development is an integral part of tumorigenesis in T cell-specific PTEN-deficient mice. *Proc. Natl. Acad. Sci. USA* 105, 2022-2027.

Yilmaz, O.H., Valdez, R., Theisen, B.K., Guo, W., Ferguson, D.O., Wu, H., & Morrison, S.J. (2006). Pten dependence distinguishes haematopoietic stem cells from leukaemia-initiating cells. *Nature* 441, 475-482.

Yoda, A., Toyoshima, K., Watanabe, Y., Onishi, N., Hazaka, Y., Tsukuda, Y., Tsukada, J., Kondo, T., Tanaka, Y., & Minami, Y. (2008). Arsenic trioxide augments Chk2/p53-mediated apoptosis by inhibiting oncogenic Wip1 phosphatase. *J. Biol. Chem.* 283, 18969-18979.

Zhang, J., Grindley, J.C., Yin, T., Jayasinghe, S., He, X.C., Ross, J.T., Haug, J.S., Rupp, D., Porter-Westpfahl, K.S., Wiedemann, L.M., et al. (2006). PTEN maintains haematopoietic stem cells and acts in lineage choice and leukaemia prevention. *Nature* 441, 518-522.

Zhang, X.P., Liu, F., & Wang, W. (2011). Two-phase dynamics of p53 in the DNA damage response. *Proc. Natl. Acad. Sci. USA* 108, 8990-8995.

Zhang, Y. & Xiong, Y. (2001). Control of p53 ubiquitination and nuclear export by MDM2 and ARF. *Cell Growth Differ.* 12, 175-186.

Zhang, Z. & Zhang, R. (2008). Proteasome activator PA28 gamma regulates p53 by enhancing its MDM2-mediated degradation. *EMBO J.* 27, 852-864.

Zhou, M., Gu, L., Findley, H.W., Jiang, R., & Woods, W.G. (2003). PTEN reverses MDM2-mediated chemotherapy resistance by interacting with p53 in acute lymphoblastic leukemia cells. *Cancer Res.* 63, 6357-6362.